Vitamin D and Rickets

Endocrine Development

Vol. 6

Series Editor

Martin O. Savage London

KARGER

Vitamin D and Rickets

Volume Editor

Ze'ev Hochberg Haifa

66 figures, 5 in color, and 23 tables, 2003

KARGER

Basel · Freiburg · Paris · London · New York · Bangalore · Bangkok · Singapore · Tokyo · Sydney

Ze'ev Hochberg, MD, DSc
Pediatric Endocrinology, Meyer Children's Hospital
Rambam Medical Center
POB 9602, Haifa 31096, Israel
Tel./Fax +972 4 854215
E-Mail z_hochberg@rambam.health.gov.il

Library of Congress Cataloging-in-Publication Data

Vitamin D and rickets / Ze'ev Hochberg, volume editor.
p. cm. – (Endocrine development ; v. 6)
Includes bibliographical references and index.
ISBN 3–8055–7582–3 (hbk.)
1. Rickets. 2. Vitamin D–Metabolism–Disorders. I. Hochberg, Z. II. Series.
RJ396.V55 2003
616.3′95–dc21 2003047691

Bibliographic Indices. This publication is listed in bibliographic services, including Current Contents® and Index Medicus.

Drug Dosage. The authors and the publisher have exerted every effort to ensure that drug selection and dosage set forth in this text are in accord with current recommendations and practice at the time of publication. However, in view of ongoing research, changes in government regulations, and the constant flow of information relating to drug therapy and drug reactions, the reader is urged to check the package insert for each drug for any change in indications and dosage and for added warnings and precautions. This is particularly important when the recommended agent is a new and/or infrequently employed drug.

www.karger.com
Printed in Switzerland on acid-free paper by Reinhardt Druck, Basel
ISSN 1421–7082
ISBN 3–8055–7582–3

Contents

Foreword

This volume is a very welcome addition to the *Endocrine Development* series because it brings a much needed focus to the importance of Rickets as a continuing global health problem and presents new scientific information underlying its pathogenesis. I am grateful to Ze'ev Hochberg and his distinguished cast of contributors, who are experts in clinical paediatrics, vitamin D and calcium physiology, molecular biology and bone metabolism. The result of their contributions is a volume of high quality, which bridges scientific advances and clinical medicine, thus maintaining the aim of this series. The book comprises a fascinating range of current knowledge from the original clinical descriptions of Rickets to the latest molecular advances in vitamin D and calcium physiology and pathophysiology.

This volume aims to be helpful to both scientists and clinicians who are still grappling with the difficult challenge of Rickets in the 21st century.

Martin O. Savage
London, April 2003

Preface

In 1650, Francis Glisson wrote his first book on rickets, 'De Rachitide Sive Morbo Puerili, Qui Vulgo'. In 1668, Glisson felt that so much had been revealed in the previous 18 years that he wrote a second book on the same topic 'A Treatise of the Rickets Being a Disease Common to Children'. Ever since the 17th century discoveries, books on rickets have been published periodically; the last of them being 'Rickets', edited by Francis Glorieux and published in 1991. In the footsteps of Glisson, I can humbly assert that so much has been revealed in the past 12 years that the present book on the same topic contains scores of recent revelations that shed innovative light on a long-standing theme.

Rickets is a disease of the growing child and it is illuminated in this volume from different perspectives. The basis for understanding rickets is rooted in the concepts of mineral metabolism and its control mechanisms in the growing fetus, infant and child. We now understand that rickets is not only vitamin D deficiency, but we also realize that vitamin D and calcium deficiency are still prevalent in developing countries, as well as in affluent societies, where children are not exposed to as much sunlight as they need. The rapid growth of molecular biology has been exemplified in the application of subcellular technologies to studying vitamin D and rickets in human and animal models.

Hopefully, this volume will provide an integration of important basic and clinical advances in our understanding of rickets.

Ze'ev Hochberg, Haifa

Hochberg Z (ed): Vitamin D and Rickets.
Endocr Dev. Basel, Karger, 2003, vol 6, pp 1–13

Introduction

Rickets – Past and Present

Ze'ev Hochberg

Pediatric Endocrinology, Meyer Children's Hospital,
Rambam Medical Center, Haifa, Israel

Contents

The name 'rickets' is from the Old English wrickken, to twist. The more technical medical term, rachitis, which comes from Greek, the spine, was suggested by Francis Glisson in 1650, both from similarity of sound and from the part of the body which he thought was one of the first to be affected.

At the turn of the industrial revolution, 'the English disease', resulting from vitamin D deficiency, spread among city-dwelling poor children and became endemic in cities. At the turn of the Internet revolution it appears to be endemic again. The increase in the incidence of vitamin D deficiency is paralleling the primacy of breast-feeding in Western societies as human milk contains only minute amounts of vitamin D. It is more prevalent in black or children of darker complexion and in those who escape well-baby clinics. The three main risk factors are nutritional status [1], breast-feeding and dark skin.

Is Vitamin D a Vitamin or a Hormone?

Vitamin D is not a vitamin in the strict definition because it can be produced by exposure of the skin to sunlight. As such, animals and humans do not have a dietary requirement for vitamin D when sufficient sunlight is available. However, nutritional vitamin D becomes essential when sunlight is insufficient to meet daily needs. This has become particularly acute as more people reside in urban centers where they are exposed to sub-optimal levels of sunlight. Air pollution, clothes, tall buildings, indoor dwelling, and sunscreens block ultraviolet light from the sun and these factors all reduce the ability of the skin to synthesize vitamin D_3. Moreover, people living far north (or south) of the equator obtain little purposeful ultraviolet radiation during the winter months. The same is true for Middle-Eastern women who remain indoors or cover their entire body from sunlight. Under these conditions vitamin D, and its hormone derivative calcitriol, can be considered a bona fide vitamin in that it must be supplied in the diet [2].

The Unit Definition of Vitamin D

The World Health Organization has defined the ‘International Unit’ of vitamin D_3 as the activity of 0.025 μg of the international standard preparation of crystalline vitamin D_3. Thus, 1 IU of vitamin D_3 is 0.025 μg, or 65 pmol. The unit definition of the active metabolite calcitriol was set to be equivalent in molar terms to that of the parent vitamin D_3. Thus, 1 unit is 65 pmol of calcitriol; as such the unit of calcitriol is much more active than the unit of vitamin D itself. The vitamin D requirements for children or adults have not been precisely defined. Historically, it was defined on the basis of the vitamin D content in a teaspoon of fish oil, a quantity shown to be sufficient to prevent rickets. A more rigorous scientific definition is unavailable.

Rickets Is a Disease of Growing Children

Osteomalacia, the bone disease in rickets, results from a defect in the mineralization of bone matrix with increased bone mass. It is to be distinguished from osteoporosis where bone mass is decreased, from hypophosphatemic osteopenia of premature infants, and from renal osteodystrophy, which is partly due to calcitriol renal deficiency, but also due to hyperphosphatemic hyperparathyroidism.

When osteomalacia wrecks the growth plate of a growing child, it impairs longitudinal bone growth, producing widening and disorganization of its structure. These result from extensive compensatory proliferation of growth plate cartilage cells, mostly in the periphery of the plate, to give the cup-shaped metaphysis. Whereas cartilage mineralization is excessive, showing as a wide hazy layer on top of the metaphysis, the latter exhibits insufficient mineralization. This type of ‘epiphyseal dysplasia’ is defined as ‘rickets’.

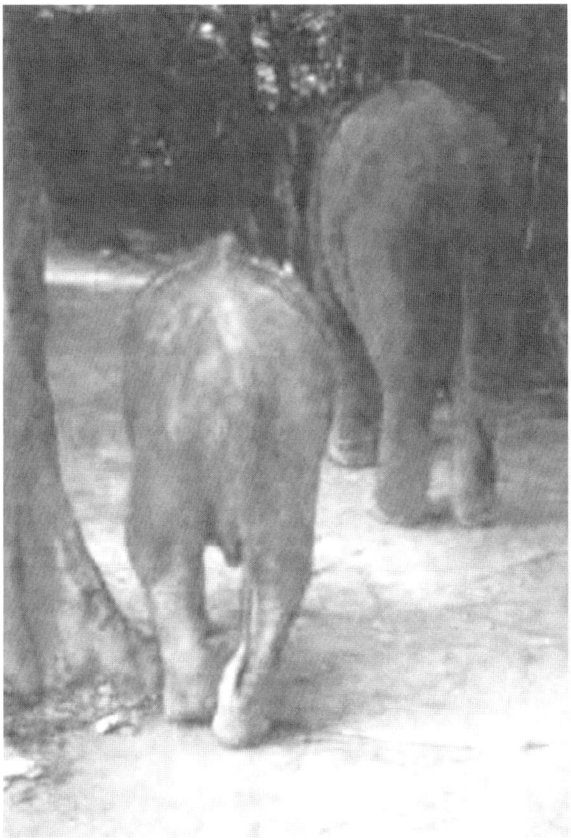

Fig. 1. An elephant mother's milk is the richest of all mammalian milks. Cow's milk is much less nutritious. When captive baby elephants lose their mothers, they are usually fed on powdered cow's milk mixed with rice and bananas. Often, the result is poorly developed bones. This 6-month-old calf has rickets [32].

From the 1911 1st Edition Encyclopedia [3]

'*Rickets*, a constitutional disease of childhood characterized chiefly by a softened condition of the bones and by other evidences of perverted nutrition… The symptoms, which precede the outward manifestation of the disease, are marked disorders of the digestive and alimentary functions. The child's appetite is diminished, and there is frequent vomiting, together with diarrhoea or irregularity of the bowels, the evacuations being clay-coloured and unhealthy. Along with this there is a falling away in flesh. Importance is to be attached to certain other symptoms present in the early stages, namely, profound

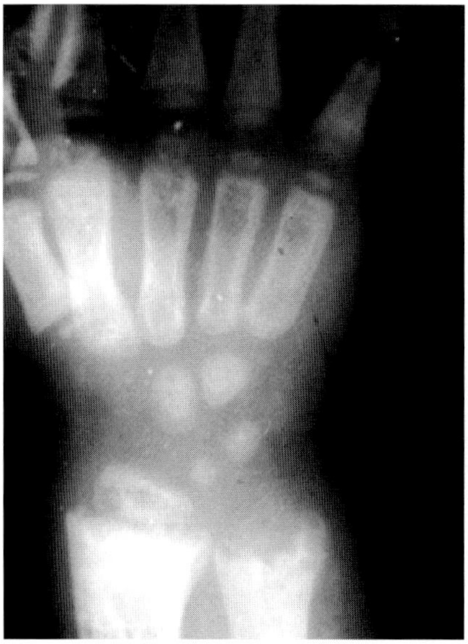

Fig. 2. Severe rickets in a child with vitamin D receptor loss-of-function.

sweating of the head and upper parts of the body, particularly during sleep, with at the same time dry heat of the lower parts and a tendency in the child to kick off all coverings and expose the limbs. At the same time there is great tenderness of the bones, as shown by the pain produced on moving or handling the child. Gradually the changes in the shape of the bones become visible, at first chiefly noticed at the ends of the long bones, as in those of the arm, causing enlargements at the wrists, or in the ribs, producing a knobbed appearance at the junction of their ends with the costal cartilages. The bones also from their softened condition tend to become distorted and misshapen, both by the action of the muscles and by the superincumbent weight of the body. Those of the limbs are bent outwards and forwards, and the child becomes "bowlegged" or "in-kneed" often to an extreme degree. The trunk of the body likewise shows various alterations and deformities owing to curvatures of the spine, the flattening of the lateral curves of the ribs, and the projection forwards of the sternum. The cavity of the chest may thus be contracted and the development of the thoracic organs interfered with as well as their functions more or less embarrassed. The pelvis undergoes distortion, which may reduce its capacity to a degree that in the female may afterwards lead to serious difficulties in parturition. The head of the rickety child is large-looking in its upper part, the individual bones of the cranium sometimes remaining long ununited, while the face is small and ill-developed, and the teeth appear late and fall out or decay early. The constitutional conditions of ill health continue, and the nutrition and

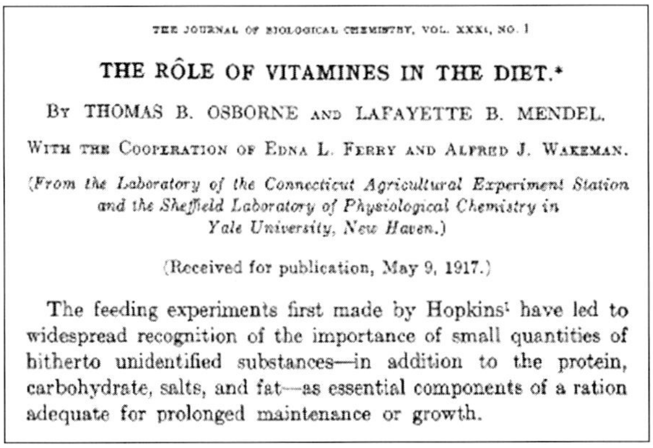
THE JOURNAL OF BIOLOGICAL CHEMISTRY, VOL. XXXI, NO. 1

THE RÔLE OF VITAMINES IN THE DIET.*

BY THOMAS B. OSBORNE AND LAFAYETTE B. MENDEL.

WITH THE COOPERATION OF EDNA L. FERRY AND ALFRED J. WAKEMAN.

(*From the Laboratory of the Connecticut Agricultural Experiment Station and the Sheffield Laboratory of Physiological Chemistry in Yale University, New Haven.*)

(Received for publication, May 9, 1917.)

The feeding experiments first made by Hopkins[1] have led to widespread recognition of the importance of small quantities of hitherto unidentified substances—in addition to the protein, carbohydrate, salts, and fat—as essential components of a ration adequate for prolonged maintenance or growth.

Fig. 3. The 1917 report on the role of vitamins in growth.

development of the child are greatly retarded. The disease may terminate in recovery, with more or less of deformity and dwarfing, the bones although altered in shape becoming firmly ossified, and this is the common result in the majority of instances. On the other hand, during the progress of the disease, various intercurrent ailments are apt to arise which may cause death, such as the infectious fevers, bronchitis and other pulmonary affections, chronic hydrocephalus, convulsions, laryngismus, stridulus, etc. An acute form of rickets of rare occurrence (*really a form of scurvy, Z.H.*) has been described by writers on diseases of children, in which all the symptoms are of more rapid development and progress, the result in many instances being fatal. The treatment of rickets is necessarily more hygienic than medicinal, and includes such preventive measures as may be exercised by strict attention to personal health and nutrition on the part of mothers, especially where there appears to be any tendency to a rickety development in any members of the family. Very important also is the avoidance of too prolonged nursing, which by its weakening effects upon the mother's health is calculated to engender the disease in any succeeding children. "At the same time it must be admitted that, when the mother is healthy, her milk abundant, and nursing discontinued before the lapse of the first year, there is no better means of preventing the occurrence of rickets than this method of feeding an infant; the disease, as is well known, being far more frequently met with in children brought up by hand." The management of the child exhibiting any tendency to rickets is of great importance, but can only be alluded to in general terms. The digestive disorders characteristic of the setting in of the disease render necessary the greatest care and watchfulness as to diet. Thus, if the child be not nursed but fed artificially, fresh milk should be almost the only article of diet for at least the first year, and the chief element for the next. When not digested well, as may at times be shown by its appearance as a curd in the evacuations, it may be diluted with water or limewater, or else discontinued for a short time; carefully-made gruel or barley water being substituted. Many of the so-called "infants' foods" which are now so extensively used appear to be well adapted for their purpose, but when employed too abundantly and to the exclusion of the due amount of milk are often productive of digestive and intestinal disorders, probably from their containing a greater amount of starchy matter than can be utilized. From the end of the first year light animal soups may occasionally be given with advantage. The medicinal remedies most to be relied on are those which improve the digestive functions and minister to nutrition, and include such "agents" as the preparations of iron, quinine, and especially cod-liver oil and phosphorus, and the cautious use of extract of thyroid gland has been advocated by Henoch. Of no less importance, however, are abundance of fresh air, cleanliness, warm clothing, and attention to the general hygiene of the child and to regularity in all its functions. When the disease is showing evidence of advancing, it is desirable to restrain the child from walking, as far as possible. But this precaution may be to some extent rendered unnecessary by the use of splints and other apparatus as supports for the limbs and body, enabling the child to move about without the risk of bending and deformity of the bones which otherwise would probably be the result.'

Historical Background

The origin of vitamin D dates backs 500–750 million years, as it was made by plant plankton. It is transferred along the food chain into animal plankton and into the seafood, where it is stored and concentrated – hence the importance of oil-rich fish and cod liver oil as a source of vitamin D. The physiologic function of vitamin D in these early organisms is unknown. It became important many years later in the evolution of animals with calcified eggs and skeleton.

In terms of human evolution, the original Africoid races required minimal substrate and storage of vitamin D in the tropical environment. Under excessive exposure to sunlight and ultraviolet-B radiation, pre-vitamin D is photoisomerized to biologically inert isomers. In the ice-age environment, white skin was better adapted to vitamin D production. In a frigid northern climate, with many sunless days and shorter hours of daylight, dark or black skin became a liability. Inbreeding within the albinoid group, which continually heightened the albinoid characteristics, made the development of this new human stock possible.

In terms of human history of vitamin D and rickets, the Greek historian, Herodotus (485–426 BC), observed that Persian warriors had much softer skulls than Egyptian warriors and attributed it to the turbans worn by Persians [4] and Hippocrates described a disease resembling rickets in 130 AD. The majority of Roman children in the first century AD seem to have been afflicted with rickets. Soranus of Ephesus (98–138 AD) in 'A Treatise on the Diseases of Women' gave a more complete description [5].

As people began to crowd in narrow streets and sunless, polluted cities, the incidence of rickets increased. Over 90% of children working in mines and many city dwellers were affected with leg bowing. Around 1645 a group of fellows of the Caius College in Cambridge began to exchange notes on rickets, thought to have been recently spread in England. They were Glisson, Sheaf, Bate, Regemorter, Pagett, Goddard and Trench. Bate, and Regemorter were assigned to publish a book on the subject. The investigation of the essential nature of the disease fell to Glisson, who impressed his co-workers so much that they entrusted him with drafting the whole book, into which their own observations and possibly those of authors like Daniel Whistler were incorporated [6]. 'Tractatus de Rachitide Sive Morbo Puerilii' appeared in 1650 with Glisson as the author [7], Bate and Regemorter as his associates, and with five, additional contributors. As early as 1668, he realized that this was a disease of children [8] with devastating consequences in young women with deformed pelvis, resulting in maternal mortality. It was then known as *the English disease*, *morbus anglicus, morbus anglorum* and *rachitic* [9].

A hundred years later, the French scholar Levacher de la Feutrie (1738–1790) wrote his book on rickets [10]. The text begins with a history of rickets, followed by sections on the nature of the disease, the parts of the body affected, those most at risk, a refutation of other opinions on the disease, the foundations of theories on rickets, description of the disease and it's diagnosis, the various causes, warning signs of the disease, a short explanation of the curving and swelling of the bones associated with rickets, a general prognosis for victims, treatments and remedies, and, finally, some observations on therapeutic treatments for rickets. At the end of the text he depicts orthopedic devices developed specifically for the treatment of rickets-deformed bones, including leg braces, corsets, and instruments to realign the spine.

In 1822, Sniadecki [11] observed that Warsaw city children had much higher rate of rickets than children from the country and suggested for the first time that this bone disease was caused by lack of sunshine. Two years later, Schutte [12] first reported of the value of cod-liver oil in the treatment of rickets. In the 1890s Palm made recommendations that children sunbath to prevent rickets. He had no idea what healing power was in the rays, but whatever it was, he surmised, these children needed it.

The turn of the 20th century was marked by a debate on small quantities of hitherto unidentified substances that are needed in addition to the protein, carbohydrate, salts and fat for prolonged maintenance of growth [13]. This was difficult to accept at the time and in 1915 the *Journal of Biological Chemistry* published the opinion that 'The assumption that some unknown substances are indispensable for growth is a convenient device for explaining experiments that result in failure – a device that becomes superfluous as soon as the experiment succeeds' [14].

Vitamin D became classified as a vitamin through a historical accident. It was in 1919/20 that Sir Edward Mellanby, working with dogs raised exclusively indoors, devised a diet that allowed him to unequivocally establish that their bone disease, rickets was caused by a deficiency of a trace component present in the diet. In 1921 he wrote, 'The action of fats in rickets is due to a vitamin or accessory food factor which they contain, probably identical with the fat-soluble vitamin' [15]. Shortly thereafter, McCollum [16] observed that by bubbling oxygen through a preparation of the 'fat-soluble vitamin', they were able to distinguish between vitamin A (which was inactivated) and vitamin D (which retained activity) and predicted several years later that the latter was a vitamin which promotes calcium deposition. A year later, this chapter was concluded when Goldblatt and Soames [17] identified that when a precursor of vitamin D in the skin was irradiated with sunlight or ultraviolet light, a substance equivalent to the fat-soluble vitamin was produced and Hess et al. [18] prevented rickets in rats by exposing them to sunlight.

The chemical structure of vitamin D was determined in the 1930s by Windaus et al. [19] in Göttingen, Germany. They discovered that vitamin D_2 is produced by ultraviolet irradiation of ergosterol and vitamin D_3 resulted from the ultraviolet irradiation of 7-dehydrocholesterol. This concept was then utilized by adding vitamin D precursor to milk and other food products, to be irradiated by a mercury arc lamp [20].

As our understanding of mineral and vitamin D metabolism grew, we also learned about possible defects in these events and the advent of molecular biology in this field enhanced our options to diagnose rare forms of rickets. The term 'rickets resistant to vitamin D' was coined in 1937 by Albright et al. [21], as the patients they described presented with changes in mineral metabolism that could only be overcome by very large daily doses of vitamin D.

But how does vitamin D affect calcium deposition to build strong bones? Since the 1950s, scientists had been puzzling over the implications of two findings related to this question [22]. In the early part of that decade, the Swedish researcher Arvid Carlsson (2000 Nobel laureate for his work on signal transduction in the nervous system) made the startling discovery that vitamin D can actually remove calcium from bones when the body needs it. At about the same

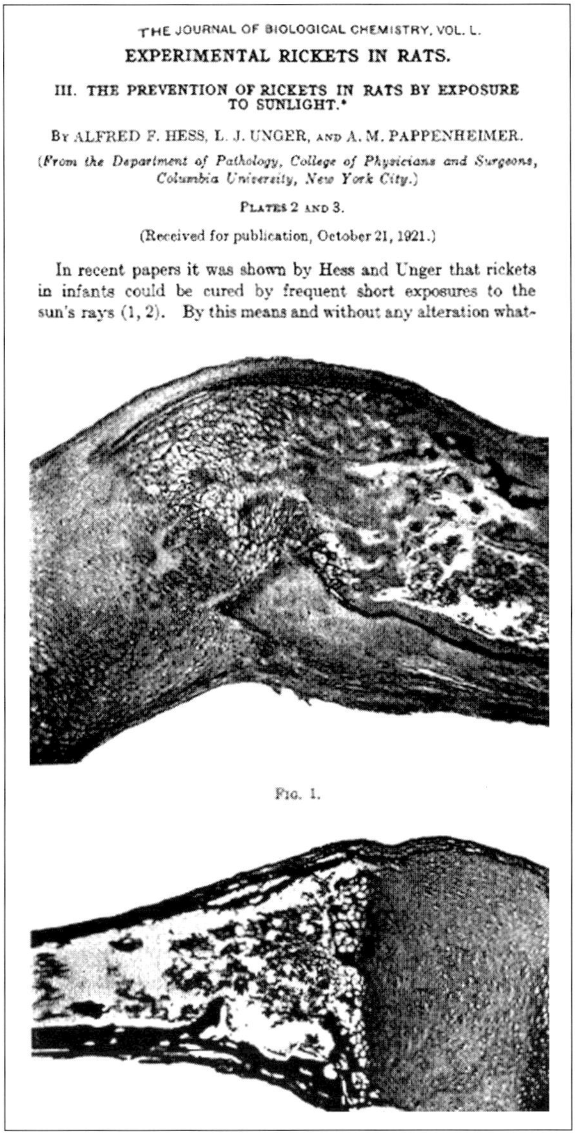
THE JOURNAL OF BIOLOGICAL CHEMISTRY, VOL. L.

EXPERIMENTAL RICKETS IN RATS.

III. THE PREVENTION OF RICKETS IN RATS BY EXPOSURE TO SUNLIGHT.*

BY ALFRED F. HESS, L. J. UNGER, AND A. M. PAPPENHEIMER.

(From the Department of Pathology, College of Physicians and Surgeons, Columbia University, New York City.)

PLATES 2 AND 3.

(Received for publication, October 21, 1921.)

In recent papers it was shown by Hess and Unger that rickets in infants could be cured by frequent short exposures to the sun's rays (1, 2). By this means and without any alteration what-

FIG. 1.

Fig. 4. The 1921 description of the healing effect of sunshine in rickets.

time, the Norwegian biochemist R. Nicolaysen, who had been testing different diets on animals for years, concluded that the uptake of calcium from food is guided by some unknown 'endogenous factor' that alerts the intestines to the body's calcium needs [23].

Table 1. Classification of rickets

	Calcium deficiency	Phosphate deficiency
Nutritional rickets	Calcium deprivation Vitamin D deficiency	Neonatal rickets Antacid misuse Phosphate binders
Absorptive rickets	Malabsorption diseases Bile salts depletion Phenytoin therapy	
Renal rickets	Renal insufficiency Renal tubular acidosis	Fanconi's syndromes (types 1 and 2, secondary) X-linked recessive hypophosphatemic rickets (Dent's disease) Hypercalciuric hypophosphatemic rickets
Metabolic rickets	25OHD-1α-hydroxylase deficiency (vitamin D-dependent rickets) End-organ resistance (hereditary vitamin D-resistant rickets)	X-linked hypophosphatemic rickets Autosomal-dominant hypophosphatemic rickets Tumor-induced osteomalacia

Answers began to emerge with the experiments tracing the activation of Vitamin D. In 1961, Prader et al. [24] reported several examples of a condition for which they coined the term 'hereditary pseudo-deficiency' rickets. Scientists did not have the tools to follow vitamin D metabolism in living subjects until the advent, in the mid-1960s, of new techniques using radioactively labeled substances. Between 1968 and 1971, researchers made great progress in understanding the metabolic processing of vitamin D and its physiological activity. In 1968, a team headed by Hector DeLuca at the University of Wisconsin isolated an active substance identified as 25-hydroxyvitamin D_3, which the team later proved to be produced in the liver [25]. Two years later, Kodicek and David R. Fraser showed that a second active metabolite is produced in the kidney. Finally, in 1971 the chemical structure of this metabolite was identified as 1,25-dihydroxyvitamin D_3 [26], now termed calcitriol. It was now clear that the liver changes vitamin D_3 to 25-hydroxy vitamin D_3, the major circulating form of the vitamin. The kidneys then convert 25-hydroxyvitamin D_3 to 1,25-dihydroxyvitamin D_3, the active form of the vitamin. It turned out that the pseudo-deficiency rickets of Prader et al. [27] was a defect in this last step of renal conversion, and it was termed 'vitamin D-dependent rickets'. The understanding that the kidneys metabolize vitamin D into its active form calcitriol raised the issue whether this was really a vitamin or a hormone. In 1997,

Table 2. Milestones in the history of vitamin D and rickets

750–500 million years ago – vitamin D in plant plankton
300–500 million years ago – calcified skeletons and eggs
2nd century AD – Soranus of Ephesus's describes rickets in Roman children
1645 – Glisson describes the English disease in city children
1822 – Sniadecki identifies the healing power of sunshine
1912 – Hopkins describes the vitamins
1921 – Mellanby describes the fat-soluble vitamin D
1923 – Goldblatt and Soames showed the conversion of a precursor to vitamin D in the skin under the effect of ultraviolet light
1930 – Windaus reports the chemical structure of vitamin D
1937 – Albright describes vitamin D-resistant rickets
1950s – Carlsson and Nicolaysen associate vitamin D with uptake of calcium from food
1968 – DeLuca identifies liver 25-hydroxyvitamin D
1970 – Kodicek and Fraser identify renal calcitriol
1975 – Haussler binds vitamin D to a nuclear receptor
1988 – Baker clones the vitamin D receptor
1997 – Fu et al. clone 25OHD-1α-hydroxylase

Table 3. Antique books on rickets

Whistler D: Morbo puerili Anglorum, quem patrio idiomate indigenae vocant. Lugduni Batavorum, 1645.
Arnold Boate (Bootius, de Boot): Observationes medicae de affectibus omissis. London, Whittaker, 1649.
Glisson F: De Rachitide sive morbo puerili, qui vulgo. The Rickets diciteur. London, 1650.
Glisson F: A Treatise of the Rickets Being a Disease Common to Children. London, 1668.
Levacher de la Feutrie T: Traite du rakitis, ou l'art de redresser les enfants contrefaits. Paris, Lacombe, 1772.
Levacher de la Feutrie T: Du rakitis, ou abrege de son historie: Suivi de propositions aphoristiques sur cette maladie. Paris, Lacombe, 1803.

the group of Walter Miller in UCSF cloned and sequenced the P450c1-alpha cDNA from human keratinocytes [28].

The most recent chapter of vitamin D and rickets started when, in 1975, Mark Haussler at the University of Arizona made the discovery of a protein receptor that binds calcitriol to the nucleus of cells in the intestine [29]. The role of the vitamin D receptor in vitamin D-dependent rickets type-2 was realized in 1982 [30] and in 1988, the group of Bert O'Malley from California Biotechnology Inc. cloned the vitamin D receptor [31].

References

1 Lulseged S, Fitwi G: Vitamin D deficiency rickets: Socio-demographic and clinical risk factors in children seen at referral hospital in Addis Ababa. East Afr Med J 1999;76:457–461.
2 Utiger RD: The need for more vitamin D. N Engl J Med 1998;228:828–829.
3 http://91.1911encyclopedia.org/R/RI/RICKETS.htm
4 Herodotus, The Histroies, 525 BC.
5 Soranus of Ephesus: Why the Majority of Roman Children Are Distorted; in: Treatise on the Diseases of Women, 98–138 AD.
6 Whistler D: Morbo puerili Anglorum, quem patrio idiomate indigenae vocant The Rickets. Lugduni Batavorum 1645, pp 1–13.
7 Glisson F. De Rachitide sive morbo puerili, qui vulgo The Rickets diciteur. London, 1650, pp 1–416.
8 Glisson F: A Treatise of the Rickets Being a Disease Common to Children. London, 1668, pp 1–373.
9 http://www.whonamedit.com/index.cfm
10 Levacher de la Feutrie T: Traite du rakitis, ou l'art de redresser les enfants contrefaits. Paris, Lacombe, 1772.
11 Mozolowski W. Jedrzej Sniadcki: On the cure of rickets. Nature 1939;143:121.
12 Schutte D: Beobachtungen über den Nutzen des Berger Leberthrans (Oleum jecoris Aselli, von *Gadus asellus* L). Arch Med Erfahr Geb Prakt Med Chir Geburtsh Staatsarzneik 1824;2:79.
13 Hopkins FJ. J Physiol 1912;xliv:425.
14 McCollum EV, Davies M. J Biol Chem 1915;xxiii:181.
15 Mellanby E: An experimental investigation in rickets. Lancet 1919;i:407.
16 McCollum EV, Simmonds N, Becker JE, Shipley PG: Studies on experimental rickets. XXI. An experimental demonstration of the existence of a vitamin which promotes calcium deposition. J Biol Chem 1922;53:293.
17 Goldblatt H, Soames KN: A study of rats on a normal diet irradiated daily by the mercury vapor quartz lamp or kept in darkness. Biochem J 1923;17:294.
18 Hess AF, Unger LJ, Pappenheimer AM: Experimental rickets in rats. III. The prevention of rickets in rats by exposure to sunlight. J Biol Chem 1921;L:77.
19 Windaus A, Linsert O, Luttringhaus A, Weidlinch G: Über das krystallistierte Vitamin D_2. Justis Liebigs Ann Chem 1932;492:226.
20 Hess AF, Weinstock M: Antirachitic imparted to inert fluids and green vegetables by ultraviolet irradiation. J Biol Chem 1924;62:301.
21 Albright F, Butler AM, Bloomberg E: Rickets resistant to vitamin D therapy. Am J Dis Child 1937;54:529.
22 http://www.beyonddiscovery.org/content/
23 Nicolaysen R, Eeg-Larsen N. Vitamin Horm 1953;11:29.
24 Prader A, Illig R, Weierli E: Eine besondere Form der primaere Vitamin D resitenden Rachitis mit Hypocalcaemi und autosomal-dominantem Erbgang: Die herediaere pseudo-mangel Rachitis. Helv Paediatr Acta 1961;16:452.
25 Blunt JW, Tanaka Y, DeLuca HF: Biological activity of 25-hydroxycholecalciferol, a metabolite of vitamin D_3. Proc Natl Acad Sci USA 1968;61:1503.
26 Lawson DE, Fraser DR, Kodicek E, et al: Identification of 1,25-dihydroxycholecalciferol, a new kidney hormone controlling calcium metabolism. Nature 1971;230:228.
27 Fraser D, Kooh SW, Kind HP, et al: Pathogenesis of hereditary vitamin-D-dependent rickets: An inborn error of vitamin D metabolism involving defective conversion of 25-hydroxyvitamin D to 1α,25-dihydroxyvitamin D. N Engl J Med 1973;289:817.
28 Fu GK, Lin D, Zhang MYH, et al: Cloning of human 25-hydroxyvitamin D-1-α-hydroxylase and mutations causing vitamin D-dependent rickets type 1. Molec Endocr 1997;11:1961.

29 Brumbaugh PF, Haussler MR: Specific binding of 1α,25-dihydroxycholecalciferol to nuclear components of chick intestine. J Biol Chem 1975;250:1588.
30 Feldman D, Chen T, Cone C, et al: Vitamin D resistant rickets with alopecia: cultured skin fibroblasts exhibit defective cytoplasmic receptors and unresponsiveness to $1,25(OH)_2D_3$. J Clin Endocrinol Metab 1982;55:1020.
31 Baker AR, McDonnell DP, Hughes M, et al: Cloning and expression of full-length cDNA encoding human vitamin D receptor. Proc Natl Acad Sci USA 1988;85:3294.
32 http://www.artbyelephants.com/background.html

Ze'ev Hochberg, MD, DSc
Pediatric Endocrinology
Meyer Children's Hospital, Rambam Medical Center
POB 9602, Haifa 31096 (Israel)
Tel./Fax +972 4 8542157, E-Mail z_hochberg@rambam.health.gov.il

Hochberg Z (ed): Vitamin D and Rickets.
Endocr Dev. Basel, Karger, 2003, vol 6, pp 14–33

Normal Mineral Homeostasis

Interplay of Parathyroid Hormone and Vitamin D

Michael A. Levine

Division of Pediatric Endocrinology, The Johns Hopkins University School of Medicine, Baltimore, Md., USA

Contents

Normal mineral metabolism and skeletal development depend upon an intricate interplay of parathyroid renal and skeletal factors. Crucial in this respect is parathyroid hormone (PTH) which is synthesized and secreted from the parathyroid glands and at a rate inversely proportional to the serum ionized calcium concentration. Hormone secretion is tightly regulated through the interaction of extracellular calcium with specific calcium-sensing receptors (CaSRs) [1–3] that are present on the surface of the parathyroid cell. In turn PTH regulates mineral metabolism and skeletal homeostasis through its actions on specialized target cells in bone and kidney that express specific type 1 PTH receptors. Most importantly in the kidney PTH activates synthesis of calcitriol (1,25-dihydroxyvitamin D) the active metabolite of vitamin D. The integrated actions of PTH and calcitriol on their target tissues provide a precise system of control to maintain the serum concentrations of calcium and phosphate within a narrow range that is critical for many physiological processes, including the mineralization of the skeleton. Although only a small fraction of the total body calcium and phosphate is located in the plasma, it is the plasma concentrations of ionized calcium and inorganic phosphate that are under hormonal control.

Because the concentrations of ionic calcium and phosphate in extracellular fluid are at, or exceed, their solubility product constant, elaborate controls have also been developed to keep calcium-phosphate from precipitating in tissues and to allow the controlled deposition of calcium-phosphate as hydroxyapatite in bone. For example, proteins such as matrix Gla protein inhibit the precipitation of calcium-phosphate in blood vessels, whereas alkaline phosphatase expressed on the osteoblast plasma membrane facilitates the deposition of minerals on the bone surface.

In this chapter, we review the hormonal control of mineral metabolism in order to provide a framework for understanding the genetic and nutritional defects that account for rickets. This control is mediated primarily by PTH and calcitriol, which affect intestinal absorption, bone formation and resorption, and urinary excretion of minerals. The physiologic roles of other hormones such as calcitonin, estrogens, and growth hormone in the regulation of calcium and phosphate balance are incompletely understood and will not be discussed.

Parathyroid Physiology and Pathophysiology

The concentration of extracellular ionized calcium is tightly regulated by PTH and 1,25-dihydroxyvitamin D (1,25$(OH)_2$D; calcitriol). PTH is synthesized in the four parathyroid glands as a preprohormone (115 amino acids), converted to a prohormone (90 amino acids) as it is transported across the rough endoplasmic reticulum, and stored in secretory granules as the mature 84-amino acid hormone. PTH is secreted at a rate inversely proportional to the ambient serum ionized calcium concentration. Secretion, as well as synthesis, of PTH is tightly regulated through the interaction of extracellular calcium (and to a lesser extent other divalent cations) with specific calcium-sensing receptors (CaSRs) that are expressed on the surface of parathyroid cells. These receptors are also present on several other cell types that are involved in regulating mineral ion homeostasis [1–3], including the calcitonin-secreting C-cells of the thyroid and renal tubular cells. The CaSR is a member of a large family of plasma membrane receptors that can bind hormones, neurotransmitter, cytokines, light photons, and taste and odor molecules. These receptors consist of a single polypeptide chain that is predicted by hydrophobicity plots to span the plasma membrane seven times (i.e. heptahelical), forming three extracellular and three or four intracellular loops and a cytoplasmic carboxyl-terminal tail. The heptahelical receptors are coupled by heterotrimeric ($\alpha\beta\gamma$) G proteins [4] to signal effector molecules (e.g. adenylyl cyclase, phospholipase C, potassium channels) that are localized to the inner surface of the plasma membrane [see, 5, 6, for reviews].

Binding of extracellular calcium to the CaSR activates the receptor and facilitates its interaction and activation of G proteins that stimulate phospholipase C activity (G_q and G_{11}) and inhibit adenylyl cyclase (G_i) [7]. Activation of phospholipase C leads to the generation of the second messengers inositol 1,4,5-trisphosphate and diacylglycerol, which increase levels of cytosolic calcium via release from intracellular stores and stimulate protein kinase C activity, respectively. These second messenger systems mediate the parathyroid cell's responses to elevated concentrations of extracellular calcium, which include inhibition of PTH release, suppression of PTH gene expression, and accelerated intracellular degradation of PTH. By contrast, PTH secretion is acutely increased when the extracellular calcium concentration is low. Over time, persistent hypocalcemia leads to reduced intracellular degradation of PTH, increased *PTH* gene expression, and parathyroid cell hypertrophy and proliferation.

PTH has direct effects on bone to regulate calcium exchange at osteocytic sites and to enhance osteoclast-mediated bone resorption. In the kidney, PTH directly enhances distal tubular reabsorption of calcium, decreases the proximal tubular reabsorption of phosphate, and stimulates the metabolic conversion of 25-hydroxyvitamin D (25(OH)D) to calcitriol, the active vitamin D metabolite. Calcitriol acts on bone to enhance bone resorption and on the gastrointestinal mucosa to increase absorption of dietary calcium (tables 1, 2; fig. 1).

PTH action first requires binding of the hormone to specific G protein coupled receptors that are expressed on the plasma membrane of specialized target cells. The classical PTH receptor is a ~75-kD glycoprotein that is often referred to as the PTH/PTHrP receptor or type 1 PTH receptor (type 1 PTH-r). Molecular cloning of cDNAs encoding PTH receptors from several species [8–11] has indicated that the type 1 receptor expressed on bone and kidney cells is identical. The type 1 PTH-r binds both PTH and parathyroid hormone-related protein (PTHrP), a factor made by diverse tumors that cause humorally mediated hypercalcemia, with equivalent affinity, which accounts for the similar activities of both hormones. The type 1 PTH-r is most abundantly expressed in the physiological target tissues for PTH action (i.e. kidney and bone), but it is also found in a wide variety of fetal and adult tissues where it appears to mediate the paracrine/autocrine signaling pathways of PTHrP rather than the endocrine actions of PTH. By contrast, a second PTH receptor, termed the type 2 receptor protein, interacts with PTH but not PTHrP [12, 13], and has a very restricted tissue distribution that does not include classical PTH target tissues (i.e. bone and kidney). Recently, a hypothalamic peptide termed TIP39 has been identified as the physiological ligand for the type 2 PTH receptor [13–15], but the biological functions mediated by this receptor remain largely unknown.

Table 1. Sites and modes of PTH action

Site	Effect	Action
Bone osteoblast	direct	PTH acts on stromal osteoblasts in the bone marrow to stimulate the secretion of cytokines which act on the osteoclasts to promote demineralization and Ca^{2+} release PTH also activates Ca^{2+} pumps within the surface osteoblasts to move Ca^{2+} out of bone fluid and into the extracellular fluid (i.e. osteocytic osteolysis)
Kidney	direct	PTH acts on the proximal tubules in the renal cortex and stimulates reabsorption of Ca^{2+}; this effect is mediated intracellularly by increased activity of protein kinase A and protein kinase C PTH increases calcium reabsorption in distal nephron PTH acts at the proximal renal tubule to decrease reabsorption of phosphate PTH favors metabolic acidosis by inhibiting Na^+/H^+ exchange PTH stimulates the biosynthesis of 1,25-dihydroxyvitamin D_3 (calcitriol) by increasing the activity of 1α-hydroxylase
Intestine	indirect	PTH-stimulated production of calcitriol promotes absorption of calcium (and phosphorous) in intestinal epithelium tissue

The type 1 PTH receptor couples to G proteins [16] that stimulate adenylyl cyclase (Gs) and phospholipase C (Gq/11) to activate protein kinase A and protein kinase C signaling pathways, respectively. Thus, receptor activation leads to rapid generation of the second messengers cAMP [17, 18], inositol 1,4,5-trisphosphate and diacylglycerol [19, 20], and cytosolic calcium [21–24]. PTH action is dependent upon the membrane localization of the receptors: basolateral PTH receptors activate protein kinase A and protein kinase C, whereas apical PTH receptors activate protein kinase C [25]. PTH decreases renal reabsorption of phosphate by controlling the concentration of the type 2a sodium-phosphate cotransporter (NPT2a) on the brush border membrane located at the apical surface of proximal tubular cells. PTH rapidly induces dislocation of NPT2a from the plasma membrane on endocytic vesicles, which route NPT2a to lysosomes for destruction [26]. Over longer time periods, PTH may decrease the levels of NPT2a messenger RNA (mRNA) and thus the synthesis of NPT2a protein [26]. Consequently, both the capacity of the proximal tubule to reabsorb phosphate and the blood level of phosphate fall.

Table 2. Sites and modes of calcitriol action

Site	Effect	Action
Intestine	direct	enhanced calcium and phosphorous absorption from the gut epithelium by stimulating synthesis of a Ca^{2+}-binding protein (CaBP) or by affecting Ca^{2+} transport directly
Bone osteoclasts	indirect	increased bone demineralization by activation of osteoclastogenesis via interaction of calcitriol with osteoblasts
Kidney	direct	stimulation of tubular Ca^{2+} reabsorption possibly by the action of CaBP

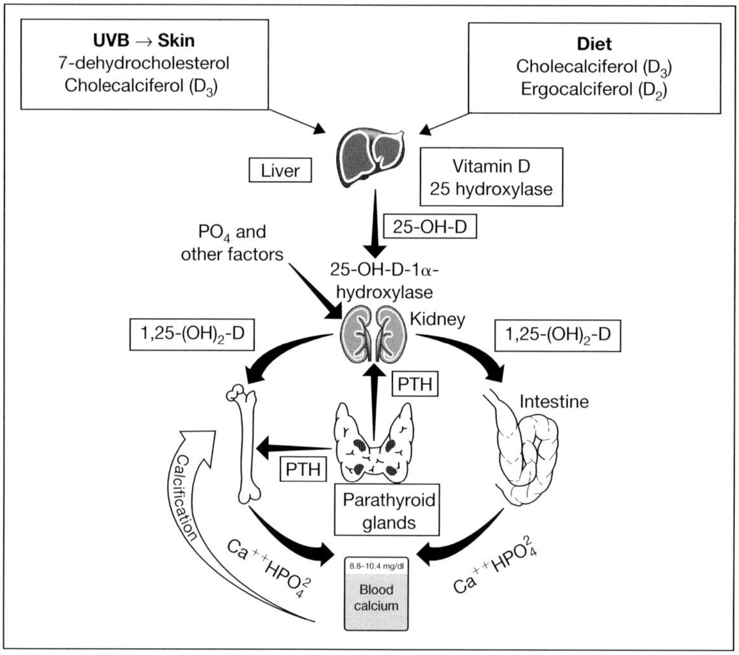

Fig. 1. Integrated control of calcium and phosphate metabolism. The four parathyroid glands located in proximity to the thyroid gland are depicted. Vitamin D from the diet or synthesized in the skin is activated by a series of hydroxylations that occur in the liver and kidney. See text.

In states of functional hypoparathyroidism, in which PTH secretion or action is deficient, the normal effects of PTH on bone and kidney are absent. Bone resorption, and release of calcium from skeletal stores, is diminished. Renal tubular reabsorption of calcium is decreased, but because of hypocalcemia and low filtered load, urinary calcium excretion is low. In the absence of PTH action, urinary clearance of phosphate is decreased, and hyperphosphatemia occurs. The deficiency of PTH action and the hyperphosphatemia together impair renal synthesis of calcitriol, and absorption of calcium from the intestine is markedly impaired. $1,25(OH)_2D$ is also a potent stimulator of bone resorption, and its absence also decreases the availability of calcium from bone.

Vitamin D Physiology

Cholecalciferol (vitamin D_3) is a secosteroid produced via opening the B-ring of 7-dehydrocholesterol (fig. 2). In humans, this reaction is driven by solar ultraviolet B (UVB; 290–315 nm) irradiation of cells in the basal layers of the epidermis, where 7-dehydrocholesterol is transformed to previtamin D. Once formed, previtamin D slowly undergoes a thermal isomerization and is transformed to vitamin D_3. Sunscreens with an SPF of 8 (fig. 3a) and the skin pigment melanin (fig. 4) can compete with 7-dehydrocholesterol for UVB photons, and can thereby decrease the amount of cholecalciferol synthesized in the skin in response to sunlight exposure. Aging is also associated with reduced cutaneous production of vitamin D_3 (fig. 3b), but this effect is primarily the result of decreased concentrations of 7-dehydrocholesterol in the epidermis [27–29].

It is unlikely that excessive sunlight exposure can lead to vitamin D intoxication, as previtamin D can be degraded by further UVB irradiation to the inert photoproducts lumisterol and tachysterol and vitamin D_3 can be photoisomerized to suprasterol and other biologically inactive products. Ergocalciferol (vitamin D_2) is produced via opening the B-ring of ergosterol, a sterol found in plants and fungi. Plants do not contain significant amounts of ergocalciferol, but this chemical is commercially synthesized in bulk for use as a nutritional supplement. Humans obtain calciferols either endogenously through metabolism of precursors in the skin, or exogenously as a dietary component or dietary supplement. For practical purposes, the metabolism and actions of vitamin D_3 and vitamin D_2 are similar in humans, although slight distinctions in the processing of these two steroids in the have been recently noted [30, 31].

Cholecalciferol and ergocalciferol are inert when exposed directly to calciferol target tissues. They must be hydroxylated at positions 25- and 1α- to become maximally active (fig. 2). The initial hydroxylation at carbon-25 is

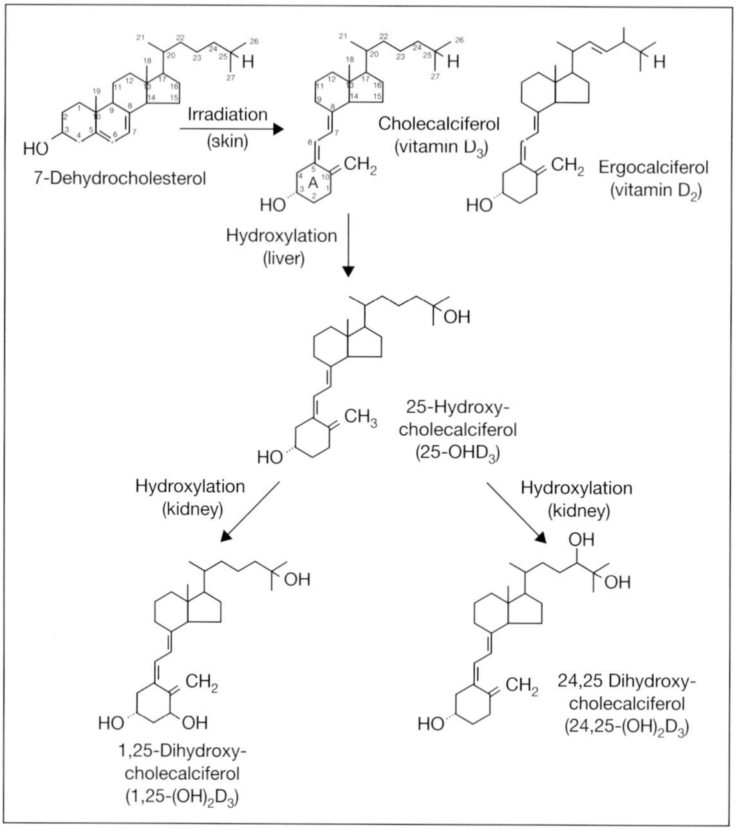

Fig. 2. Metabolism of vitamin D. Vitamin D can be metabolized to the active form, 1α 25-dihydroxyvitamin D or to an inactive form, 24,25-dihydroxyvitamin D.

carried out only in the liver by a mitochondrial cytochrome P450 mono-oxygenase [32]. 25-hydroxylation of vitamin D is not highly regulated; the principal determinant of its rate is the circulating level of vitamin D. Therefore, measurement of circulating concentrations of 25(OH) vitamin D provides a useful index of vitamin D status.

25(OH)D is 1α-hydroxylated to 1α-25$(OH)_2$D or 24-hydroxylated to 24, 25$(OH)_2$D by enzyme systems in the kidney (fig. 2). 25$(OH)D_3$ 1α-hydroxylase activity is also found in the placenta, in normal and pathological parathyroid glands, cultured cells of diverse origin, and in certain pathologic tissues (such as granulomas and malignant T cells) [33, 34]. Virtually all 1α-25$(OH)_2$D normally in blood comes from the kidney. Expression and activity of the renal 1α-hydroxylase enzyme is stringently regulated. Parathyroid hormone activates

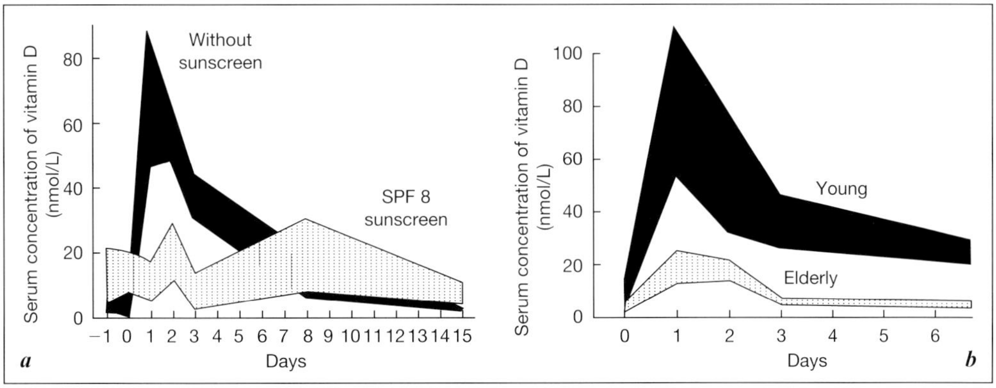

Fig. 3. Circulating concentrations of vitamin D in response to a whole body exposure to one minimal erythemal dose in healthy young subjects with and without a sunscreen (***a***) and in healthy young and elderly subjects (***b***). Adapted from refs [27] and [28].

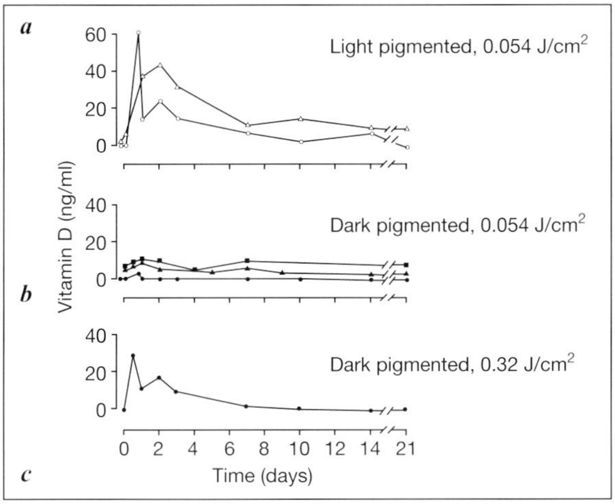

Fig. 4. Circulating concentrations of vitamin D in response to whole body exposure to simulated sunlight in healthy young subjects of differing skin pigments. Darker skin subjects require approximately six times as much ultraviolet irradiation as light-skinned subjects to generate similar amounts of vitamin D. Adapted from ref. [29].

it in the renal proximal tubule through a cyclic AMP mediated pathway. Enzyme activity is also stimulated directly by calcitonin and indirectly by growth hormone and prolactin. 1α-$25(OH)_2D$, phosphate, and calcium can inhibit the expression of the 1α-hydroxylase gene.

25(OH)D, 1α-25$(OH)_2$D, and other metabolites are substrates for 24-hydroxylation. Many similarities between the 1-hydroxylase and 24-hydroxylase systems suggest that they share certain components. Both are mitochondrial enzymes containing cytochrome P450. Both are modulated (though in opposing directions) by cAMP and by 1α-25$(OH)_2$D. Their normal anatomical distributions differ; the 1α-hydroxylase is expressed in the proximal renal tubule and the collecting tubule [35, 36], but the 24-hydroxylase is found in a wide range of tissues. The role of 24-hydroxylase has not been fully determined; it may be the only route to a group of calciferols with unique actions not obtainable with 1α-25$(OH)_2$D (see below), and it might be the most important step in 1α-25$(OH)_2$D removal. Expression of the 24-hydroxylase is reciprocally regulated by 1α-25$(OH)_2$D and inhibited by PTH in the kidney [37]; 1α-25$(OH)_2$D induces expression of 24-hydroxylase at the transcriptional level, suggesting an important role in terminating the action of 1α-25$(OH)_2$D (fig. 2).

All calciferols are fat-soluble and circulate principally bound to an α-globulin of 58,000 Daltons [38]. It contains one high-affinity sterol binding site with the following order of affinities: 25$(OH)D_3$–26,23-lactone $>$ 25(OH)D $=$ 24,25$(OH)_2$D $>$ 1α-25$(OH)_2$D $\gg$ vitamin D. It is a major component of plasma protein (normal concentration 10^{-5} *M*) that has multiple isoforms [39] extensively studied for their genetic diversity long before a function in calciferol transport was recognized. The messenger RNA for this vitamin D binding protein, also known as group-specific component, or Gc, has been sequenced and is homologous to that for albumin and α-fetoprotein [40].

Most of the body pool of vitamin D is in fat, compared to only a small fraction of the pools of 25(OH)D or 1α-25$(OH)_2$D [41]. In the circulation more than 99% of each metabolite is bound to proteins. Normal turnover of vitamin D is approximately 30 μg per day; most of this is cleared through catabolic pathways with only 1 μg per day being cleared as 1α-25$(OH)_2$D.

1α-25$(OH)_2$D acts by binding to a high-affinity intracellular receptor, analogous to the receptors for other steroid hormones [42–44]. The human 1α-25$(OH)_2$D receptor (VDR), a 50-kD protein, has been cloned and sequenced [43]. The VDR belongs to the steroid hormone-thyroid hormone-retinoic acid receptor gene superfamily, that includes the receptors for other steroid hormones, the receptor for triiodothyronine, the receptor for retinoic acid, and a product of the v-ERB-A oncogene, which act as a regulators of gene transcription [45, 46]. The VDR has a hormone-binding domain at the C-terminus for the binding of 1α-25$(OH)_2$D and a DNA-binding domain with two 'zinc fingers' at the amino terminus. The VDR must complex with the retinoic acid X receptor (RXR) to form a heterodimeric complex with 1α-25$(OH)_2$D [47–49].

After 1α-25$(OH)_2$D binds to the hormone binding domain of the VDR, the DNA-binding domain is then able to bind to a vitamin D response element (VDRE) in target genes, thereby regulating gene transcription [49].

The VDR is found in small intestine and bone, the major target tissues, but also in other tissues including testis, ovary, pituitary, parathyroid, skin, breast, muscle, lymphocytes and some tumor cell lines [45]. The VDR can be induced by cell proliferation, by exposure to 1α-25$(OH)_2$D and by the ontogenetic state. 1α-$(OH)_2$D is the most potent natural calciferol metabolite, with a binding affinity that is approximately 1,000-fold greater than that of 25(OH)D in most test systems. Because of differing concentration ranges for metabolites, the receptor may be activated in vivo by a mixture of agonists including 1α-25$(OH)_2$D, 25(OH)D3 and 5,6-*trans*-25(OH)D.

The recent identification of allelic variations of the *VDR* gene has stimulated interest in examining possible relationships between VDR genotypes and a variety of traditional as well as nontraditional potential vitamin D target effects, including bone mineral density, bone turnover, and parathyroid function, as well as immune function, propensity to urolithiasis, and risk of certain malignancies [45, 50–63]. These allelic variants, which represent polymorphisms for the recognition sites of the restriction endonucleases *Bsm*I, *Taq*I, *Fok*I, and *Apa*I, generate specific genotypes in most populations studied. Although initial studies showed a strong association between *VDR* gene polymorphisms, bone mass, and bone turnover [59], more recent studies have been conflicting, and suggest a lesser role for *VDR* alleles in the determination of the heritable component of bone density.

1α-25$(OH)_2$D binds to the VDR hormone-binding domain in target tissues, enabling the VDR DNA-binding domain to bind to hormone response elements (HREs) in target genes, thereby regulating gene transcription of many proteins (table 2). The details of this process, such as the nature of the HREs are now beginning to become clear, and some of the target genes are known (e.g. intestinal calcium-binding protein, osteocalcin, osteopontin, and calmodulin). 1α-25$(OH)_2$D also has some cellular effects that are not mediated by a genomic pathway. Evidence for these non-genomic mechanisms includes extremely rapid effects, interaction with receptor proteins that are localized to the plasma membrane, and dependency on normal receptor genes [64–67].

The most important physiologic action of 1α-25$(OH)_2$D is stimulation of active calcium transport across the duodenum from lumen to bloodstream [68]. Surprisingly, few details are known about the molecular basis of this process. Vitamin D compounds are believed to increase calcium absorption by inducing a calcium channel (epithelial calcium transporter or calcium transporter-1 [CaT1]) on the luminal membrane, a calcium-binding protein (Calbindin D9k) in the cytosol, and a calcium pump (plasma membrane calcium adenosine triphosphatase-1 [PMCA1]) on the basolateral membrane. There are at least two calbindin genes; one codes for the 9-kD protein concentrated in the duodenum, the other for a homologous 28-kD protein concentrated in kidney, brain, and many other tissues [69].

Most of the antirachitic actions of calciferols are secondary to maintenance of calcium and phosphate concentrations in extracellular fluid adequate for bone mineralization. 1α-25$(OH)_2$D inhibits proliferation and collagen synthesis in fetal bone and in fetal osteoblasts, whereas in osteoblast-like cells from adult humans 1α-25$(OH)_2$D stimulates collagen synthesis. Differing effects on alkaline phosphatase have been reported in several systems; however, there is general agreement that in rapidly growing osteoblast-like cells alkaline phosphatase levels are low and that they rise in response to 1α-25$(OH)_2$D.

In vivo and in organ culture, 1α-25$(OH)_2$D is a potent activator of osteoclasts. 1α-25$(OH)_2$D induces monocyte stem cells in the bone marrow to differentiate to osteoclasts. Once osteoclasts have matured they no longer respond directly to 1α-25$(OH)_2$D and do not contain VDRs. Osteoclastic activity is stimulated indirectly by 1α-25$(OH)_2$D through its action on osteoblasts and osteocytes, which produce a variety of cytokines, including a factor termed osteoclast differentiation/inhibitory factor (ODIF, also termed RANK ligand). RANK ligand (RANKL) is a member of the tumor necrosis factor (TNF) superfamily that plays an essential role in osteoclastogenesis, as well as the activation and survival of mature osteoclasts. This factor is expressed on osteoblasts, stromal cells, B-lymphoid lineage cells and activated T cells as a transmembrane ligand and it also exists in a biologically active soluble form [70–74]. RANKL acts through its receptor RANK, which is expressed on osteoclast precursors, mature osteoclasts, as well as dendritic cells [75, 76]. Osteoprotegerin (OPG) is a soluble decoy receptor, which binds RANKL and blocks its interaction with RANK [75, 76].

Calcium Homeostasis

A normal adult may ingest 1,000 mg of elemental calcium per day, of which roughly 400–500 mg may be absorbed. However, 300 mg of calcium from digestive secretions is lost in the stool, resulting in the net absorption of only 100–200 mg. In the steady state, this quantity of calcium is excreted in the urine (fig. 5a).

The regulation of body calcium content is primarily by way of the gastrointestinal tract. Calcium absorption occurs by active transport primarily in the

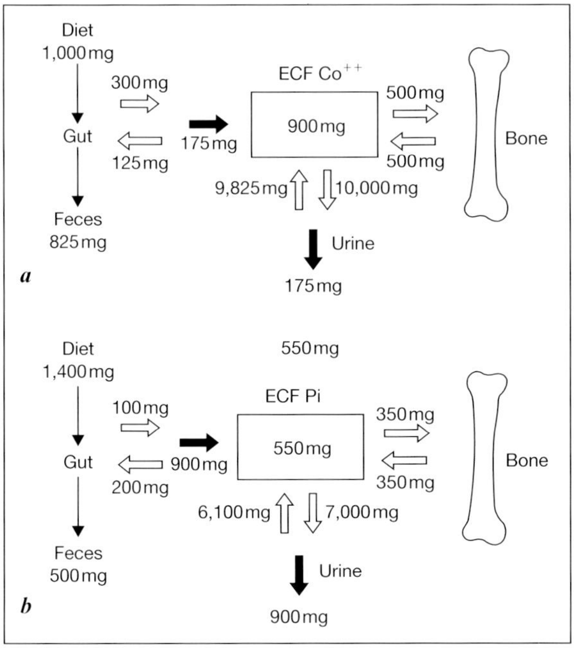

Fig. 5. Normal mineral homeostasis. The daily fluxes of calcium (***a***) and phosphorous (***b***) in a normal adult in zero mineral ion balance are shown.

duodenum, there is also absorption by passive diffusion. Variations in endogenous (intestinal secretory) losses of calcium can markedly affect measures of true percent calcium absorption. The efficiency of calcium absorption is affected by the calcium and vitamin D status of the body and by physiological states such as growth, old age and pregnancy. The efficiency of calcium absorption is much greater from the duodenum/jejunum segments of the intestine than from the ileum. A more important factor may be the residence time of the calcium in the segments of the intestine. The intestinal calcium absorption occurs by two processes, a saturable, active transfer in the upper and mid section of the small intestine and a nonsaturable, diffusional transfer. The latter, along the entire small intestine, is independent of the vitamin D status. In preterm infants, as calcium intake increases, so does the intestinal absorption of calcium. Human milk fed and formula fed infants supplemented with vitamin D exhibit significantly greater absorption of calcium compared with their unsupplemented counterparts. Intestinal maturation with regard to vitamin D responsiveness is accelerated by preterm delivery. Although the above does not establish the relative importance of passive and active mechanisms or the timing of intestinal vitamin D responsiveness with regard to calcium absorption, they do indicate that absorption of calcium is not a limiting issue for the preterm infant. With proper attention to dietary manipulation, adequate calcium balance should be attained.

Most of the body calcium and much of the phosphate exist as hydroxy-apatite, $Ca_{10}(PO_4)_6(OH)_2$, the main mineral component of bone. Phosphate also is present in high concentration in the cells. Within the plasma, both calcium and phosphate circulate in different forms. Of the plasma calcium, roughly 40% is bound to albumin, 15% is complexed with citrate, sulfate, or phosphate, and 45% exists as the physiologically important ionized (or free) Ca^{2+}. Plasma phosphorus, in comparison, consists of phospholipids, ester phosphates, and inorganic phosphates. The latter are completely ionized, circulating primarily as HPO_4^{2-} or $H_2PO_4^-$ in a ratio of 4:1 at a plasma pH of 7.40.

Albumin is the major calcium-binding serum protein, and hypoalbuminemia, rather than a decrease in the concentration of ionized calcium, accounts for most cases of low total serum calcium in hospitalized patients. Because reliable direct measurement of ionized serum calcium is not always readily available, a number of algorithms have been proposed, which are based on albumin or total protein concentrations, for the 'correction' of total serum calcium. None of these correction factors should be regarded as absolutely accurate, but they are useful as general indicators of the concentration of ionized calcium in serum. One widely used algorithm estimates that total serum calcium declines by approximately 0.8 mg/dl for each 1-g/dl decrease in albumin concentration, without a change in ionized calcium.

Sudden changes in the distribution of calcium between ionized and bound fractions may cause symptoms of hypocalcemia, even in patients who have normal hormonal mechanisms for the regulation of the ionized calcium concentration. Increases in the extracellular fluid concentration of anions, such as phosphate, citrate, bicarbonate, or edetic acid, will increase the proportion of bound calcium and decrease ionized calcium until intact regulatory mechanisms normalize ionized calcium. Extracellular fluid pH also affects the distribution of calcium between ionized and bound fractions. Acidosis increases the ionized calcium, whereas alkalosis decreases it.

Phosphorous Homeostasis

Phosphorus plays a critical role in skeletal development, mineral metabolism, and diverse cellular functions involving intermediary metabolism and energy-transfer mechanisms. It is a vital component of bone mineralization, phospholipids in membranes, nucleotides that provide energy and serve as components of DNA and RNA, and phosphorylated intermediates in cellular signaling. Compared to calcium, much less is known about the intestinal absorption of inorganic phosphate. The absorption of inorganic phosphate occurs throughout the entire small intestine, but the jejunum exhibits the highest rate of transport. Both active and passive processes are involved in the movement of inorganic phosphate from the intestinal mucosa to the serosa (fig. 5b).

The regulation of intestinal inorganic phosphate appears to be centered on the co-transport of sodium and inorganic phosphate. With restriction of dietary inorganic phosphate, fractional intestinal absorption of inorganic phosphate increases. Dietary inorganic phosphate restriction increases the production of 1α-$25(OH)_2D$ and thereby augments the active component of inorganic phosphate absorption. There is also an increase in intestinal absorption of inorganic phosphate in response to dietary restriction that is independent of vitamin D. The intestinal absorption is enhanced when the intraluminal environment is somewhat acidic. In contrast, metabolic acidosis, which should decrease intracellular pH, markedly decreases inorganic phosphate uptake.

In preterm and term infants inorganic phosphate is well absorbed from the gastrointestinal tract regardless of the type of feeding given and generally independent of the intake of vitamin D. The percentage of inorganic phosphate absorbed increases as inorganic phosphate intake decreases, but the absolute absorption of inorganic phosphate increases proportionally with increasing intake. In infants fed soy-based formula, the intestinal absorption of inorganic phosphate is lower than infants fed cow's milk-base formula. It appears that by increasing the calcium and inorganic phosphate content of soy formula, this problem may be overcome.

Phosphorus exists in the plasma in an inorganic form and an organic form. Approximately 20% of the plasma inorganic phosphorus is protein bound, and the remainder circulates as free phosphate ions HPO_4^{2-} or $H_2PO_4^-$. Phosphorus in the form of the phosphate ions circulates in the blood and is filtered at the glomerulus. However, measurement of the plasma and urine phosphate content is expressed in terms of elemental phosphorus. Thus arises the interchangeable use of phosphorus and phosphate concentrations.

Similar to calcium, the serum phosphate level is maintained within a narrow range through a complex interplay between intestinal absorption, exchange with intracellular and bone storage pools, and renal tubular reabsorption. Hypophosphatemia stimulates calcitriol synthesis via the 25(OH)D-1α-hydroxylase in the kidney, leading to increased calcium and phosphorus absorption in the intestine and enhanced mobilization of calcium and phosphorus from bone. In addition, hypophosphatemia is a potent stimulator of an increase in maximal tubular reabsorption of phosphate (TmP/GFR). The resultant increased serum calcium inhibits PTH secretion with a subsequent increase in urinary calcium excretion and increases tubular reabsorption of phosphate. Thus, normal serum calcium levels are maintained and serum phosphorus levels are returned to normal.

The principal organ that regulates phosphate homeostasis is the kidney. Serum inorganic phosphorus (P_i) is filtered by the glomerulus, and 80% of the filtered load is reabsorbed predominantly along the proximal nephron. Regulation of proximal renal tubular reabsorption of phosphate is achieved through changes in the activity, number, and intracellular location of the brush border membrane type IIa sodium-phosphate co-transporter (NPT2). In mice, *Npt2* is the major sodium-phosphate (Na^+/P_i) co-transporter in the renal proximal tubule and comprises 84% of the sodium phosphate co-transporters [77]. Transgenic mice, in which both copies of *Npt2* have been disrupted, develop marked renal phosphate wasting that is associated with an 80% loss in proximal renal tubular absorptive capacity [78].

Many hormones and cytokines influence phosphorous reabsorption in the proximal renal tubule. GH, IGF-I, insulin, epidermal growth factor, thyroid hormone, calcitriol, and dietary phosphate depletion stimulate renal phosphorous reabsorption. PTH, PTHrp, calcitonin, atrial naturetic factor, TGF-α and -β, and glucocorticoids all inhibit renal phosphorous reabsorption.

PTH is the best-characterized physiological regulator of phosphate reabsorption, but its principal function is to maintain calcium homeostasis. PTH increases urinary phosphate excretion via cAMP-dependent inhibition of NPT2 expression. This effect is rapid and is achieved by endocytic retrieval of NPT2 molecules from the brush border membrane and enhanced lysosomal degradation [79–81]. By contrast, both acute and chronic phosphorous deprivation initiates an adaptive increase in brush border membrane sodium phosphate transport through microtubule-dependent recruitment of Npt2 protein to the apical membrane surface [82].

The role of FGF23 as a putative regulator of phosphate homeostasis is emerging from studies of acquired and genetic syndromes of hypophosphatemic rickets [83]. FGF-23, the largest member of the FGF family, contains 251 amino acids, including a 24 amino acid hydrophobic amino terminus that is a signal sequence [84]. FGF-23 has a distinct carboxy-terminus that is not homologous to other members of the FGF family. FGF-23 is most similar to FGF-21 and FGF-19 (24 and 22% amino acid identities, respectively) [84]. FGF-23 lacks several heparin-binding residues that are conserved in other FGFs and, thus, FGF-23 may be more soluble and more likely to circulate than other FGFs.

Missense mutations in one of two arginine residues at positions 176 or 179 have been identified in affected members of four unrelated ADHR families [85]. This clustering of missense mutations suggests that they are activating mutations. Furthermore, the mutated arginine residues, located in the consensus proteolytic cleavage RXXR motif, prevent the degradation of FGF-23 and, thus, may result in prolonged or enhanced FGF-23 action [86, 87]. Thus far, FGF-23 is the only known FGF that is associated with a human disease.

Preliminary reports [88] demonstrate that FGF-23 binds to the FGFR2 and FGFR4 receptors, both of which are expressed in the kidney. Interestingly, the FGF-23 (R179Q) mutant binds preferentially to FGFR4. Identifying a specific receptor for FGF-23 is an area of intense interest, and although the entire FGF family shares four receptors, the distinctive structural properties of FGF-23 suggest that it may have a unique receptor.

FGF-23 has been proposed to have either paracrine and/or endocrine roles. Decreased FGF-23 secretion could represent an endocrine response to dietary phosphate restriction, and, thus, circulating FGF-23 might provide a closed feedback loop between a putative phosphate sensor and renal phosphate reabsorption. By analogy to PTHrp, a paracrine factor that was initially recognized as the humoral mediator of malignancy-associated hypercalcemia, FGF-23 may function physiologically as a locally-acting factor, but may also function pathophysiologically when secreted in excess into the circulation, where it can cause marked renal loss of phosphorous.

Conclusion

Acquired and genetic disorders of mineral metabolism can impair skeletal mineralization and result in rickets and osteomalacia. These conditions can reveal important physiological intersections between the effects of nature and nurture on the developing and growing skeleton, and point to important metabolic pathways that involve known as well as yet unknown regulatory hormones and cytokines. Insights gained from elucidating the molecular defects in calciopenic and hypophosphatemic disorders will further augment our understanding of these regulatory pathways.

References

1 Hebert SC, Brown EM: The extracellular calcium receptor (review; 64 refs.). Curr Opin Cell Biol 1995;7:484–492.

2 Brown EM, Gamba G, Riccardi D, Lombardi M, Butters R, Kofor O, Sun A, Hediger MA, Lytton J, Hebert SC: Cloning and characterization of an extracellular Ca^{2+}-sensing receptor from bovine parathyroid. Nature 1993;366:575–580.

3 Chattopadhyay N, Mithal A, Brown EM: The calcium-sensing receptor: a window into the physiology and pathophysiology of mineral ion metabolism. Endocr Rev 1996;17:289–307.

4 Neer EJ: Heterotrimeric G proteins: Organizers of transmembrane signals. Cell 1995;80:249–257.

5 Gudermann T, Nurnberg B, Schultz G: Receptors and G proteins as primary components of transmembrane signal transduction. 1. G-protein-coupled receptors: Structure and function. J Mol Med 1995;73:51–63.

6 Nurnberg B, Gudermann T, Schultz G: Receptors and G proteins as primary components of transmembrane signal transduction. 2. G proteins: Structure and function. J Mol Med 1995;73:123–132.

7 Yamaguchi T, Chattopadhyay N, Brown EM: G protein-coupled extracellular Ca^{2+} ($Ca^{2+}o$)-sensing receptor (CaR): Roles in cell signaling and control of diverse cellular functions. Adv Pharmacol 2000;47:209–253.

8 Schipani E, Karga H, Karaplis AC, Potts JT Jr, Kronenberg HM, Segre GV, Abou-Samra AB, Juppner H: Identical complementary deoxyribonucleic acids encode a human renal and bone parathyroid hormone (PTH)/PTH-related peptide receptor. Endocrinology 1993;132:2157–2165.

9 Abou Samra AB, Juppner H, Force T, Freeman MW, Kong XF, Schipani E, Urena P, Richards J, Bonventre JV, Potts JT Jr, et al: Expression cloning of a common receptor for parathyroid hormone and parathyroid hormone-related peptide from rat osteoblast-like cells: A single receptor stimulates intracellular accumulation of both cAMP and inositol trisphosphates and increases intracellular free calcium. Proc Natl Acad Sci USA 1992;89:2732–2736.

10 Juppner H, Abou Samra AB, Freeman M, Kong XF, Schipani E, Richards J, Kolakowski LF Jr, Hock J, Potts JT Jr, Kronenberg HM, et al: A G protein-linked receptor for parathyroid hormone and parathyroid hormone-related peptide. Science 1991;254:1024–1026.

11 Adams AE, Pines M, Nakamoto C, Behar V, Yang QM, Chorev M, Rosenblatt M, Levine MA, Suva LJ: Probing the bimolecular interaction of parathyroid hormone (PTH) and the human PTH/PTHrP receptor. II. Cloning, characterization of and photoaffinity crosslinking to the recombinant human PTH/PTHrP receptor. Biochemistry 1995;34:10553–10559.

12 Behar V, Pines M, Nakamoto C, Greenberg Z, Bisello A, Stueckle SM, Bessalle R, Usdin TB, Chorev M, Rosenblatt M, et al: The human PTH2 receptor: Binding and signal transduction properties of the stably expressed recombinant receptor. Endocrinology 1996;137:2748–2757.

13 Usdin TB, Gruber C, Bonner TI: Identification and functional expression of a receptor selectively recognizing parathyroid hormone, the PTH2. J Biol Chem 1995;270:15455–15458.

14 Usdin TB: Evidence for a parathyroid hormone-2 receptor selective ligand in the hypothalamus. Endocrinology 1997;138:831–834.

15 Hoare SR, Clark JA, Usdin TB: Molecular determinants of tuberoinfundibular peptide of 39 residues (TIP39) selectivity for the parathyroid hormone-2 (PTH2) receptor: N-terminal truncation of TIP39 reverses PTH2 receptor/PTH1 receptor binding selectivity. J Biol Chem 2000;275:27274–27283.

16 Schwindinger WF, Fredericks J, Watkins L, Robinson H, Bathon JM, Pines M, Suva LJ, Levine MA: Coupling of the PTH/PTHrP receptor to multiple G-proteins: Direct demonstration of receptor activation of Gs, Gq/11, and Gi(1) by [α-32P]GTP-gamma-azidoanilide photoaffinity labeling. Endocrine 1998;8:201–209.

17 Melson GL, Chase LR, Aurbach GD: Parathyroid hormone-sensitive adenyl cyclase in isolated renal tubules. Endocrinology 1970;86:511–518.

18 Chase LR, Fedak SA, Aurbach GD: Activation of skeletal adenyl cyclase by parathyroid hormone in vitro. Endocrinology 1969:84:761–768.

19 Civitelli R, Reid IR, Westbrook S, Avioli LV, Hruska KA: PTH elevates inositol polyphosphates and diacylglycerol in a rat osteoblast-like cell line. Am J Physiol 1988;255:E660–E667.

20 Dunlay R, Hruska K: PTH receptor coupling to phospholipase C is an alternate pathway of signal transduction in bone and kidney. Am J Physiol 1990;258:F223–F231.

21 Gupta A, Martin KJ, Miyauchi A, Hruska KA: Regulation of cystosolic calcium in fibroblasts from normal and pseudohypoparathyroid patients. Endocrinology 1991;128:2825–2836.

22 Civitelli R, Martin TJ, Fausto A, Gunsten SL, Hruska KA, Avioli LV: Parathyroid hormone-related peptide transiently increases cytosolic calcium in osteoblast-like cells: Comparison with parathyroid hormone. Endocrinology 1989;125:1204–1210.

23 Reid IR, Civitelli R, Halstead LR, Avioli LV, Hruska KA: Parathyroid hormone acutely elevates intracellular calcium in osteoblast-like cells. Am J Physiol 1987;253:E45–E51.

24 Yamaguchi DT, Hahn TJ, Iida-Klein A, Kleeman CR, Muallem S: Parathyroid hormone-activated calcium channels in an osteoblast-like clonal osteosarcoma cell line. J Biol Chem 1987;262: 7711–7718.

25 Kaufmann M, Muff R, Stieger B, Biber J, Murer H, Fischer JA: Apical and basolateral parathyroid hormone receptors in rat renal cortical membranes. Endocrinology 1994;134:1173–1178.

26 Kempson SA, Lotscher M, Kaissling B, Biber J, Murer H, Levi M: Parathyroid hormone action on phosphate transporter mRNA and protein in rat renal proximal tubules. Am J Physiol 1995;268: F784–F791.

27 Matsuoka LY, Ide L, Wortsman J, MacLaughlin JA, Holick MF: Sunscreens suppress cutaneous vitamin D_3 synthesis. J Clin Endocrinol Metab 1987;64:1165–1168.

28 Holick MF, Matsuoka LY, Wortsman J: Age, vitamin D, and solar ultraviolet. Lancet 1989; ii:1104–1105.

29 Holick MF: Vitamin D – new horizons for the 21st century. Am J Clin Nutr 1994;60:619–630.

30 Goode JL: Bone disease: A primer. I. Clinical differences among vitamin D hormone compounds. Nephrol News Issues 2001;15:22–23.

31 Bailie GR, Johnson CA: Comparative review of the pharmacokinetics of vitamin D analogues. Semin Dial 2002;15:352–357.

32 Saarem K, Bergseth S, Oftebro H, Pedersen JI: Subcellular localization of vitamin D_3 25-hydroxylase in human liver. J Biol Chem 1984;259:10936–10940.

33 Zehnder D, Bland R, Williams MC, McNinch RW, Howie AJ, Stewart PM, Hewison M: Extrarenal expression of 25-hydroxyvitamin d(3)-1 alpha-hydroxylase. J Clin Endocrinol Metab 2001; 86:888–894.

34 Segersten U, Correa P, Hewison M, Hellman P, Dralle H, Carling T, Akerstrom G, Westin G: 25-hydroxyvitamin D(3)-1alpha-hydroxylase expression in normal and pathological parathyroid glands. J Clin Endocrinol Metab 2002;87:2967–2972.

35 Zehnder D, Bland R, Walker EA, Bradwell AR, Howie AJ, Hewison M, Stewart PM: Expression of 25-hydroxyvitamin D_3−1alpha-hydroxylase in the human kidney. J Am Soc Nephrol 1999; 10:2465–2473.

36 Bland R, Zehnder D, Hewison M: Expression of 25-hydroxyvitamin D_3−1alpha-hydroxylase along the nephron: New insights into renal vitamin D metabolism. Curr Opin Nephrol Hypertens 2000;9:17–22.

37 Zierold C, Mings JA, DeLuca HF: Regulation of 25-hydroxyvitamin D3–24-hydroxylase mRNA by 1,25-dihydroxyvitamin D_3 and parathyroid hormone. J Cell Biochem 2003;88:234–237.

38 Haddad JG, Kowalski MA, Sanger JW: Actin affinity chromatography in the purification of human, avian and other mammalian plasma proteins binding vitamin D and its metabolites (Gc globulins). Biochem J 1984;218:805–810.

39 Coppenhaver DH, Sollenne NP, Bowman BH: Post-translational heterogeneity of the human vitamin D-binding protein (group-specific component). Arch Biochem Biophys 1983;226:218–223.

40 Cooke NE, David EV: Serum vitamin D-binding protein is a third member of the albumin and alpha fetoprotein gene family. J Clin Invest 1985;76:2420–2424.

41 Lawson DE, Douglas J, Lean M, Sedrani S: Estimation of vitamin D_3 and 25-hydroxyvitamin D_3 in muscle and adipose tissue of rats and man. Clin Chim Acta 1986;157:175–181.

42 MacDonald PN, Dowd DR, Haussler MR: New insight into the structure and functions of the vitamin D receptor. Semin Nephrol 1994;14:101–118.

43 Baker AR, McDonnell DP, Hughes M, Crisp TM, Mangelsdorf DJ, Haussler MR, Pike JW, Shine J, O'Malley BW: Cloning and expression of full-length cDNA encoding human vitamin D receptor. Proc Natl Acad Sci USA 1988;85:3294–3298.

44 Haussler MR, Mangelsdorf DJ, Komm BS, Terpening CM, Yamaoka K, Allegretto EA, Baker AR, Shine J, McDonnell DP, Hughes M, et al: Molecular biology of the vitamin D hormone. Recent Prog Horm Res 1988;44:263–305.

45 Haussler MR, Haussler CA, Jurutka PW, Thompson PD, Hsieh JC, Remus LS, Selznick SH, Whitfield GK: The vitamin D hormone and its nuclear receptor: molecular actions and disease states. J Endocrinol 1997;154(suppl):S57–S73.

46 Whitfield GK, Hsieh JC, Jurutka PW, Selznick SH, Haussler CA, MacDonald PN, Haussler MR: Genomic actions of 1,25-dihydroxyvitamin D_3. J Nutr 1995;125:1690S–1694S.

47 Pathrose P, Barmina O, Chang CY, McDonnell DP, Shevde NK, Pike JW: Inhibition of 1,25-dihydroxyvitamin D_3-dependent transcription by synthetic LXXLL peptide antagonists that target the activation domains of the vitamin D and retinoid X receptors. J Bone Miner Res 2002;17: 2196–2205.

48 Jin CH, Kerner SA, Hong MH, Pike JW: Transcriptional activation and dimerization functions in the human vitamin D receptor. Mol Endocrinol 1996;10:945–957.

49 Sone T, Kerner S, Pike JW: Vitamin D receptor interaction with specific DNA: Association as a 1,25-dihydroxyvitamin D_3-modulated heterodimer. J Biol Chem 1991;266:23296–23305.

50 Hustmyer FG, DeLuca HF, Peacock M: *Apa*I, *Bsm*I, *Eco*RV and *Taq*I polymorphisms at the human vitamin D receptor gene locus in Caucasians, blacks and Asians. Hum Mol Genet 1993;2:487.

51 Peacock M, Hustmyer FG, Hui S, Johnston CC, Christian J: Vitamin D receptor genotype and bone mineral density: Evidence conflicts on link. BMJ 1995;311:874–875.

52 Ferrari S, Rizzoli R, Bonjour JP: Genetic aspects of osteoporosis. Curr Opin Rheumatol 1999; 11:294–300.

53 Gennari L, Becherini L, Falchetti A, Masi L, Massart F, Brandi ML: Genetics of osteoporosis: role of steroid hormone receptor gene polymorphisms. J Steroid Biochem Mol Biol 2002;81:1–24.

54 Eckstein M, Vered I, Ish-Shalom S, Shlomo AB, Shtriker A, Koren-Morag N, Friedman E: Vitamin D and calcium-sensing receptor genotypes in men and premenopausal women with low bone mineral density. Isr Med Assoc J 2002;4:340–344.

55 Laaksonen M, Karkkainen M, Outila T, Vanninen T, Ray C, Lamberg-Allardt C: Vitamin D receptor gene *Bsm*I-polymorphism in Finnish premenopausal and postmenopausal women: its association with bone mineral density, markers of bone turnover, and intestinal calcium absorption, with adjustment for lifestyle factors. J Bone Miner Metab 2002;20:383–390.

56 Zajickova K, Zofkova I, Bahbouh R, Krepelova A: Vitamin D receptor gene polymorphisms, bone mineral density and bone turnover: *Fok*I genotype is related to postmenopausal bone mass. Physiol Res 2002;51:501–509.

57 Morrison NA, Yeoman R, Kelly PJ, Eisman JA: Contribution of trans-acting factor alleles to normal physiological variability: Vitamin D receptor gene polymorphism and circulating osteocalcin. Proc Natl Acad Sci USA 1992;89:6665–6669.

58 Hustmyer FG, Peacock M, Hui S, Johnston CC, Christian J: Bone mineral density in relation to polymorphism at the vitamin D receptor gene locus. J Clin Invest 1994;94:2130–2134.

59 Morrison NA, Qi JC, Tokita A, Kelly PJ, Crofts L, Nguyen TV, Sambrook PN, Eisman JA: Prediction of bone density from vitamin D receptor alleles. Nature 1994;367:284–287.

60 White CP, Morrison NA, Gardiner EM, Eisman JA: Vitamin D receptor alleles and bone physiology. J Cell Biochem 1994;56:307–314.

61 Sambrook PN, Kelly PJ, Morrison NA, Eisman JA: Genetics of osteoporosis. Br J Rheumatol 1994;33:1007–1011.

62 Riggs BL, Nguyen TV, Melton LJ III, Morrison NA, O'Fallon WM, Kelly PJ, Egan KS, Sambrook PN, Muhs JM, Eisman JA: The contribution of vitamin D receptor gene alleles to the determination of bone mineral density in normal and osteoporotic women. J Bone Miner Res 1995;10:991–996.

63 Curran JE, Vaughan T, Lea RA, Weinstein SR, Morrison NA, Griffiths LR: Association of A vitamin D receptor polymorphism with sporadic breast cancer development. Int J Cancer 1999;83:723–726.

64 Baran DT: Nongenomic actions of the steroid hormone 1 alpha 25-dihydroxyvitamin D_3. J Cell Biochem 1994;56:303–306.

65 Baran DT, Quail JM, Ray R, Leszyk J, Honeyman T: Annexin II is the membrane receptor that mediates the rapid actions of 1alpha 25-dihydroxyvitamin D(3). J Cell Biochem 2000; 78:34–46.

66 Barsony J, Marx SJ: Rapid accumulation of cyclic GMP near activated vitamin D receptors. Proc Natl Acad Sci USA 1991;88:1436–1440.

67 Boland R, de Boland AR, Buitrago C, Morelli S, Santillan G, Vazquez G, Capiati D, Baldi C: Non-genomic stimulation of tyrosine phosphorylation cascades by 1 25(OH)(2)D(3) by VDR-dependent and -independent mechanisms in muscle cells. Steroids 2002;67:477–482.

68 Christakos S, Barletta F, Huening M, Dhawan P, Liu Y, Porta A, Peng X: Vitamin D target proteins: Function and regulation. J Cell Biochem 2003;88:238–244.

69 Li YC, Bolt MJ, Cao LP, Sitrin MD: Effects of vitamin D receptor inactivation on the expression of calbindins and calcium metabolism. Am J Physiol Endocrinol Metab 2001;281:E558–E564.

70 Yasuda H, Shima N, Nakagawa N, Yamaguchi K, Kinosaki M, Mochizuki S, Tomoyasu A, Yano K, Goto M, Murakami A, et al: Osteoclast differentiation factor is a ligand for osteoprotegerin/ osteoclastogenesis-inhibitory factor and is identical to TRANCE/RANKL. Proc Natl Acad Sci USA 1998;95:3597–3602.

71 Nakagawa N, Kinosaki M, Yamaguchi K, Shima N, Yasuda H, Yano K, Morinaga T, Higashio K: RANK is the essential signaling receptor for osteoclast differentiation factor in osteoclastogenesis. Biochem Biophys Res Commun 1998;253:395–400.
72 Lacey DL, Timms E, Tan HL, Kelley MJ, Dunstan CR, Burgess T, Elliott R, Colombero A, Elliott G, Scully S, et al: Osteoprotegerin ligand is a cytokine that regulates osteoclast differentiation and activation. Cell 1998;93:165–176.
73 Burgess TL, Qian Y, Kaufman S, Ring BD, Van G, Capparelli C, Kelley M, Hsu H, Boyle WJ, Dunstan CR, et al: The ligand for osteoprotegerin (OPGL) directly activates mature osteoclasts. J Cell Biol 1999;145:527–538.
74 Manabe N, Kawaguchi H, Chikuda H, Miyaura C, Inada M, Nagai R, Nabeshima Y, Nakamura K, Sinclair AM, Scheuermann RH, et al: Connection between B lymphocyte and osteoclast differentiation pathways. J Immunol 2001;167:2625–2631.
75 Hofbauer LC, Heufelder AE: Role of receptor activator of nuclear factor-kappaB ligand and osteoprotegerin in bone cell biology. J Mol Med 2001;79:243–253.
76 Hofbauer LC, Khosla S, Dunstan CR, Lacey DL, Boyle WJ, Riggs BL: The roles of osteoprotegerin and osteoprotegerin ligand in the paracrine regulation of bone resorption. J Bone Miner Res 2000;15:2–12.
77 Tenenhouse HS, Roy S, Martel J, Gauthier C: Differential expression, abundance, and regulation of Na^+-phosphate cotransporter genes in murine kidney. Am J Physiol 1998;275:F527–F534.
78 Beck L, Karaplis AC, Amizuka N, Hewson AS, Ozawa H, Tenenhouse HS: Targeted inactivation of Npt2 in mice leads to severe renal phosphate wasting, hypercalciuria, and skeletal abnormalities. Proc Natl Acad Sci USA 1998;95:5372–5377.
79 Hernando N, Forster IC, Biber J, Murer H: Molecular characteristics of phosphate transporters and their regulation. Exp Nephrol 2000;8:366–375.
80 Murer H, Hernando N, Forster I, Biber J: Proximal tubular phosphate reabsorption: molecular mechanisms. Physiol Rev 2000;80:1373–1409.
81 Murer H, Hernando N, Forster I, Biber J: Regulation of Na/Pi Transporter in the Proximal Tubule. Annu Rev Physiol 2003;65:531–542.
82 Pfister MF, Hilfiker H, Forgo J, Lederer E, Biber J, Murer H: Cellular mechanisms involved in the acute adaptation of OK cell Na/P_i-cotransport to high- or low-P_i medium. Pflügers Arch 1998; 435:713–719.
83 Jan de Beur SM, Levine MA: Molecular pathogenesis of hypophosphatemic rickets. J Clin Endocrinol Metab 2002;87:2467–2473.
84 Yamashita T, Yoshioka M, Itoh N: Identification of a novel fibroblast growth factor, FGF-23, preferentially expressed in the ventrolateral thalamic nucleus of the brain. Biochem Biophys Res Commun 2000;277:494–498.
85 The ADHR Consortium: Autosomal dominant hypophosphataemic rickets is associated with mutations in FGF23. Nat Genet 2000;26:345–348.
86 White KE, Carn G, Lorenz-Depiereux B, Benet-Pages A, Strom TM, Econs MJ: Autosomal-dominant hypophosphatemic rickets (ADHR) mutations stabilize FGF-23. Kidney Int 2001;60:2079–2086.
87 Bowe AE, Finnegan R, Jan de Beur SM, Cho J, Levine MA, Kumar R, Schiavi SC: FGF-23 inhibits renal tubular phosphate transport and is a PHEX substrate. Biochem Biophys Res Commun 2001;284:977–981.
88 Jonsson KB, Pragnell M, Larsson T, White K, Econs M, Schiavi S: Recombinant FGF-23 interacts in vitro with FGF receptors 2 and 4 (abstract). J Bone Miner Res 2001;16:S251.

Michael A. Levine, MD
Division of Pediatrics
The Children's Hospital at The Cleveland Clinic Foundation
Crile Building, A120, 9500 Euclid Avenue
Cleveland, OH 44195 (USA)
Tel. +1 216 444 6717, Fax +1 216 445 3523, E-Mail levinem@ccf.org

Hochberg Z (ed): Vitamin D and Rickets.
Endocr Dev. Basel, Karger, 2003, vol 6, pp 34–49

Maternal, Fetal and Neonatal Vitamin D and Calcium Metabolism during Pregnancy and Lactation

Yosef Weisman

Bone Disease Unit, Tel-Aviv Sourasky Medical Center, Tel-Aviv, and Sackler Faculty of Medicine, Tel-Aviv University, Tel-Aviv, Israel

Contents

The placental translocation of large amounts of calcium from the pregnant woman to the fetus and, subsequently, the accretion of calcium in the fetal skeleton mandate significant hormone-mediated alterations in vitamin D and calcium metabolism in both the mother and fetus during pregnancy. In the neonatal period and during lactation, the newborn must quickly adjust to the loss of placental calcium supply while continuing to undergo rapid skeletal growth and the mother must continue to supply the daily calcium needs of the growing infant throughout the lactation period. These adjustments in calcium metabolism take place with minimal long-term consequences to the maternal skeleton.

This is a review of the present understanding of human calcium metabolism and the vitamin D endocrine system during normal pregnancy, the neonatal period and lactation. Since the subject of this book is rickets, the focus of this review is mainly on the vitamin D status and physiology in the mother and its effects on the vitamin D status and physiology in the fetus and newborn.

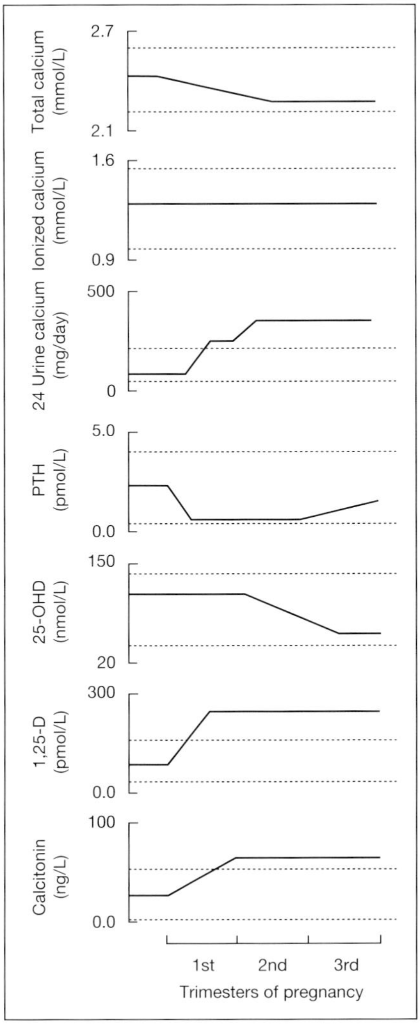

Fig. 1. Schematic illustration of the longitudinal changes in calcium and calcitropic hormones that occur during pregnancy. Data adapted from references [4] and [37]. Normal adult ranges are indicated by dashed lines.

Maternal Vitamin D and Calcium Metabolism during Pregnancy (fig. 1)

The normal fetus accumulates about 20–30 g calcium by the end of gestation. Approximately 80% of this calcium accumulates during the third trimester when the fetal skeleton is rapidly mineralized, i.e. at a daily rate of 250–300 mg [1, 2]. Theoretically, the maternal adaptations to meet the calcium needs of the developing fetus could involve: increased intestinal absorption of calcium, increased resorption of calcium from the maternal skeleton and decreased renal excretion of calcium. Accumulating evidence indicates that alterations in vitamin D metabolism during pregnancy is the major maternal adaptive mechanism, although increased resorption from the maternal skeleton may also play a part. The main characteristic of vitamin D metabolism during pregnancy is the 2- to 3-fold rise in maternal serum free and total $1,25(OH)_2D$ levels [3–7] (fig. 1). This increase starts as early as at 10–12 weeks of gestation and continues throughout the entire pregnancy. The rise in serum $1,25(OH)_2D$ concentration apparently causes increased intestinal expression of the vitamin D-dependent calcium binding protein, calbindin 9 k/D and, subsequently, a 2-fold increase in calcium absorption in the gut [4]. The rise in calcium absorption from the intestines causes a 2-fold increase in the 24-hour urinary calcium excretion [4, 5]. Although it was originally believed that these changes were caused by a state of physiologic hyperparathyroidism [8], it has been now become apparent from the results of the two-site immunoradiometric assays that the concentrations of parathyroid hormone (PTH) in the mother during pregnancy is at the lower end of normal for the non-pregnant values [5, 9, 10]. This is in contrast to previous high PTH levels obtained by the old radioassays, which were later shown to also measure biologically inactive PTH fragments. Despite the increase in intestinal calcium absorption, there is a progressive decrease in the maternal total serum calcium concentration during pregnancy [2]. This fall in total calcium is due to increased plasma volume, hemodilution and drop in serum albumin concentration [2]. Indeed, ionized calcium concentration is unchanged or slightly elevated during pregnancy [4]. It appears, therefore, that pregnancy is a state of physiologic absorptive hypercalciuria [4] and not a state of physiological maternal hyperparathyroidism. The question arises as to why maternal serum $1,25(OH)_2D$ increases so significantly when the PTH levels remain normal or low. PTH is the major stimulator of 25-hydroxyvitamin D-1α-hydroxylase activity in the kidneys of non-pregnant women, but the low PTH concentrations during pregnancy make PTH an unlikely candidate for stimulation of $1,25(OH)_2D$ production in the maternal kidney. It has been suggested that other tissues, such as the decidua, placenta and fetal kidney may also contribute to the elevated maternal $1,25(OH)_2D$ levels in pregnancy. Several lines of evidence support the notion that those tissues are apparently significant sources of increased $1,25(OH)_2D$ in the maternal serum: (1) in vivo experiments have shown that when $[^3H]$-25-hydroxyvitamin D is injected into anephric pregnant rats, $[^3H]$-$1,25(OH)_2D$ appears in both the fetal and maternal serum [11]; (2) in vitro studies have shown that $1,25(OH)_2D$ is produced by the human decidua and placenta as well as by the human fetal kidney [12–15]; (3) women with pseudo-hypoparathyroidism who, before pregnancy, had hypocalcemia, markedly elevated PTH levels and low $1,25(OH)_2D$ levels, remained normocalcemic during pregnancy, even without calcium and vitamin D therapy, while their serum 1,25$(OH)_2$D increased by 2-fold and their PTH levels were half of what they had been before pregnancy [14, 16], and (4) uremic rats with secondary hyperparathyroidism had increased levels of 1,25$(OH)_2$D and their elevated PTH levels decreased to normal levels on becoming pregnant. The state of hyperparathyroidism returned after parturition [17]. The relative contribution and amounts of 1,25$(OH)_2$D produced in the maternal kidney, the decidua, placenta and fetal kidney are unknown at present. While the decidua and placenta may add significant amounts of 1,25$(OH)_2$D to the maternal compartment, the contribution of the fetal kidney is probably negligible, since 1,25$(OH)_2$D production and fetal serum levels are low [18]. The increase in the maternal 1,25$(OH)_2$D concentration, while the PTH level is in the normal range, suggests that PTH does not mediate the up-regulation of 1,25$(OH)_2$D production. Another potential regulator of 1α-hydroxylase activity during pregnancy might be parathyroid hormone-related protein (PTHrP) whose levels rise during pregnancy in the mother and the placenta [19, 20]. Other regulating factors may include: prolactin, placental lactogen, estradiol and IGF-1, all of which have been shown to stimulate 1α-hydroxylase activity [21–24].

Serum 25(OH)D and 24,25$(OH)_2$D levels are unchanged or slightly lower in pregnant women than in non-pregnant ones [25]. The reduction of serum 25(OH)D levels may be due to hemodilution during pregnancy, but the major factor that determines 25(OH)D levels is the maternal exposure to sunlight, which depends on the season, the geographical location and the degree of covering of the body in accord with religious or cultural requirements [26–28].

Seasonal differences between the highest and lowest monthly means of serum 25(OH)D levels in pregnant women range from 10 to 20 ng/ml in various northern countries [26, 29] and may reach levels associated with osteomalacia in the winter and spring. Even in a sunny country such as Israel, seasonal variations in 25(OH)D serum levels were found in pregnant women and also expressed in cord serum [30] (fig. 2). It is now well recognized that pregnant Asian and Moslem women living in Britain [31, 32] and in other northern countries [33] are particularly at risk of vitamin D deficiency. The main causes are said to be underexposure to ultraviolet light due to religious modest dress codes of Moslems and the practice of vegetarianism [31] among Hindus. It is interesting that in sunny countries such as Israel [28] and the Arab countries [34], orthodox Jewish and Moslem religious traditions that require modest dress codes may result in maternal vitamin D deficiency during pregnancy. Human skeletal calcium metabolism during pregnancy and its contribution to maternal calcium homeostasis and to maternal fetal calcium transfer have been relatively unexplored. One histomorphometric study on women who electively terminated a pregnancy in the first trimester yielded biopsy evidence of

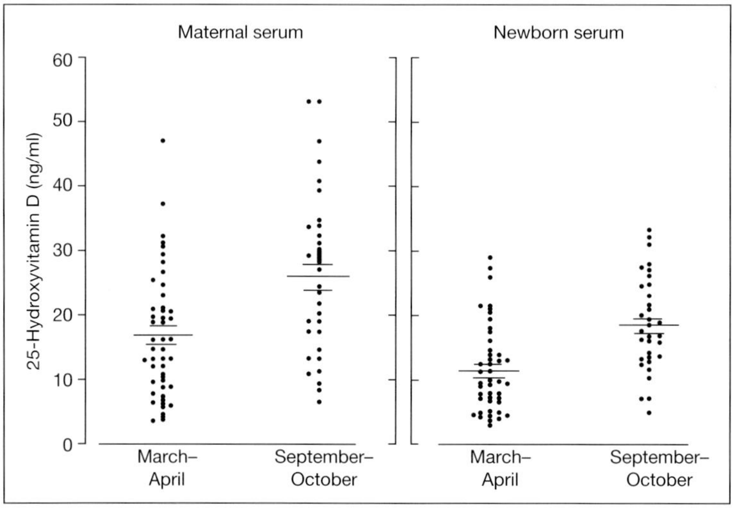

Fig. 2. 25-Hydroxyvitamin D levels in maternal and newborn serum in the spring and autumn [adapted from ref. 30].

increased bone resorption and decreased bone formation [35]. Measurement of bone markers demonstrated increased bone turnover as early as the 10th week of gestation and during the second trimester, but there is no evidence for accelerated resorption during the third trimester at the time of peak maternal-fetal calcium transfer. Studies using dual-energy X-ray absorptiometry (DXA) before conception and after delivery obtained conflicting results [36]. Therefore, the question remains unsettled as to whether there is a significant loss of bone mineral during human pregnancy. At present, there is no evidence to show that changes in bone metabolism during pregnancy cause long-term changes in bone mineral content.

Fetal Placental Vitamin D and Calcium Metabolism

The fetus obtains large amounts of calcium and vitamin D from the mother, particularly during the third trimester. Despite the absolute dependence of these materials from the mothers, the calcium and vitamin D metabolism in the fetus is relatively independent and except for extreme conditions is not affected by the nutritional state of the mother. Maternal primary hyperparathyroidism may cause adverse outcomes in the fetus, including abortion, stillbirth and neonatal tetany and untreated maternal hypoparathyroidism may cause secondary hyperparathyroidism in the fetus and newborn. However, fetal calcium homeostasis remains unaffected in most cases of maternal hypocalcemia, hypercalcemia or vitamin D deficiency. Furthermore, the mineralization of the skeleton proceeds normally [37]. The fetal total and ionized calcium concentrations are maintained at a level significantly higher than that of the mother [38, 39]. The hypercalcemia of the fetus can be measured even at 15–20 weeks of gestation [40]. It is not yet clear what is the reason or the mechanism for the raising of calcium concentration in the blood of the fetus. It is probably not a requisite for normal skeletal mineralization or fetal growth, since skeletal mineral content in the PTHrP knockout fetal mice (in which the fetal calcium is low and not significantly different from that of the mother) is probably normal [41]. The fetus does not keep a constant gradient of calcium relative to the mothers but rather establishes for itself a high concentration of calcium, irrespective of the maternal level of calcium. When the mother is hypocalcemic, the calcium gradient increases and the high fetal calcium level remains unchanged.

We still do not know what determines the transplacental calcium transport. Receptors for $1,25(OH)_2D$ are present in the placenta [42] and pharmacological doses of $1,25(OH)_2D$ increased calcium transport across the placenta in placental perfusion models [43, 44]. It is tempting, therefore, to suggest that the $1,25(OH)_2D$ that is formed in the decidua and placenta [12, 13] may act in a paracrine fashion to stimulate the transport of calcium from the mother to the fetus, by analogy to its function in the intestinal tract. To date, however, there is no proof that vitamin D plays a major role in human placental calcium transport. Furthermore, 25-hydroxyvitamin D 1α-hydroxylase activity in the placenta and decidua is significantly higher in the first and second trimesters than in the third trimester of pregnancy, while calcium transport is much higher in the third trimester [45]. The authors of that study suggested that $1,25(OH)_2D$ production by the placenta and decidua has an autocrine/paracrine immunomodulatory function and a role in the implantation/placentation processes during early pregnancy. This assumption is supported by the observations that cytokines, such as TNF-α and γ-interferon stimulated $1,25(OH)_2D$ production in those tissues [Weisman, unpubl. data].

It has been suggested that PTHrP is the principal stimulator of the placental calcium transport from the mother to the fetus. PTHrP cord levels are significantly higher than its level in the maternal concentration while the concentration of PTH is only about 25% of the maternal levels [46]. PTHrP is produced in many sites in the developing fetus including fetal parathyroid glands [47], the skeletal growth plate [48] and the placenta amnion and chorion [20, 49]. All these sources may contribute to the high concentration of PTHrP in the fetus. Experiments performed in sheep and mice indicate that PTHrP (particularly the mid-molecular fragment PTHrP-67–86) is important in the placental transport of calcium [51, 52], but there are still no data for humans.

The cord levels of 25(OH)D and 24,25$(OH)_2D$ are between two-thirds and three-quarters that of the mother and correlate significantly with those found in the maternal circulation [52, 53]. These data are consistent with easy passive or facilitative placental transfer of 25(OH)D and 24,25$(OH)_2D$ and indicate that maternal stores of vitamin D and 25(OH)D comprise the critical factor which determines the newborn's vitamin D status at birth. Studies in rats have demonstrated that vitamin D, 25(OH)D and 24,25$(OH)_2D$ and, to a lesser degree, 1,25$(OH)_2D$ pass through the placenta during pregnancy and support the data obtained from paired human maternal and cord sera [54]. Since breast milk is a poor source of vitamin D [55], it is likely that vitamin D and 25(OH)D, which pass through the placenta during the third trimester of gestation, and stored in the fetus furnish the main vitamin D requirement of the newly born infant in its first months of life. This assumption is supported by the observation that vitamin D deficiency rickets in infants is associated with mothers whose diets were inadequate or with mothers who were underexposed to sunlight during pregnancy due to the dress code required by religious tradition or mothers with dark pigmentation of the skin [28, 31–34, 56]. Hypovitaminosis D in the mother and fetus is probably not a major limiting factor on bone linear growth in utero [57]. Frank rickets is very rare at birth and is seen only in fetuses of mothers with severe vitamin D deficiency [58, 59]. Nevertheless, there is presumably some interference in normal skull ossification, since larger fontanelles and craniotabes were found in infants born to mothers with vitamin D deficiency [57, 60]. Seasonal variations in vitamin D status during pregnancy may also affect bone mineral content of the fetus; low total body bone mineral content and high bone resorption were demonstrated in Korean winter-born versus summer-born newborn infants [29]. Supplementary vitamin D (1,000 IU/day) administered during the third trimester to vitamin D-deficient Asian women living in London and to French women living in Lyon resulted in significantly higher calcium concentrations and elimination of symptomatic hypocalcemia in newborns of treated mothers [57, 61]. Therefore, it was recommended that 400 IU/day should be given during pregnancy in countries where dairy products are not supplemented with vitamin D or in countries where sunshine exposure is low. A dose of 1,000 IU/day may be administered during the last trimester to women at risk to develop vitamin D deficiency [62].

Fetal blood levels of 1,25$(OH)_2D$ are lower than maternal levels in humans [18, 63, 64] and, unlike 25(OH)D and 24,25$(OH)_2D$, it does not readily cross the placenta in rats [65]. In humans, the free placental transport of 1,25$(OH)_2D$ is also unresolved; in some studies, no correlation between fetal and maternal concentrations was observed [18, 63] whereas a significant correlation was found in other studies [66]. It appears that the fetus has an independent 1,25(OH)$_2$D metabolism and that circulating levels of 1,25(OH)$_2$D in the fetus are largely derived and maintained by fetal sources. In rats and humans, the placenta [12, 13] and the kidney [15, 54] possess 1α-hydroxylase activity. The contribution of the fetal kidney must be significant since the cord plasma concentrations of 1,25(OH)$_2$D in infants with agenesis of the kidney (Potter syndrome) are one-third of those observed in healthy newborns [62] and since fetal nephrectomy in sheep [67] and rats [68] significantly reduced the fetal 1,25(OH)$_2$D levels. Receptors for 1,25(OH)$_2$D are present in the fetal intestine as early as 13 weeks of gestation [62] and in cultured amniotic fluid cells, skin fibroblasts and kidney cells obtained at mid-gestation [15]. Cultured amniotic fluid cells, skin fibroblasts and kidney cells obtained between 17–22 weeks' gestation also responded to 1,25(OH)$_2$D stimulation by increased 25(OH)D-24-hydroxylase activity [15]. These observations confirm the integrity of the 1,25(OH)$_2$D receptor effecter system in human fetal tissues at mid-gestation. Despite these observations in humans and the widespread expression of 1,25(OH)$_2$D receptor early in rat fetal skeleton development [69], the role of 1,25(OH)$_2$D in fetal calcium homeostasis and particularly in skeletal development and mineralization has not yet been determined. Furthermore, there are observations that support the notion that 1,25(OH)$_2$D is not essential for normal fetal calcium and bone metabolism: fetal mice that lack the gene encoding the receptor for 1,25(OH)$_2$D are born with a normal skeleton [70] and human fetuses with hereditary end-organ resistance to 1,25(OH)$_2$D due to mutations of the vitamin D receptor (vitamin D-dependent rickets type II) are also born with a normal skeleton [71] and develop hypocalcemia and rickets several months later.

Neonatal Vitamin D and Calcium Metabolism (table 1)

After the umbilical cord has been cut the neonate loses the transplacental supply of calcium and must adapt rapidly to ensure normal calcium homeostasis and skeletal growth and mineralization. The newborn is dependent on intestinal absorption and, therefore, must quickly stimulate the synthesis of PTH and 1,25(OH)$_2$D, which had been suppressed in the fetus. Total and ionized calcium levels decrease significantly within 24–48 h after birth [38, 72, 73]. Calcium concentrations usually return to normal by days 5–8 after birth. Serum PTH levels which are low at birth increase within the first 24–48 h, probably in response to the decrease in serum calcium [72, 74]. Subsequently, 1,25(OH)$_2$D levels rise to adult levels within a few days [63]. Serum calcitonin rises 2- to 10-fold over cord blood levels within the first 48 h [75]. Hypocalcemic,

Table 1. Serum calcium, intact PTH, 25-OHD and 1,25$(OH)_2$D in full-term and preterm infants

	Cord blood	24 h	48 h	96–120 h	30 days
Calcium, nmo/l					
Full-term	2.42 ± 0.08	2.17 ± 0.10	2.16 ± 0.08	2.22 ± 0.12	2.52 ± 0.08
Preterm	2.28 ± 0.09	1.91 ± 0.06	1.86 ± 0.07	2.08 ± 0.11	2.43 ± 0.06
Intact PTH, pg/ml					
Full-term	5.1 ± 3	33 ± 8	30 ± 5	28 ± 16	
Preterm	4.5 ± 3	72 ± 17	56 ± 20	36 ± 14	
25(OH)D, ng/ml					
Full-term	13 ± 3	12 ± 2		12 ± 2	17 ± 1
Preterm	10 ± 3	8 ± 2		12 ± 2	17 ± 2
1,25$(OH)_2$D, pg/ml					
Full-term	38 ± 4	74 ± 9		100 ± 5	61 ± 4
Preterm	37 ± 6	62 ± 9		128 ± 29	108 ± 13

Values of calcium and vitamin D are the mean ± SEM.

Values of PTH are the mean ± SD.

Data have been compiled from the following sources: Calcium – author's lab; PTH – reference [74]; 25(OH)D and 1,25$(OH)_2$D – reference [98].

premature and asphyxiated newborns have the highest levels of postnatal calcitonin. Therefore, it has been suggested that high serum calcitonin may be a major cause of neonatal hypocalcemia. Other studies, however, have indicated that calcitonin plays a minor role in calcium homeostasis of the neonate [37, 75]. The intestinal absorption of calcium is based on both a vitamin D-dependent mechanism and on passive transport of calcium. In newborn rat pups, intestinal calcium absorption is largely a passive process and one not dependent on 1,25$(OH)_2$D until weaning. The situation in humans is not known. There are indications, however, that the passive non-vitamin D dependent absorption of calcium is important, at least in preterm babies [76]. Nonetheless, vitamin D supplementation of preterm infants increased the absorption of calcium by 2–4 weeks after birth [77]. Furthermore, neonates with hypocalcemia responded to treatment with 1-α-hydroxyvitamin D or with 1,25$(OH)_2$D by increasing their calcium levels [78, 79]. These observations indicate the integrity of the 1,25$(OH)_2$D receptor-effector system in the newborn intestine.

As described above, mild or moderate vitamin D deficiency during pregnancy has little effect on the development and mineralization of the human fetus in utero, mainly because the transplacental supply of calcium and phosphorus satisfy the requirements of the developing fetus. Indeed, frank congenital rickets is rare and seen only in newborns of mothers with severe vitamin D deficiency [58, 59]. Although large fontanelles and craniotabes are early features of rickets [57, 60], the effects of vitamin D deficiency during gestation become prominent only 2–3 months after birth when rickets develops, probably because intestinal vitamin D-dependent calcium transport becomes essential for the supply of calcium to the developing skeleton. Since breast milk is a poor source of vitamin D [55], vitamin D and 25(OH)D which pass through the placenta and are stored in the fetus furnish the main vitamin D requirements of the neonate in its first months of life. Vitamin D deficiency in the pregnant woman may reduce vitamin D stored in the fetus and subsequently may result later in vitamin D deficiency rickets in the infant. Supplementation of vitamin D to the pregnant woman affects postnatal calcium homeostasis: the decreases of serum calcium in the first 4 days of life is less marked in infants of supplemented mothers [61, 62]. Similarly, breast-fed infants who received 400 IU of vitamin D daily had higher bone mineral content and serum 25-hydroxyvitamin D concentration than did control infants [80].

Premature infants, particularly those born with a low birth weight, are prone to develop hypocalcemia in the first 1–3 days of life. The hypocalcemia is usually of short duration and asymptomatic in many infants. It has been suggested that early hypocalcemia in premature infants results from a combination of immaturity of the PTH and the vitamin D endocrine systems as well as transient end-organ resistance to hormonal effects [62]. Premature infants also tend to develop rickets which usually appears by 2 months of age [81]. This form of rickets is caused by the loss of placental calcium and phosphorus transport at a time when the rate of fetal mineral accretion is at its peak and the inability of intestinal dietary supply and absorption of calcium and phosphorus to meet the requirements of the mineralizing neonatal skeleton [62, 82, 83]. Special oral formulas that are high in calcium and phosphorus usually correct bone metabolism and allow normal mineralization and healing of the rickets. Although rickets of prematurity appears to be the result of inadequate calcium and phosphorus supply, the vitamin D status of preterm infants at birth is related to the length of gestation and maternal stores and may be insufficient. Therefore, while there is now widespread agreement that inadequate calcium and phosphorus and not vitamin D nutritional status or metabolism is the major cause of rickets in preterm infants, the need for vitamin D supplementation should be taken into consideration. It has been recommended by the American Academy of Pediatrics that preterm infants receive ≥400 IU vitamin D per day. The European Society of Pediatric

Gastroenterology recommended a dose of 1,000 IU vitamin D per day to breast-fed preterm infants [84, 85].

Maternal Vitamin D and Calcium Metabolism during Lactation

During lactation, the mother still has to provide calcium to the newborn via her milk and the amounts have to be between 300 and 400 mg per day [86, 87]. To adapt to this situation, she has to change her strategy of calcium metabolism. She uses temporary demineralization of the skeleton as the main mechanism to maintain calcium homeostasis and to satisfy the calcium requirement of suckling infants. Whereas during pregnancy, serum 1, $25(OH)_2D$ concentration and intestinal calcium absorption are increased 2- to 3-fold higher than those in non-pregnant women, maternal free and bound $1,25(OH)_2D$ levels fall to normal levels and remain within normal range throughout lactation within days of delivery [5, 6]. Subsequently to the fall in $1,25(OH)_2D$ levels, intestinal absorption of calcium in lactating women decreases from the high amounts measured in pregnancy to those obtained in non-pregnant women [4, 88]. Renal excretion of calcium is also significantly reduced to low levels [89]. Intact PTH levels, as determined by two-site immunoradiometric assays, has been found to be low or low-normal [90]. Despite the normal serum levels of $1,25(OH)_2D$ and the low levels of PTH, total and ionized calcium levels of lactating women have been found to be higher than those of normal controls [91]. The question arises which are the hormones or factors that regulate calcium metabolism during lactation. It has been suggested that PTHrP, which is significantly higher in lactating women than that in non-pregnant controls is the major regulator of calcium homeostasis during lactation [37, 92]. The main source of PTHrP in the plasma of lactating women may be the breasts since PTHrP concentration in breast milk is about 5,000–10,000 times higher than that found in normal plasma [93, 94]. Small, but biologically effective amounts of PTHrP produced in the breasts may reach the maternal circulation and stimulate bone resorption and increase renal tubular reabsorption of calcium. The importance of PTHrP to calcium metabolism during lactation is emphasized by the observations that in women with hypoparathyroidism $1,25(OH)_2D$ requirements fall early in the postpartum period and hypercalcemia may occur if $1,25(OH)_2D$ dosage is not reduced [95]. This phenomenon does not occur in women with pseudohypoparathyroidism who have resistance to the action of the amino-terminal site of both PTH and PTHrP.

As indicated above, a temporary demineralization of the maternal skeleton seems to be the main mechanism by which lactating women meet the calcium requirements of their infants [96]. Indeed, excretion of urinary markers of bone resorption have been reported to be 2- to 3-fold higher in lactating women than in pregnant women [36, 70] and measurements of bone density during lactation by DXA have demonstrated a 3–10% decrease in mineral content at the lumbar spine and femoral neck [36, 96]. The high bone turnover and decrease in bone mineral content comprise a normal physiological phenomenon and may not be significantly changed by calcium supplementation [90, 97]. It has been suggested that the combination of increased plasma PTHrP levels and estrogen deficiency form the major mechanism of the loss of skeletal calcium during lactation. Although elevated serum calcitonin levels may protect the maternal skeleton from excessive resorption in rats, its functional role in humans is unknown. The bone density losses during lactation are usually reversed during weaning and do not cause a long-term effect on bone density or increased fracture risk in the future [37, 98]. The mechanism by which bone mineral content is restored after weaning is not known but it may be relevant to our understanding of bone metabolism and development of new modes of treatment for osteoporosis in the future.

References

1 Givens MH, Macy IC: The chemical composition of the human fetus. J Biol Chem 1933;102: 7–17.

2 Pitkin RM: Calcium metabolism in pregnancy and the prenatal period: a review. Am J Obstet Gynecol 1985;151:99–101.

3 Kumar R, Cohen WR, Silva P, Epstein FH: Elevated 1,25-dihydroxyvitamin D levels in normal human pregnancy. J Clin Invest 1979;6:342–344.

4 Gertner JM, Coustan DR, Kliger AS, Mallette LE, Ravin N, Broadus AE: Pregnancy as a state of physiologic absorptive hypercalciuria. Am J Med 1986;81:451–456.

5 Seely EM, Brown EM, DeMaggio DM, Weldon DK, Graves SW: A prospective study of calciotropic hormones in pregnancy and post partum: Reciprocal changes in intact parathyroid hormone and 1,25-dihydroxyvitamin D. Am J Obstet Gynecol 1997;176:214–217.

6 Wilson SG, Retallack RW, Kent JC, Work GK, Gutteridge DH: Serum free 1,25-dihydroxyvitamin D and the free 1,25-dihydroxyvitamin D index during longitudinal study of human pregnancy and lactation. Clin Endocrinol (Oxf) 1990;32:613–622.

7 Bouillon R, VanAssche FA, VanBaelen H, Heyns W, DeMoor P: Influence of the vitamin D-binding protein on the serum concentration of 1,25-diyhdroxyvitamin D. J Clin Invest 1981;67: 589–596.

8 Cushard WG Jr, Creditor MA, Canterbury JM, Reiss E: Physiological hyperparathyrodism in pregnancy. J Clin Endocrinol Metab 1972;34:767–771.

9 Davis OK, Hawkins DS, Rubin LP, Posillico JT, Brown EM, Schiff I: Serum parathyroid hormone (PTH) in pregnant woman determined by an immunoradiometric assay for intact PTH. J Clin Endocrinol Metab 1988;67:850–852.

10 Seki K, Makimura N, Mitsui C, Hirata J, Nagata I: Calcium regulating hormones and osteocalcin levels during pregnancy: A longitudinal study. Am J Obstet Gynecol 1991;164:1248–1252.

11 Weisman Y, Vargas A, Duckett G, Reiter E, Root AW: Synthesis of 1,25-dihydroxyvitamin D in the nephrectomized pregnant rat. Endocrinology 1978;103:1992–1996.

12 Weisman Y, Harell A, Edelstein S, David M, Spirer Z, Golander A: 1,25-Dihydroxyvitamin D_3 and 24,25-dihydroxyvitamin D_3 in vitro synthesis by human decidua and placenta. Nature 1979;281: 317–319.

13 Delvin EE, Arabian A, Glorieux FH, Mamer OA: In vitro metabolism of 25-hydroxycholecalciferol by isolated cells from human decidua. J Clin Endocrinol Metab 1985;60:880–885.
14 Zerwekh JE, Breslau NA: Human placental production of 1α-25-dihydroxyvitamin D: Biochemical characterization and production in normal subjects and patients with pseudo hypoparathyroidism. J Clin Endocrinol Metab 1986;62:192–196.
15 Weisman Y, Jaccard N, Legum C, Spirer Z, Yedwab G, Even L, Edelstein S, Kay AM, Hochberg Z: Prenatal diagnosis of vitamin D dependent rickets type II: Response to 1,25-dihydroxyvitamin D in amniotic fluid cells and fetal tissues. J Clin Endocrinol Metab 1990:17:937–943.
16 Breslau NA, Zerwekh JE: Relationship of estrogen and pregnancy to calcium homeostasis in pseudohypoparathyroidisim. J Clin Endocrinol Metab 1986;62:45–51.
17 Blum M, Weisman Y, Turgeman C, Cabili Y, Wollman Y, Peer G, Stern N, Silverber D, Schwartz D, Iaina A: Pregnancy decreases immunoreactive parathyroid hormone level in rats with chronic renal failure. Clin Sci 1999;96:427–430.
18 Fleishman AR, Rosen JF, Cole J, Smith CM, DeLuca HF: Maternal and fetal serum 1,25-dihydroxyvitamin D. J Pediatr 1980;97:640–642.
19 Gallacher SJ, Fraser WD, Owens OJ, Dryburgh FJ, Logue FC, Jenkins A, Kennedy J: Charges in calciotrophic hormones and biochemical markers of bone turnover in normal human pregnancy. Eur J Endocrinol 1994;131:369–374.
20 Dvir R, Golander A, Jaccard N, Yedwab G, Otremski I, Spirer Z, Weisman Y: Amniotic fluid and plasma levels of parathyroid hormone-related protein and hormonal modulation of its secretion by amniotic fluid cells. Eur J Endocrinol 1995;133:277–282.
21 Beksi SN, Kenny AD: Acute effect of estradiol on the renal vitamin D hydroxylases in Japanese quail. Biochem Pharmacol 1978;27:2765–2768.
22 Spanos E, Brown DJ, Stevenson JC, MacIntyre I: Stimulation of 1,25-dihydroxycholecalciferol production by prolactin and related peptides in intact renal cell preparations in vitro. Biochim Biophys Acta 1981;672:7–15.
23 Halhali A, Diaz L, Sanchez I, Garabedin M, Bourges H, Larsea F: Effects of IGF-1 on placenta in culture. Mol Hum Reprod 1999;5:771–776.
24 Diaz L, Arranz C, Avila E, Halhali A, Vilchis F, Larrea F: Expression and activity of 25-hydroxyvitamin D-1α-hydroxylase are restricted in cultures of human syncytiotrophoblast cells from preeclamptic pregnancies. J Clin Endocrinol Metab 2002;87:3876–3882.
25 Reiter EO, Brounstein GD, Vargas A, Root AW: Changes in 25-hydroxyvitamin D and 24,25-dihydroxyvitamin D during pregnancy. Am J Obstet Gynecol 1979;135:227–230.
26 Verity CM, Burman D, Beadle PC, Holton JB, Morris A: Seasonal changes in perinatal vitamin D metabolism: Maternal and cord blood biochemistry in normal pregnancies. Arch Dis Child 1981;55:943–948.
27 Hillman LS, Haddad JG: Prenatal vitamin D metabolism III factors influencing late gestational human serum 25-hydroxyvitamin D. Am J Obstet Gynecol 1976;125:196–199.
28 Mukamel MN, Weisman Y, Somech R, Eisenberg Z, Landman J, Shapira I, Spirer Z, Jurgenson U: Vitamin D deficiency and insufficiency in orthodox and non-orthodox Jewish mothers in Israel. IMAJ 2001;3:419–421.
29 Namgung R, Tsong RC, Lee C, Han DG, Ho ML, Sierra R: Low total body bone mineral content and high bone resorption in Korean winter born versus summer born newborn infants. J Pediatr 1998;132:421–424.
30 Nehama H, Wientroub S, Eisenberg Z, Birger A, Milbauer B, Weisman Y: Seasonal variation in paired maternal- newborn serum 25-hydroxyvitamin D and 24,25-dihydroxyvitamin D concentrations in Israel. Isr J Med Sci 1987;23:274–277.
31 Brooke OG, Brown IRF, Cleeve HJW, Sood A: Observations on the vitamin D state of pregnant Asian women in London. Br J Med Obstet Gynecol 1981;88:18–26.
32 Heckmatt JZ, Peacock M, Davies AEJ, McMurray J, Isherwood DM: Plasma 25-hydroxyvitamin D in pregnant Asian women and their babies. Lancet 1979;ii:546–549.
33 Henriksen C, Brunvand L, Stoltenberg C, Trigg K, Haug E, Pedersen J: Diet and vitamin D status among pregnant Pakistani women in Oslo. Eur J Clin Nutr 1995;49:211–218.
34 Elidrissy ATH, Sedrani SH, Lawson DEM: Vitamin D deficiency in mothers of rachitic infants. Calcif Tissue Int 1984;36:266–270.

35 Purdie DW, Aaron JE, Selby PL: Bone histology and mineral homeostasis in human pregnancy. Br J Obstet Gynecol 1988;95:849–854.
36 Kovacs CS: Calcium and bone metabolism in pregnancy and lactation. J Clin Endocrinol Metab 2001;86:2344–2348.
37 Kovacs CS, Kronenberg HM: Maternal fetal calcium and bone metabolism during pregnancy puerperium and lactation. Endocr Rev 1997;18:832–872.
38 Schauberger CW, Pitkin RM: Maternal perinatal calcium relationships. Obstet Gynecol 1979;53: 74–76.
39 Delivoria papadopoulos M, Battaglia FC, Bruns PD, Meschia G: Total protein bound and ultrafilterable calcium in maternal and fetal plasmas. Am J Physiol 1967;213:363–366.
40 Moniz CF, Nicolaides KH, Tzannatos C, Rodeck CH: Calcium homeostasis in second trimester fetuses. J Clin Pathol 1986;39:838–841.
41 Karaplis AC, Luz A, Glowacki J, Bronson RT, Tybulewicz VL, Kronenberg HM, Mulligon RC: Lethal skeletal dysplasia from targeted disruption of the parathyroid hormone related peptide gene. Genes Dev 1994;8:277–289.
42 Tanamura A, Nomura S, Kurauchi O, Furui T, Mizutani S, Tomoda Y: Purification and characterization of 1,25$(OH)_2D_3$ receptor from human placenta. J Obstet Gynecol 1995;21:631–639.
43 Durand D, Braithwaite GD, Barlet JP: The affect of 1α-hydroxycholecalciferol on the placental transfer of calcium and phosphate in the sheep. Br J Nutr 1983;49:475–480.
44 Care AD: The placental transfer of calcium. J Dev Physiol 1991;15:253–257.
45 Zehnder D, Evans KN, Kilby MD, Bulmes JN, Innes BA, Stewart PM, Hewison M: The ontogeny of 25-hydroxyvitamin D_3 1α-hydroxylase expression in human placenta and decidua. Am J Pathol 2002;161:105–114.
46 Seki K, Wada S, Nagata I: Parathyroid hormone related protein during pregnancy and the perinatal period. Gynecol Obstet Invest 1994;37:83–86.
47 Abbas SK, Pickarad DW, Illingworth, Storer J, Purdi DW, Moniz C, Dixit M, Caple IW, Ebeling PR, Rodda CP: Measurement of parathyroid hormone related protein in extracts of fetal parathyroid glands and placental membranes. J Endocrinol 1990;124:319–325.
48 Lee K, Deeds JD, Segre GV: Expression of parathyroid hormone related peptide and its receptor messenger ribonucleic acids during fetal development of rats. Endocrinology 1995;136: 453–463.
49 Bowden SJ, Emly JF, Hughes SV, Powell G, Ahmed A, Whittle MJ, Ratcliffe JG, Ratcliffe WA: Parathyroid hormone related protein in human term placenta and membranes. J Endocrinol 1994;142:217–224.
50 Care AD, Abbas SK, Pickard DW, Barri M, Drinkhill M, Findlady JB, White IR, Caple IW: Stimulation of ovine placental transport of calcium and magnesium by mid-molecule fragments of human parathyroid hormone related protein. Exp Physiol 1990;75:605–608.
51 Kovacs CS, Lanske B, Hunzelman JL, Gose J, Karaplis AC, Kronenberg HM: Parathyroid hormone related peptide (PTHrP) regulated fetal placental calcium transport through a receptor distinct from the PTH/PTHrP receptor. Proc Natl Acad Sci USA 1996;93:15233–15238.
52 Hillman LS, Haddad JG: Human perinatal vitamin D metabolism. I. 25-Hydroxyvitamin D in maternal and cord blood. J Pediatr 1974;84:742–749.
53 Weisman Y, Occhipinti M, Knox G, Reiter G, Root A: Concentrations of 24,25-dihydroxyvitamin D and 25-hydroxyvitamin D in paired maternal cord sera. Am J Obstet Gynecol 1978;130: 704–707.
54 Weisman Y, Sapir R, Harell A, Edelstein S: Maternal perinatal interrelationship of vitamin D metabolism in rats. Biochim Biophys Acta 1976;428:388–395.
55 Weisman Y, Bawnik JC, Eisenberg Z, Spirer Z: Vitamin D metabolites in human milk. J Pediatr 1982;100:745–748.
56 Dent CE, Gupta MM: Plasma 25-hydroxyvitamin D levels during pregnancy in Caucasians and in vegetarians and non-vegetarians. Lancet 1975;2:1057–1060.
57 Brooke OG, Brown IRF, Bone CDM, Carter ND, Cleeve HJW, Maxwell JD, Robinson VP, Winder SM: Vitamin D supplements in pregnant Asian women: Effects on calcium status and fetal growth. Br Med J 1980;1:751–754.
58 Moncrieff M, Fadahunsi TO: Congenital rickets due to maternal vitamin D deficiency. Arch Dis Child 1974;49:810–811.

59 Ford JA, Davidson DC, McIntosh WB, Fyfe WB, Dunnigan MG: Neonatal rickets in Asian immigrant populations. Br Med J 1973;3:211–212.
60 Reif S, Katzir Y, Eisenberg Z, Weisman Y: Serum 25-hydroxyvitamin D levels in congenital craniotabes. Acta Pediatr Scand 1988;77:167–178.
61 Delvin EE, Salle BL, Glorieux FH, Adeleine P, David LS: Vitamin D supplementation during pregnancy: Effect on neonatal calcium homeostasis. J Pediatr 1986;109:328–334.
62 Salle BL, Delvine EE, Lapillonne A, Bishop NJ, Glorieux FH: Perinatal metabolism of vitamin D. Am J Clin Nutr 2000;71(suppl):317s–324s.
63 Steichen JJ, Tsang RC, Grattom TL, Hamstra A, Deluca HF: Vitamin D homeostasis in the perinatal period: 1,25-dihydroxyvitamin D in maternal cord and neonatal blood. N Engl J Med 1980;302:315–319.
64 Seki K, Furuya K, Makmura N, Mitsui C, Hirata J, Nagata I: Cord blood levels of calcium regulating hormones and osteocalcin in premature infants. J Perinat Med 1994;22:189–194.
65 Noff D, Edelstein S: Vitamin D and its hydroxylated metabolites in the rat. Placental and lacteal transport subsequent metabolic pathways and tissue distribution. Horm Res 1978;9:292–300.
66 Gertner JM, Glassman MS, Coustan DR, Goodman BPG: Fetomaternal vitamin D relationships at term. J Pediatr 1980;97:637–639.
67 Ross R, Care AD, Robinson JS, Pickard DW, Weatherlay AJ: Perinatal 1,25-dihydroxycholicalicifrol in the sheep and its role in the maintenance of the transplacental calcium gradient. J Endocrinol 1980;87:17–18.
68 Chalon S, Garel JM: Plasma calcium control in the rat fetus. II. Influence of fetal hormones. Biol Neonate 1985;48:323–328.
69 Johnson JA, Grande JP, Roche PC, Kumar R: Ontogeny of the 1,25-dihydroxyvitamin D_3 receptor in fetal rat bone. J Bone Miner Res 11:56–61.
70 Li YC, Pirro AE, Amling M, Delling G, Baron R, Bronson R, Demay MB: Targeted ablation of the vitamin D receptor: An animal model of vitamin D dependent rickets type II with alopecia. Proc Natl Acad Sci USA 1997;94:9831–9835.
71 Hochberg Z, Benderli A, Levi J, Vardi P, Weisman Y, Chen T, Feldman D: 1,25-Dihydroxyvitamin D resistance, rickets and alopecia. Am J Med 1984;77:805–811.
72 David L, Anast CS: Calcium metabolism in newborn infants: The interrelationship of parathyroid function and calcium, magnesium, and phosphorus metabolism in normal, sick and hypocalcemic newborns. J Clin Invest 1974;54:287–296.
73 Loughead JL, Mimouni F, Tsang RC: Serum ionized calcium concentrations in normal neonates. Am J Dis Child 1988;142:516–518.
74 Saggese G, Baroncelli GI, Bertelloni S, Cipalloni C: Intact parathyroid hormone levels during pregnancy in healthy term neonates and in hypocalcemic preterm infants. Acta Pediatr Scand 1991;80:36–41.
75 Mimouni F, Loughead JL, Tsang RC, Khoury J: Postnatal surge in serum calcitonin concentration: No contribution to neonatal hypocalcemia in infants of diabetic mothers. Pediatr Res 1990;28: 493–495.
76 Giles MM, Fenton MH, Shaw B, Elton RA, Clarke M, Lang M, Hume R: Sequential calcium and phosphorus balance studies in preterm infants. J Pediatr 1987;110:591–598.
77 Senterre J, Salle B: Calcium and phosphorus economy of the preterm infants and its interaction with vitamin D and its metabolites. Acta Pediatr Scand Suppl 1982;296:85–92.
78 Barak Y, Milbauer B, Weisman Y, Edelstein S, Spirer Z: Response of neonatal hypocalcemia to 1-α-hydroxyvitamin D_3. Arch Dis Child 1979;54:642–643.
79 Kooh SH, Frazer D, Toon R, DeLuca HF: Response of protracted neonatal hypocalcemia to 1α-dihydroxyvitamin D. Lancet 1976:1105–1107.
80 Greer FR, Searcy JE, Levin RS, Steichen JJ, Arch PS, Tsang RC: Bone mineral content and serum 25-hydroxyvitamin D concentration in breast-fed infants with and without supplemental vitamin D. J Pediatr 1981;98:896–701.
81 Campbell DE, Fleishman AR: Rickets of prematurity: Controversies in causation and prevention. Clin Perinatal 1988;15:879–890.
82 Steichen JJ, Gratton TL, Tsang RC: Osteopenia of prematurity: The cause and possible treatment. J Pediatr 1980;96:528–534.

83 Tsang RC, Demarini S: Rickets and calcium and phosphorus requirements in very low birth weight infants. Monatsschr Kinderheilkd 1995;143:s125–s129.
84 American Academy of Pediatrics Committee on Nutrition: Nutritional needs of low birth weight infants. Pediatrics 1985;72:177–179.
85 European Society of Pediatric Gastroenterology and Nutrition Committee on Nutrition of the Preterm Infants: Nutrition and feeding of preterm infants. Acta Pediatr Scand Suppl 1987;336:6–7.
86 Vaughan LA, Weber CW, Kemberling SR: Longitudinal changes in the mineral content of human milk. Am J Clin Nutr 1979;32:2301–2306.
87 Macy I, Kelly H, Sloan R: The Composition of Milks, publ No 254. Washington, National Research Council, 1953, p 63.
88 Kalkwarf HJ, Specker BL, Heubi JE, Viera NE, Yergey AL: Intestinal calcium absorption of women during lactation and after weaning. Am J Clin Nutr 1996;63:526–531.
89 Ritchie LD, Fung EB, Halloran BP, Turnlund JR, Van Loan MD, Cann CE, King JC: A longitudinal study of calcium homeostasis during human pregnancy and lactation and after resumption of menses. Am J Clin Nutr 1998;67:693–701.
90 Cross NA, Hillman LS, Allen SH, Krause GF, Viera NE: Calcium homeostasis and bone metabolism during pregnancy, lactation and post weaning: Longitudinal study. Am J Clin Nutr 1995;61:514–523.
91 Specter BL, Tsang RC, Ho ML: Changes in calcium homeostasis over the first year postpartum: Effect of lactation and weaning. Obstet Gynecol 1991;78:5–26.
92 Grill V, Hillary J, Ho PM, Law FM, MacIsaac RJ, MacIsaac IA, Moseley JM, Martin TJ: Parathyroid hormone-related protein: A possible endocrine function in lactation. Clin Endocrinol (Oxf) 1992;37:405–410.
93 Budayr AA, Halloran BP, King JC, Diep D, Nissenson RA, Strewler GJ: High levels of parathyroid hormone like protein in milk. Proc Natl Acad Sci USA 1989;86:7183–7185.
94 Khosla S, Johansen KL, Ory SJ, O'Brein PC, Kao PC: Parathyroid hormone related peptide in lactation and in umbilical cord blood. Mayo Clin Proc 1990;65:1408–1414.
95 Mather KJ, Chik CL, Corenblum B: Maintenance of serum calcium by parathyroid hormone related peptide during lactation in a hypoparathyroid patient. J Clin Endicrinol Metab 1999;84:424–427.
96 Sowers M: Pregnancy and lactation as risk factors for subsequent bone loss and osteoporosis. J Bone Miner Res 1996;11:1052–1060.
97 Kalkwarf HJ, Specker BL, Bianchi DD, Ranz J, Ho M: The effect of calcium supplementation on bone density during lactation and after weaning. N Engl J Med 1997;337:523–528.
98 Delmas PD, Glorieux FH, Delvin EE, Salle BL, Melki I: Perinatal serum bone Gla-Protein and vitamin D metabolites in preterm and full-term neonates. J Clin Endocrinol 1987;65:588–591.

Yosef Weisman, MD
Professor of Pediatrics, Director
Bone Disease Unit, Tel Aviv Sourasky Medical Center
6 Weizman Street, Tel Aviv 64239, (Israel)
Tel. +972 3 6974554, Fax +972 3 6973063, E-Mail golander@tasmc.health.gov.il

Hochberg Z (ed): Vitamin D and Rickets.
Endocr Dev. Basel, Karger, 2003, vol 6, pp 50–68

Vitamin D Receptor

Sachiko Yamada, Masato Shimizu, Keiko Yamamoto

Department of Molecular Recognition, Institute of Biomaterials and Bioengineering, Tokyo Medical and Dental University, Tokyo, Japan

Contents

The genomic actions of 1,25-$(OH)_2D_3$ are mediated through the vitamin D receptor (VDR, NR1I1), a member of the nuclear receptor (NR) superfamily [1] to which receptors for steroid hormones, retinoic acids, thyroid hormone, and numerous orphan receptors belong. Members of the NR family are grouped into 7 (0–6) subfamilies according to similarities in their sequences [2] and the VDR belongs to the same subfamily (subfamily 1) as the receptors for all-trans-retinoic acid (RAR), thyroid hormone (TR), and the receptors regulating lipid metabolism (PPAR), cholesterol homeostasis (LXR and FXR) and oxidation of xenobiotics (PXR and CAR). All NRs function by regulating the transcription of target genes through a common mechanism. Figure 1 shows schematically the function of the VDR/vitamin D system, which demonstrates the generally accepted mechanism of the action of NRs. Vitamin D transported to a target cell enters by diffusion into the cytoplasm and binds to the VDR. The VDR that has nuclear localization signals (NLS) can enter the nucleus. Alternatively, vitamin D enters the nucleus by diffusion and binds the VDR there. Upon binding to the ligand 1,25-$(OH)_2D_3$, the VDR changes its conformation to a transcriptionally active form and interacts with the 9-cis-retinoic acid receptor (RXR) forming a heterodimer. The VDR/RXR heterodimer binds to specific DNA sequences termed vitamin D-responsive

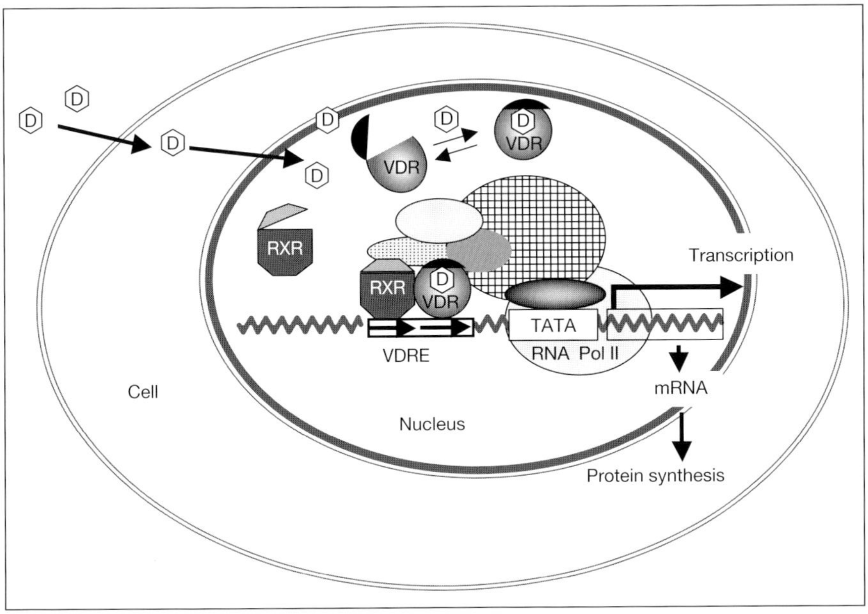

Fig. 1. Mechanism of the action of vitamin D_3 mediated by nuclear VDR.

elements (VDRE) in the promoter region of target genes. Recruitment of coactivator proteins occurs on the active form of the VDR, binding its ligand, and this triggers complex events that lead to transactivation.

The existence of a chromosomal receptor for vitamin D was suggested as early as 1969 [3] and was unequivocally demonstrated in 1974 [4]. The tissue distribution of the VDR has been studied extensively by autoradiographic and immunoradiometric analyses, and the presence of the VDR has been demonstrated in most tissues except for skeletal muscle, cerebrum and cerebellum [5, 6].

Molecular cloning of the cDNA encoding chick VDR was achieved for the first time in 1987 by McDonnell et al. [7], and this led to the successful cloning of the cDNA encoding the human VDR [8] in 1988. Now VDR sequences of nine species are known including the rat [9], mouse [10], Japanese quail [11] and *Xenopus* VDRs [12].

Chromosomal Vitamin D Receptor Gene

Unlike many of the other NR family members, which are the products of multiple genes, the VDR is the product of a single gene. The human VDR gene lies on chromosome 12 and comprises 11 exons that, together with the associated

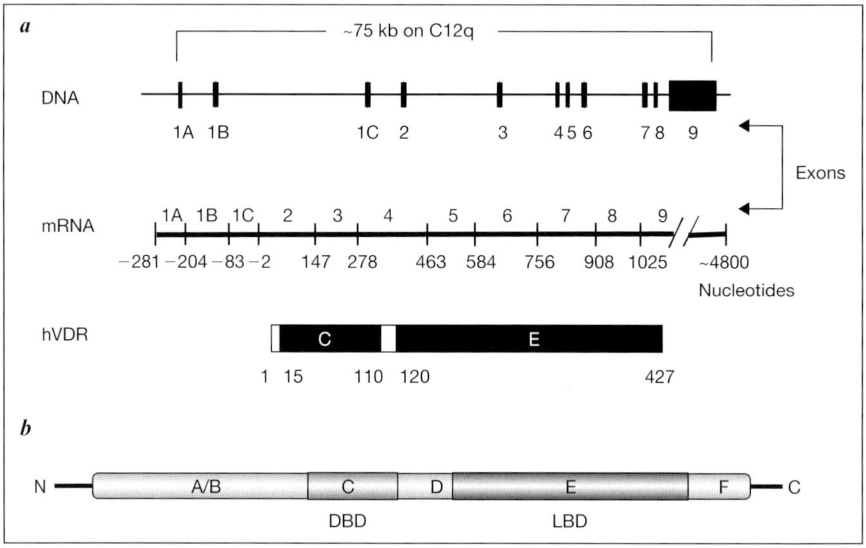

Fig. 2. Organization map of the chromosomal hVDR gene (***a***) and modular structure of nuclear receptors (***b***).

introns, cover approximately 75 kb of DNA (fig. 2) [8, 13]. Three exons, 1A, 1B and 1C, make up the 5′-noncoding leader sequence of the hVDR mRNA and the other eight exons (exons 2–9) encode the structural portion of the gene product. There are two translation start sites in the mRNA of hVDR, codons 1 and 4, and a polymorphism associated with these start sites has been identified [14, 15]. One corresponds to the mRNA sequence wherein the translation starts at codon 1, and the other, in which T in the codon 1 (ATG) is converted to C, begins translation at codon 4. The translations of these mRNAs result in proteins of 427 and 424 amino acids, respectively. The ACG allele is the more common form in the human population and is correlated with higher bone density in several human female populations [14, 15]. It is also known that the DNA encoding the shorter protein exhibits greater transcriptional activity [15].

Promoter of the hVDR gene: The sequence of the promoter region of the hVDR gene has been analyzed in detail and shown to contain potential binding sites for a variety of transcriptional regulators including SP-1, AP-1, AP-2, NFκB, GATA-1, Pit-1 and C/EBP [13]. However, no VDR binding site has been detected, suggesting that the autoregulatory actions of vitamin D may be indirect. Miyamoto et al. evaluated the transcriptional capacity of the hVDR promoter using the luciferase reporter gene and suggested that the proximal region (−103 to −34) imparts more than 80% of promoter activity and the upstream regions (−586 to −464) may be responsible for negative regulations [13].

Structure and Function of the VDR

Assembly of hVDR: Members of the NR family exhibit a common modular structure consisting of domains A–F [1] (fig. 2b). A/B domain: A variable NH_2-terminal region containing an autonomous transcriptional activation function (termed AF-1). C domain: A highly conserved DNA-binding domain (DBD). D domain: A hinge region. E domain: A moderately conserved ligand-binding domain (LBD), which functions in ligand-dependent transcriptional activation (termed AF-2), dimerization, and interaction with other protein factors. F domain: A variable C-terminal region.

Since the three-dimensional structures of the DBDs and LBDs of NR members have been determined by X-ray crystallography, we need to revise these domain definitions. For example, in the case of VDR, we now know that the hinge domain (D) originally defined as a domain connecting DBD and LBD covers the regions from the C-terminal extension (CTE) of the DBD to the loop between helices H1 and H3 in the LBD [16–18]. The VDR consists essentially of two domains, the DBD and LBD. The functional domains and secondary structures of VDR are mapped on the sequence of hVDR as determined by the crystallography of the DBD and LBD of hVDR (fig. 3).

Crystal structure of NRs: Three-dimensional structural data with atomic resolution obtained by X-ray crystallography are essential for understanding the mechanism of action of the functional proteins. The crystal structures of members of the NR family have been well documented: DBD/DNA complexes of GR and ER homodimers, TR/RXR and RAR/RXR heterodimers; LBDs of RXR, RAR, TR, PPAR, ER, PR, AR, GR etc.

The crystal structures of the hVDR DBD were solved recently as homodimers complexed with three different DNA sequences of VDRE [18]. The crystal structure of the VDR LBD remained elusive until recently, because the LBD contains a long and flexible insertion between helices 1 and 3 (H1 and H3: the numbering of the secondary structures follows that generally accepted for subfamily 1 members) (fig. 3) and this prohibited the formation of stable crystals. In early 2000, Moras' group [16] successfully solved the crystal structure of the hVDR LBD deletion mutant (Δ165–215) complexed with the natural hormone 1,25-$(OH)_2D_3$ by engineering the structure of loop 1–3. Meanwhile, several homology models were reported [19–22], some of which successfully predicted the 3D structure as well as the docking manner of the natural ligand [21, 22]. Because the crystal structures of the DBD and LBD overlap at the hinge region, we now know how the whole VDR is assembled. Figure 4a shows the crystal structures of the DBD homodimer/DNA (VDRE) and LBD (Δ165–215) where the two structures are overlaid at the overlapping region.

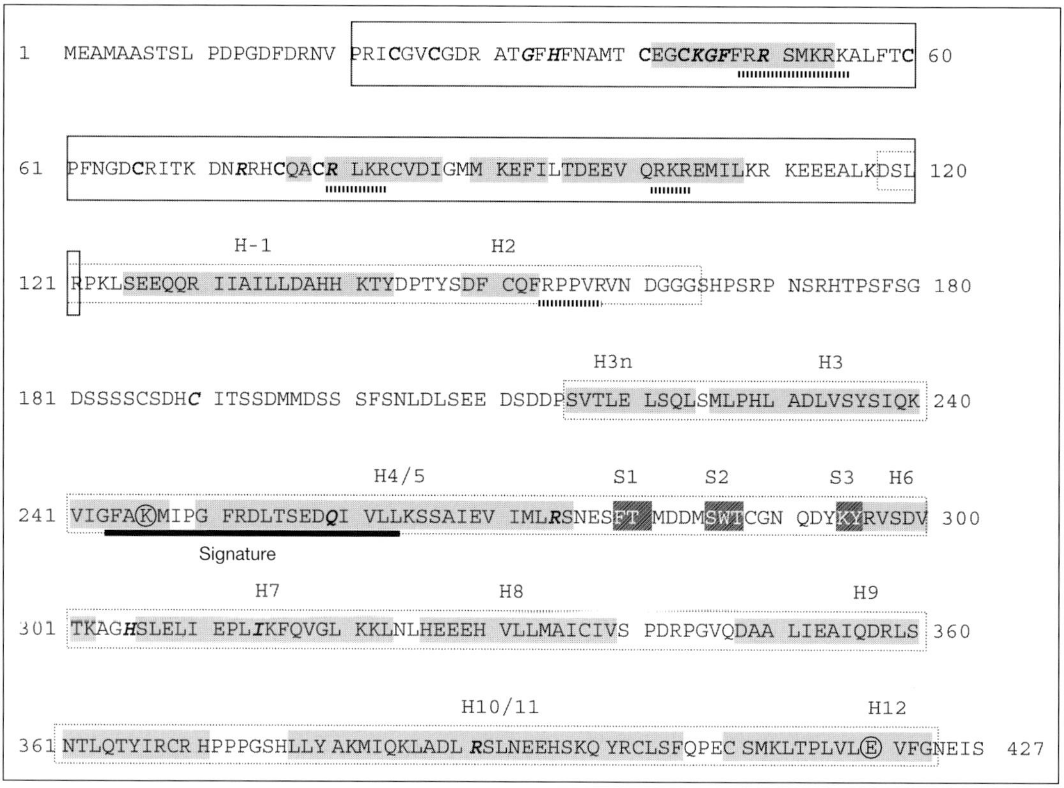

Fig. 3. Amino acid sequence and functional domains of hVDR. The X-ray crystal structures were determined at the regions boxed with solid line (DBD) and dotted lines (LBD). Secondary structure elements are shaded in light gray (α-helices) or hatched dark gray (β-strands). The cysteine (C) residues forming Zn binding motifs are indicated with boldface letters. Sequences involved in putative NLSs (broken lines) and signature region (solid line) are underlined. Residues involved in the missense mutations found in HVDRR are set in ***bold italics*** and those forming the charge clump are circled.

DNA Binding Domain

Vitamin D response element: In general, nuclear receptors bind as homo- or heterodimers to hormone-responsive elements (HREs) typically consisting of two hexameric half-sites whose consensus sequence, for the non-steroid receptors, is 5′-AGGTCA-3′ [23]. Diversity is achieved largely by varying the arrangement of the half-sites relative to one another (inverted, everted and direct repeats) and the number of neutral basepairs separating the half-site repeats [23]. The VDR binds preferentially to a direct repeat of hexameric

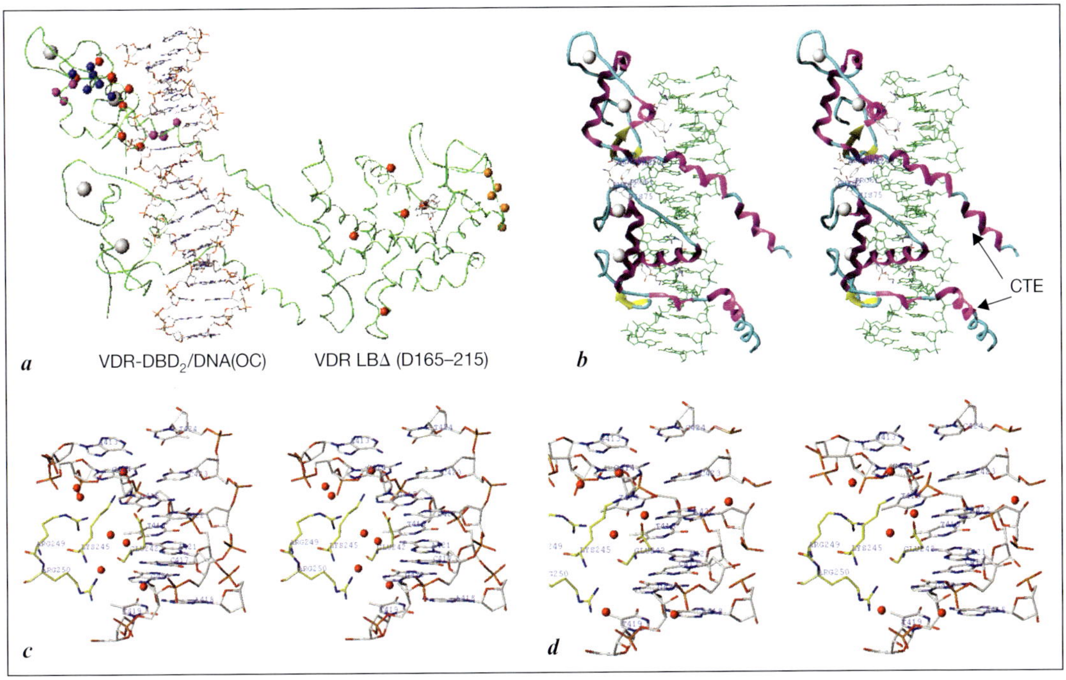

Fig. 4. Three-dimensional structures of hVDR DBD. ***a*** Three-dimensional structures of whole hVDR including the positions of mutations found in HVDRR and the putative NLSs. The crystal structures of the hVDR DBD homodimer complexed with VDRE (OC consensus sequence) and hVDR LBD (Δ165–215) are overlaid at the overlapping sequence (118–120): proteins, ribbon presentation (green); DNA and 1,25-$(OH)_2D_3$, stick model (atom type colors); Zn atoms, space-fill models (white). The positions of mutations found in HVDRR are shown with red balls and those of NLSs with magenta, blue and orange balls. ***b*** The 3D structure of hVDR-DBD homodimer/DR3 (stereoview): proteins, ribbon loop presentation; DNA, stick model (green); Zn, space-fill model (white); residues involved in the dimer and DNA interfaces, stick models (atom type colors). ***c***, ***d*** Protein-DNA contacts in the DBD complexes with DR3 (***c***) and OPN (***d***) VDRE (stereoview): DNA (atom type colors) and amino acid residues (atom type colors with C in yellow), stick model; water, red ball.

half-sites with three basepair spacers (DR3), mainly forming a heterodimer with RXR [24] and rarely forming a homodimer [25, 26]. It has been reported that, when the VDR/RXR heterodimer binds to VDRE, the VDR binds to the downstream half-site. The same polarity operates in TR/RXR (DR4) and RAR/RXR (DR5) heterodimers. This polarity that RXR is required to bind to the upstream half-site, may be important for the selection of response elements because the CTE of the RXR partner oriented downstream is thereby able to make contacts with the half-site spacer bases. At least 19 putative VDREs have

Table 1. Natural DR3-type VDREs [24]

VDRE	Sequence[1]	Position[2]	Gene product
Class I DR3-type VDREs			
rANF	AG**AGGTCA**TGA**AGGACA**	–907	atrial natriuretic factor
mOPN	AA**GGTTCA**CGA**GGTTCA**	–759	osteopontin
pOPN	AT**GGGTCA**TAT**GGTTCA**	–2261	osteopontin
cCAII	GA**AGGGCA**TGG**AGTTCG**	–62	carbonic anhydrase II
Class II DR3-type VDREs			
hCYP24	GG**AGTTCA**CCG**GGTGTG**	–291	24-hydroxylase
hNaPi	CA**GGGGCA**GCA**AGGGCA**	–1977	Na^--dependent P_i transporter type II
rOC	CT**GGGTGA**ATG**AGGACA**	–457	osteocalcin
rCYP24	AG**GGTTCA**GCG**GGTGCG**	–259	24-hydroxylase
hPTH	AT**GGTTCA**AAG**CAGACA**	–122	parathyroid hormone
rPTHrP1	TA**AGGTTA**CTC**AGTGAA**	–805	PTH-related peptide
Class III DR3-type VEREs			
rPTHrP2	AG**GGTGGA**GAG**GGGTGA**	–1107	PTH-related peptide
rD9k	GA**GGGTGT**CGG**AAGCCC**	–490	calbindin D_{9k}
aMyHC	GA**AGGACA**AAG**AGGGGA**	–801	slow myosin heavy chain
hGH	TG**GGGTCA**ACA**GTGGGA**	–59	growth hormone
cIntβ	GC**GAGGCA**GAA**GGGAGA**	–772	integrin β3
cPTH	GA**GGGTCA**GGA**GGGTGT**	–76	parathyroid hormone
Hp21	GT**AGGGAG**ATT**GGTTCA**	–779	$p21^{WAF1/CIP1}$

[1]Hexameric core binding motifs are shown in boldface.
[2]The position relative to the transcription start site.

been identified to date [24] and, with few exceptions, these are organized as DR3s that vary only in their precise half-site sequences. These VDREs have been classified into three groups according to their affinity for the VDR/RXR heterodimer as shown in table 1 [24]. Direct repeats with four or six spacing nucleotides (DR4- and DR6-type VDRE) and inverted palindromes with nine intervening nucleotides (IP9-type VDRE) are exceptions [27].

X-Ray Crystal Structures of the VDR-DBD Homodimer Bound to VDREs

Overall architecture: The NR DBD consists of a highly conserved core made up of two zinc-nucleated modules and two α-helices placed at right angles crossing near their midpoints [28, 29] (fig. 4b). The N-terminal α-helix, termed the recognition helix, interacts with the major glove of the half-site sequence. In addition, the DBDs of the VDR and TR have long CTE (fig. 3, 4b) (termed A helix in TR DBD) [18, 29].

The 3D structure of the VDR DBD (residues 21–121) was elucidated as homodimers complexed with three VDREs, osteopontin (OPN), canonical DR3 and osteocalcin (OC) [18]. The structure of the heterodimer with RXR has not yet been elucidated. Figure 4b shows the crystal structure of the VDR-DBD homodimer/DR3 complex. The overall folding of the VDR DBD is nearly identical to that of TR DBD [29]. Each DBD subunit engages its hexameric half-site forming a head-to-tail dimer. The relative orientation of the two subunits is determined by the spacer number and the 3-bp spacer between the two half-sites separates the two subunits with a center-to-center distance of nine basepairs and a relative azimuthal rotation of 45°.

Dimer interface: It is known that the DBDs of RXR, TR, RAR and VDR alone can direct the binding of hetero- or homodimers to properly spaced half-sites. However, DBDs alone do not dimerize in solution even at millimolar concentrations. Their assembly on the appropriate target DNA is highly cooperative, overwhelmingly favoring dimeric binding of the correct heterodimers to the properly spaced half-sites. The two subunits VDR DBD contact at P61, F62 and H75 of the upstream subunit and at N37, E92 and F93 of the downstream subunit (fig. 4b). The six interfacial residues are conserved among the nine known VDRs from various species. Mutation of residues N37, F62, H75 and F93 abolished cooperative assembly on DR3 elements [30, 31]. The association across these interfacial residues is mainly via van der Waals contacts, and is not buttressed by contact with the DNA, unlike homo- and heterodimers of other NR DBDs such as RAR/RXR [32], GR/GR [33] and TR/RXR [29].

Protein DNA interfaces: The core DBDs of all NRs bind to the consensus half-site sequence in nearly identical manner. Thus, the key interactions between the VDR DBD and the DNA half-sites are similar to those seen in previous structural determinations of NR DBD/DNA complexes [28, 29, 32, 33]: four conserved residues in the recognition helix, E42, K45, R49 and R50, make sequence-specific base contacts in the major groove of the half-site (fig. 4c, d) making roughly the same number of base and backbone contacts as RXR [29, 32], RAR [32] and TR [29] do with their response elements.

The three VDREs, OPN, DR3 and OC differ in their affinity for the DBD homodimer (table 1). The X-ray crystal structures of the complexes of the VDR DBD with these three VDREs reveal precise interactions that lead to the sequence-specific variation in affinity for DR3-type response elements [24]. For example, the substitution of a T_3-A_3 pair (OPN) (fig. 4d) for a G_3-C_3 pair (DR3) (fig. 4c) at the third position of the half-site dictates the more favorable interaction in the OPN-VDR complex: the substitution of the larger purine (A_3) for a pyrimidine (C_3) results in the formation of additional water-mediated hydrogen bonds to the DNA bases.

C-terminal extension: In contrast to the core DBD, whose 3D structure has been found to be the same in all receptor DBDs reported to date, the structure of each CTE determined so far has been unique. Moreover, each unique structure has been shown to be the key mediator of spacer discrimination. The CTE of the downstream subunit has been shown to be employed as a molecular dumper that makes severe steric clashes with the upstream subunit in the course of selecting against the wrong inter-half-site spacing. For example, for spacer lengths of less than three basepairs, the CTE helix of the downstream VDR molecule clashes with the backbone of the upstream partner [18]. The CTE of VDR strikingly resembles that of TR [29] but their interaction with the DNA response element is different: The TR CTE makes 15 direct or water-mediated hydrogen bonds with the DNA, while the VDR CTE forms only two. One reason may be that the VDR is assembled as a homodimer while the TR forms a heterodimer with the RXR, which lacks a long CTE.

Ligand Binding Domain

Overall Folding: The NR LBD adopts a common fold, the so-called antiparallel α-helical sandwich [34]. The crystal structure of the VDR-LBD was solved using a deletion mutant in which 51 amino acids were deleted in the thermally mobile loop 1–3 (amino acids 165–215) [16, 17]. This has been shown to have little effect on either biological functions such as ligand binding, dimerization with RXR and ligand-dependent transactivation of the VDR, or on the 3D structure of the rest of the LBD [35]. The VDR LBD contains 13 α-helices and a small three-stranded β-sheet, and is packed in an anti-parallel three-layered α-helical sandwich fold in which helices H4/5, H8 and H9 are sandwiched between H1 and H3 on one side, and H7 and H10/11 on the other (fig. 5a). Ligand binding is of primary importance for the function of the LBD. There is

Fig. 5. Three-dimensional structures of hVDR LBD and related NR LBDs. ***a*** The X-ray crystal structure of hVDR LBD (Δ165–215): left, front view, right, side view and center, the Connolly channel surface of the LBP (the same topology as the left figure). ***b*** The crystal structure of apo hRXR LBD as a representative model of transcriptionally inactive form. ***c*** The crystal structure of ERα-LBD/hydroxytamoxifen complex as a representative model of transcriptionally suppressive form. α-Helix, green (or red for H12) cylinder; β-sheet, blue arrow; loop, yellow tube; ligand, space-fill model (atom type colors); numbers on the cylinders, helix numbers. ***d*** Connolly surface structure of hVDR LBD (color, lipophilic potential). AF-2 surface is circled (red) and the two charge clump residues, K246 and E420, are shown with cyan (+) and red (−) disks, respectively. ***e*** The structure of 1,25-$(OH)_2D_3$ accommodated in the VDR and residues forming key hydrogen bonds with the ligand.

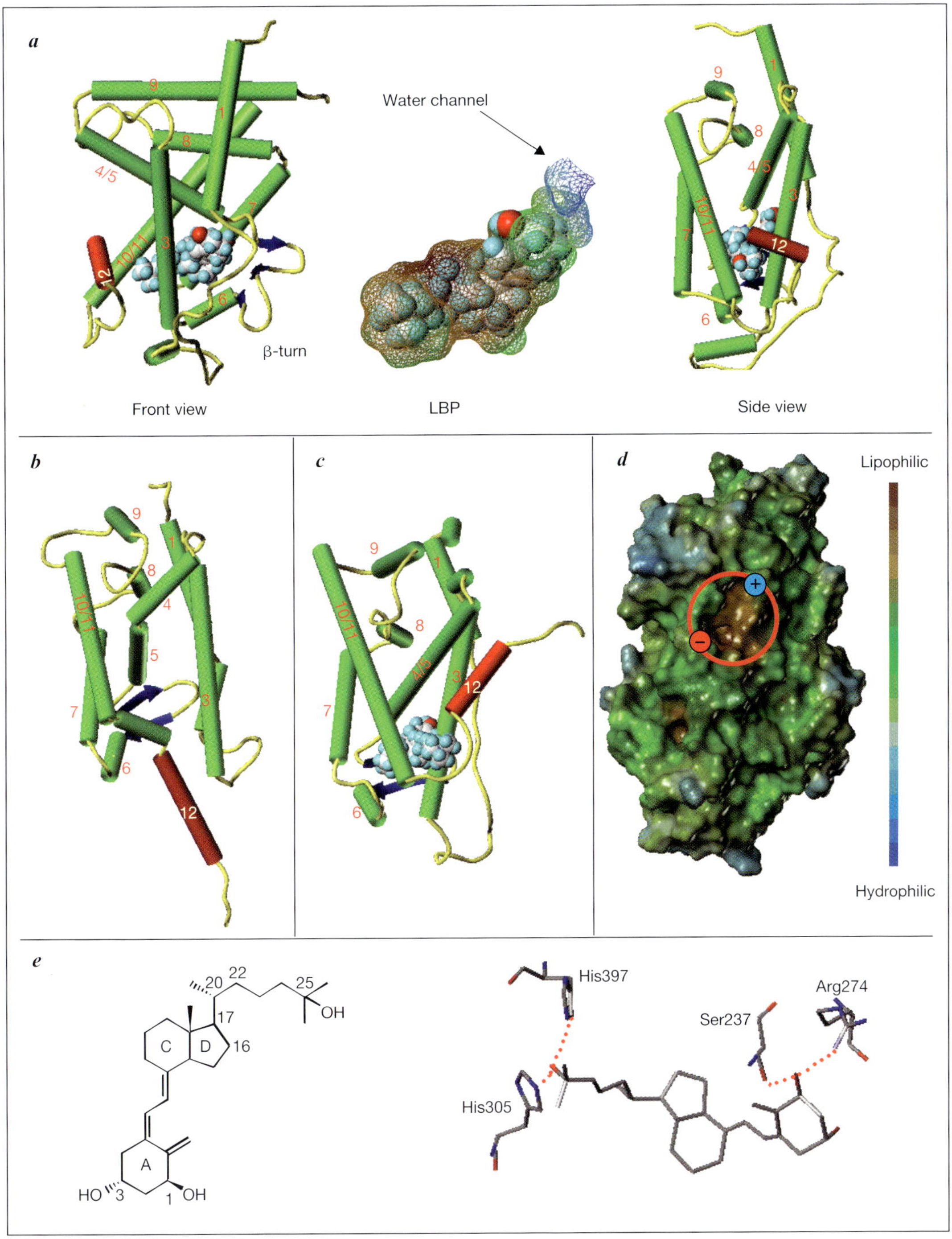
a
Water channel
β-turn
Front view
LBP
Side view
b
c
d
Lipophilic
Hydrophilic
e
20
22
25
OH
17
16
C
D
A
HO
3
1
OH
His397
Arg274
Ser237
His305

5

a hydrophobic cavity below helices 4/5 in the middle layer of the sandwich fold. This cavity serves as the ligand-binding pocket (LBP) and 1,25-$(OH)_2D_3$ is accommodated here (fig. 5a). The C-terminal helix H12 (termed AF-2 helix) has a specific role in the transactivation function (AF-2) and serves as a lid for the LBP in this conformation.

Three Major Conformations of NRs and Role of Ligands

The role of NR ligands is to change the conformation of the LBD to transcriptionally active forms; that is the ligands act as molecular switches of gene transcription. The NR LBD adopts three major conformations depending on the position of H12: (1) *Transcriptionally inactive conformation* adopted generally by apo NRs in which H12 adopts an extended conformation (fig. 5b) [36]. (2) *Transcriptionally active conformation* adopted when an agonist ligand is accommodated in the LBP [34]. The sandwich fold of NRs is tightly packed through the contact with the ligand in the LBP and is stabilized (compare fig. 5a and b). The crystal structure of the VDR LBD accommodating 1,25-$(OH)_2D_3$ adopts this active conformation (fig. 5a), in which H12 is folded back to the body of LBD and serves as a lid for the LBP. This completes the functionally important AF-2 surface to which protein factors important for the transactivation are recruited. (3) A *suppressive conformation* adopted when an antagonist is accommodated in the LBP (fig. 5c) [37, 38]. When an antagonist is accommodated in the LBP, H12 cannot adopt an active conformation and instead binds to the static AF-2 surface; its hydrophobic residues mimick the LXXLL motif of coactivators and thus prevent the binding of coactivators.

Activation function 2 (AF-2) surface of the hVDR: The AF-2 surface is composed of two parts: a *static part* made from the residues in the COOH-terminal half of H3, loop 3–4 and H4 (highly conserved region, termed the *signature domain*, see fig. 3) and the *mobile part* operated by H12. Figure 5d shows the AF-2 surface of the VDR LBD. The AF-2 surface of the VDR is quite similar to those of other NRs. It has a hydrophobic cleft in the center and two highly conserved residues termed charge clump, K246 (H3) and E420 (H12), at the opposite edges of the hydrophobic cleft. To this AF-2 surface, a coactivator is recruited [39–41], which, in turn, binds to other protein factors to allow transmission of the hormonal signal to the transcriptional machinery. An LXXLL motif of P160 coactivators binds to this hydrophobic cleft and the two polar residues of the charge clump form hydrogen bonds with the backbone amides of the LXXLL motif and its flanking regions to set the coactivator in the right position. The interactions between the AF-2 surface and coactivators have been clarified at the structural level by X-ray crystallographic analysis of the ternary complexes, such as ERα-LBD/diethylstilbestrol/GRIP1(NR Box II) [40] and PPARγ-LBD/rosiglitazone/SRC-1 [41]. P160 coactivators also have histone acetyl transferases (HAT) activity [42] and contribute to the transactivation by unraveling the chromatin and recruiting general transcription factors and RNA polymerase. The VDR interacts with various P160 coactivators [43, 44] and ligand dependent coactivator selectivity has also been reported [45]. Interaction of VDR LBD with other protein factors such as DRIP complex has also been reported [46].

Repression of gene transcription by NRs is mediated by interactions with corepressor proteins, such as SMRT and N-CoR [47], which, in turn, recruit histone deacetylases to the chromatin. The binding of corepressors to NR occurs in the unliganded state and can be stabilized by binding of antagonists. The X-ray crystal structure of the ternary complex containing PPARα LBD bound to the antagonist GW6471 and a SMRT corepressor motif has been reported [48]. The 3D structure reveals that the corepressor-binding site partly overlaps with the coactivator-binding site. The corepressor motif (LXXXIXXXL) binds to the static AF-2 surface where the H12 does not adopt the active conformation but is loosely packed against H3.

Interaction of the VDR with corepressors, SMRT and NCoR, has been investigated [49, 50]. A novel DNA selective VDR corepressor Alien has also been reported [50].

LBP and ligand docking: The LBP of the VDR is larger (697 $Å^3$) than that of the ERα (369 $Å^3$) [37] and RARγ (421 $Å^3$) [51] and the ligand 1,25-$(OH)_2D_3$ occupies 56% of the volume of the LBP. The cavity is wide at the H11 site and narrow at the β-turn site (fig. 5a). At the end of this narrow cavity there is a water channel open between the loop 1–3 and H3. The ligand 1,25-$(OH)_2D_3$ is accommodated with the side chain directed towards H11-H12 and the A-ring facing the β-turn. Twenty-seven amino acids line the LBP in an arrangement complementary to the structure of the ligand: major hydrophobic residues (16 residues) line the center of the LBP and the remaining hydrophilic residues face the two polar ends of the ligand, the A-ring and the terminal of the side chain. The ligand is anchored by hydrogen bonds and key van der Waals contacts. Two biologically important hydroxyl groups, the 1α- and 25-hydroxyl groups, are anchored to form pincer-type hydrogen bonds with R274 and S237 for the former and with H305 and H397 for the latter (fig. 5e).

The natural ligand 1,25-$(OH)_2D_3$ accommodated in the LBP adopts one of the minimum-energy conformations, though the dihedral angle at C (16, 17, 20, 22) takes less stable gauche (–) conformation. The A-ring adopts one of the stable conformations (β-form) (fig. 5e).

Dimer interface: As described above, the VDR recognizes VDRE forming a VDR/RXR heterodimer. Although NR DBDs only dimerize cooperatively with properly spaced DNA half-sites, dimerization of LBDs is DNA-independent. Thus, dimerization of LBDs has no selective role for response element recognition, but stabilizes dimer assemblies. Heterodimerization in the LBD is mediated mainly by hydrophobic interaction at H10 and additional charge interaction with H7 and H9 [52, 53]. It is known that ligand binding enhances the heterodimerization of VDR LBD.

Mutations in hVDR and Hereditary Vitamin D-Resistant Rickets

Hereditary vitamin D-resistant rickets (HVDRR) is a rare genetic disorder caused by a generalized resistance to 1,25-$(OH)_2D_3$ actions [54]. Heterogeneous mutations in the VDR that alter the function of the receptor are the molecular basis of HVDRR. Mutations that cause HVDRR are summarized in table 2 along with the assumed function of each amino acid. In addition, this table includes 10 artificial one-point mutants of functionally important residues [55, 56]. The positions of the mutations are shown in the amino acid sequence (fig. 3) and 3D structures (fig. 4a) of the hVDR.

VDR knock-out mice have been created [57], revealing apparently normal heterozygotes but severely affected homozygotes (VDR−/−), 90% of which die within 8–10 weeks. Surviving mice lose their hair and show low bone mass, hypocalcemia, hypophosphatemia, as well as a 10-fold elevation of 1,25-$(OH)_2D_3$ level coincident with extremely low 24,25-$(OH)_2D_3$.

Subcellular Localization of VDR and Its Nuclear Localization Signal

Subcellular localization of NRs has been the subject of many studies for over 20 years. In steroid hormone receptors, it was believed initially that the receptor localizes in the cytoplasm and migrates into the nucleus when the hormone binds. The availability of monoclonal antibodies has allowed immunocytochemical methods to be used in these studies. ER and PR have shown to be intranuclear, even when they are unoccupied by their hormones [58, 59]. However, the GR is mainly cytoplasmic in the absence of hormone and nuclear in the presence of the hormone [60]. The VDR was shown to be located predominantly in nuclei, with a significant presence in the cytoplasm without the ligand [61]. The proportion of the nuclear VDR increases in the presence of 1,25-$(OH)_2D_3$.

A number of nuclear localization signals (NLS) in nuclear proteins have been identified and most contain a short stretch of basic amino acids, K-K(R)-X-K(R) (X = K, R, P, V or A) [62]. Such a short sequence of basic amino acids that apparently facilitates transfer of NRs to the nucleus has been identified in several

Table 2. Missense mutations found in HVDRR

	Mutation	Position	Role of the residue	Ref. No.
DBD				
1	Gly33Asp	1st Zn motif	hold architecture of DBD	54
2	His35Gln	1st Zn motif	hold architecture of DBD	54
3	Lys45Glu	recognition helix	direct base contact	54
4	Gly46Asp	recognition helix	hold architecture of DBD	54
5	Phe47Ile	recognition helix	hold architecture of DBD	54
6	Arg50Gln	recognition helix	direct base contact	54
7	Arg73Gln	2nd Zn motif	contact with phosphate backbone	54
8	Arg80sGln	helix 2 of DBD	contact with phosphate backbone	54
LBD				
9	Cys190Trp	loop 1–3	deleted in the X-ray structure of LBD	54
10	Gln259pro	H4	AF-2 surface	54
11	Arg274Leu	H5	H-bond with 1α-OH group & VDW contacts with H1 and H3	54
12	His305Gln	loop 6–7	H-bond with 25-OH group	54
13	Ile314Ser	H7	VDW contact with residues at β-sheet	54
14	Arg391His	H10/11	VDW contact with residues at H8 and H4/5	54
	Mutation	**Position**	**Function**	
Artificial mutations				
15	Y143A	H1	H-bond with 3β-OH group	*
16	D144A	H1	folding	*
17	L233A	H3	VDW contact with ligand	55
18	I271A	H3	VDW contact with ligand and H4/5	*
19	R274A	H4/5	H-bond with 1α-OH group	55
20	W286A	β-turn	VDW contact with ligand	55
21	H397A	H11	H-bond with 25-OH group	55
22	Y401A	H11	VDW contact with H12	55
23	L417A	H12	dominant negative mutation, holds H12 in the active conformation	56
24	E420A	H12	dominant negative mutation, charge clump	56

*Unpublished results, Choi, Yamamoto and Yamada.

of the steroid hormone receptors, including GR, PR, and AR. Three putative NLS of the hVDR have been reported. Luo et al. [63] investigated the basic amino acid stretch (residues 70–111), which covers half of the second Zn-binding motif to the CTE region of the DBD. They used three peptide fragments within this region conjugated to fluorescein-labeled IgG and showed that the basic residues at both ends of fragment 79–105 were equally necessary for nuclear accumulation (fig. 3 and 4a – magenta balls). Hsieh et al. [64] focused on an array of five basic amino acids, RRSMKRK, between residues 49 and 55 (fig. 3 and 4a – blue balls). When residues within this region are mutated to nonbasic amino acids, or when this domain is deleted, the receptor no longer associates with VDRE, in vitro, and VDR-mediated transcriptional activation is abolished. Immunocytochemical studies demonstrated that mutation or deletion of this basic domain dramatically attenuates hVDR nuclear localization. Michigami et al. [65] used various deletion mutants of VDR fused to green fluorescent protein to search NLS and found a new motif RPPVR that is homologous to PPXR motif in NLS of nuclear RNA-binding proteins. Deletion of a region (117–173) containing this motif eliminated the preferential nuclear localization of VDR. This motif is located in the LBD (N-terminal part of loop 1–3) as shown in figures 3 and 4a (orange balls).

Conclusion

Elucidation of the crystal structures of the VDR is one of the most important advances in recent VDR studies. In this chapter, we described the structure and function of the VDR based on the crystal structures of the DBD and LBD of hVDR. We often referred to studies of other NR members, because the protein folding and function in target gene transcription show common features among the NR members: these are studied in much greater detail in other NRs. We did not describe phosphorylation of the VDR, although this has been a subject of intense studies, because the role of phosphorylation has not been clearly understood on a structural level. Having the precise 3D structure of the whole VDR in hand, the stage of VDR research is now set for the elucidation, on a structural level, of the mechanism of VDR mediated gene transactivation including the interaction with various protein factors and the structure-based design of selective VDR modulators [66].

References

1 Mangelsdorf DJ, Thummel C, Beato M, Herrlick P, Schutz G, Umesono K, Blumberg B, Kastner P, Mark M, Chambon P, Evans RM: The nuclear receptor superfamily: The second decade. Cell 1995;83:835–839.

2 Nuclear Receptors Nomenclature Committee: A unified nomenclature system for the nuclear receptor superfamily. Cell 1999;97:161–163.

3 Haussler MR, Norman AW: Chromosomal receptor for a vitamin D metabolite. Proc Natl Acad Sci USA 1969;62:155–162.

4 Brumbaugh PF, Haussler MR: 1,25-Dihydroxycholecalciferol receptors in intestine: Temperature-dependent transfer of the hormone to chromatin via a specific cytosol receptor. J Biol Chem 1974;249:1258–1262.

5 Sandgren ME, Brönnegärd M, DeLuca HF: Tissue distribution of the 1,25-dihydroxyvitamin D_3 receptor in the male rat. Biochem Biophys Res Commun 1991;181:611–616.

6 Stumpf WE, Sar M, DeLuca HF: Site of action of 1,25-$(OH)_2$ vitamin D_3 identified by thaw-mount autoradiography; in Cohn DV, Talmage RV, Matthews JL (eds): Hormonal Control of Calcium Metabolism. Amsterdam, Excerpta Medica, 1981, pp 222–229.

7 McDonnell DP, Mangelsdorf DJ, Pike JW, Haussler MR, O'Malley BW: Molecular cloning of complementary DNA encoding the avian receptor for vitamin D. Science 1987;235:1214–1217.

8 Baker AR, McDonnell DP, Hughes MR, Crisp TM, Mangelsdorf DJ, Haussler MR, Pike JW, Shine J: Cloning and expression of full-length cDNA encoding human vitamin D receptor. Proc Natl Acad Sci USA 1988;85:3294–3298.

9 Burmester JK, Maeda N, DeLuca HF: Isolation and expression of rat 1,25-dihydroxyvitamin D receptor cDNA. Proc Natl Acad Sci USA 1988;85:1005–1009.

10 Kamei Y, Kawada T, Fukuwatari T, Ono T, Kato S. Sugimoto E: Cloning and sequencing of the gene encoding the mouse vitamin D receptor. Gene 1995;152:281–282.

11 Elaroussi MA, Prahl JM, DeLuca HF: The avian vitamin D receptors: Primary structures and their origins. Proc Natl Acad Sci USA 1994;91:11596–11600.

12 Li YC, Bergwitz C, Juppner H, Demay MB: Cloning and characterization of the vitamin D receptor from *Xenopus laevis*. Endocrinology 1997;138:2347–2353.

13 Miyamoto K, Kesterson RA, Yamamoto H, Taketani Y, Nishiwaki E, Tatsumi S, Inoue Y, Morita K, Takeda E, Pike JW: Structural organization of the human vitamin D receptor chromosomal gene and its promoter. Mol Endocrinol 1997;11:1165–1179.

14 Harris SS, Eccleshall TR, Gross C, Dawson-Hughes B, Feldman D: The vitamin D receptor start codon polymorphism (*Fok*I) and bone mineral density in premenopausal American black and white women. J Bone Miner Res 1997;12:1043–1048.

15 Arai H, Miyamoto K-I, Taketani Y, Yamamoto H, Iemori Y, Morita K, Tonai T, Nishisho T, Mori S, Takeda E: A vitamin D receptor gene polymorphism in the translation initiation codon: Effect on protein activity and relation to bone mineral density in Japanese women. J Bone Miner Res 1997;12:915–921.

16 Rochel N, Wurtz JM, Mitschler A, Klaholz B, Moras D: The crystal structure of the nuclear receptor for vitamin D bound to its natural ligand. Mol Cell 2000;5:173–179.

17 Tocchini-Valentini G, Rochel N, Wurtz JM, Mitschler A, Moras D: Crystal structure of the vitamin D receptor complexed to superagonist 20-epi ligands. Proc Natl Acad Sci USA 2001;98:5491–5496.

18 Shaffer PL, Gewirth DT: Structural basis of VDR-DNA interactions on direct repeat response elements. EMBO J 2002;21:2242–2252.

19 Wurtz J-M, Guillot B, Moras D: 3D Model of the ligand binding domain of the vitamin D nuclear receptor based on the crystal structure of holo RARγ; in Norman AW, Bouillon R, Thomasset M (eds): Vitamin D: Chemistry, Biology and Clinical Applications of the Steroid Hormone. Riverside, University of California-Riverside Printing and Reprographics, 1997, pp 165–177.

20 Norman AW, Adams D, Collins ED, Okamura WH, Fletterick RJ: Three-dimensional model of the ligand binding domain of the nuclear receptor for 1α,25-dihydroxyvitamin D_3. J Cell Biochem 1999;74:323–333.

21 Yamamoto K, Masuno H, Choi M, Nakashima K, Taga T, Ooizumi H, Umesono K, Sicinska W, VanHooke J, DeLuca HF, Yamada S: Three-dimensional modeling of and ligand docking to vitamin D receptor ligand binding domain. Proc Natl Acad Sci USA 2000;97:1467–1472.

22 Swamy N, Xu W, Paz N, Hsieh J-C, Haussler MR, Maalouf GJ, Mohr SC, Ray R: Molecular modeling, affinity labeling, and site-directed mutagenesis define the key points of interaction between the ligand-binding domain of the vitamin D nuclear receptor and 1α,25-dihydroxyvitamin D_3. Biochemistry 2000;39:12162–12171.

23 Umesono K, Murakami KK, Thompson CC, Evans RM: Direct repeats as selective response elements for the thyroid hormone, retinoic acid and vitamin D_3 receptors. Cell 1991;65:1255–1266.

24 Toell A, Polly P, Carlberg C: All natural DR3-type vitamin D response elements show a similar functionality in vitro. Biochem J 2000;352:301–309.

25 Takeshita A, Ozawa Y, Chin WW: Nuclear receptor coactivators facilitate vitamin D receptor homodimer action on direct repeat hormone response elements. Endocrinology 2000;141: 1281–1284.

26 Freedman LP, Arce V, Perez Fernandez R: DNA sequences that act as high affinity targets for the vitamin D_3 receptor in the absence of the retinoid X receptor. Mol Endocrinol 1994;8: 265–273.
27 Carlberg C: Critical analysis of 1α,25-dihydroxyvitamin D_3 response elements; in Norman AW, Bouillon R, Thomasset M (eds): Vitamin D: Chemistry, Biology and Clinical Applications of the Steroid Hormone. Riverside, University of California-Riverside Printing and Reprographics, 1997, pp 268–275.
28 Schwabe JWR, Chapman L, Finch JT, Rhodes D: The crystal structure of the oestrogen receptor DNA-binding domain bound to DNA: How receptors discriminate between their response elements. Cell 1993;75:567–578.
29 Rastinejad F, Perlmann T, Evans RM, Sigler PB: Structural determinations of nuclear receptor assembly on DNA direct repeats. Nature 1995;375:203–211.
30 Towers TL, Luisi BF, Asianov A, Freedman LP: DNA target selectivity by the vitamin D_3 receptor: Mechanism of dimer binding to an asymmetric repeat element. Proc Natl Acad Sci USA 1993; 90:6310–6314.
31 Quack M, Szafranski K, Rouvinen J, Carlberg C: The role of the T-box for the function of the vitamin D receptor on different types of response elements. Nucl Acids Res 1998;26:5372–5378.
32 Rastinejad F, Wagner T, Zhao Q, Khorasanizadeh S: Structure of the RXR-RAR DNA-binding complex on the retinoic acid response element DR1. EMBO J 2000;19:1045–1054.
33 Luisi BF, Xu WX, Otwinowski Z, Freedman LP, Yamamoto KR, Sigler PB: Crystallographic analysis of the interaction of the glucocorticoid receptor with DNA. Nature 1991;352:497–505.
34 Moras D, Gronemeyer H: The nuclear receptor ligand-binding domain: structure and function. Curr Opin Cell Biol 1998;10:384–391.
35 Rochel N, Tocchini-Valentini G, Egea PF, Juntunen K, Garnier J-M, Vihko P, Moras D: Functional and structural characterization of the insertion region in the ligand binding domain of the vitamin D nuclear receptor. Eur J Biochem 2001;268:971–979.
36 Bourguet W, Ruff M, Chambon P, Gronemeyer H, Moras D: Crystal structure of the ligand-binding domain of the human nuclear receptor RXR-α. Nature 1995;375:377–382.
37 Brzozowski AM, Pike ACW, Dauter Z, Hubbard RE, Bonn T, Engström O, Öhman L, Greene GL, Gustafsson J-Å, Carlquist M: Molecular basis of agonism and antagonism in the oestrogen receptor. Nature 1997;389:753–758.
38 Oberfield JL, Collins JL, Holmes CP, Goreham DM, Cooper JP, Cobb JE, Lenhard JM, Hull-Ryde EA, Mohr CP, Blanchard SG, Parks DJ, Moore LB, Lehmann JM, Plunket K, Miller AB, Milburn MV, Kliewer SA, Willson TM: A peroxisome proliferator-activated receptor g ligand inhibits adipocyte differentiation. Proc Natl Acad Sci USA 1999;96:6102–6106.
39 Darimont BD, Wagner RL, Apriletti JW, Stallcup MR, Kushner PJ, Baxter JD, Fletterick RJ, Yamamoto KR: Structure and specificity of nuclear receptor-coactivator interactions. Genes Dev 1998;12:3343–3356.
40 Shiau AK, Barstad D, Loria PM, Cheng L, Kushner PJ, Agard DA, Greene GL: The structure basis of estrogen receptor/coactivator recognition and the antagonism of this interaction by tamoxifen. Cell 1998;95:927–937.
41 Nolte RT, Wisely GB, Westin S, Cobb JE, Lambert MH, Kurokawa R, Rosenfeld MG, Willson TM, Glass CK, Milburn MV: Ligand binding and co-activator assembly of the peroxisome proliferator-activated receptor. Nature 1998;395:137–143.
42 Chen H, Lin RJ, Xie W, Wilpitz D, Evans RM: Regulation of hormone-induced histone hyper-acetylation and gene activation via acetylation of an acelylase. Cell 1999;98:675–686.
43 Rachez C, Freedman LP: Mechanisms of gene regulation by vitamin D_3 receptor: A network of coactivator interactions. Gene 2000;246:9–21.
44 Herdick M, Bury Y, Quack M, Uskokovic MR, Polly P, Carsten Carlberg C: Response element and coactivator-mediated conformational change of the vitamin D_3 receptor permits sensitive interaction with agonists. Mol Pharmacol 2000;57:1206–1217.
45 Takeyama K, Masuhiro Y, Fuse H, Endoh H, Murayama A, Kitanaka S, Suzawa M, Yanagisawa J, Kato S: Selective interaction of vitamin D receptor with transcriptional coactivators by a vitamin D analog. Mol Cell Biol 1999;19:1049–1055.

46 Rachez C, Lemon BD, Suldan Z, Bromleigh V, Gamble M, Naar AM, Erdjument-Bromage H, Tempst P, Freedman LP: Ligand-dependent transcription activation by nuclear receptors requires the DRIP complex. Nature 1999;398:824–828.

47 Perissi V, Staszewski LM, McInerney EM, Kurokawa R, Krones A, Rose DW, Lambert MH, Milburn MV, Glass CK, Rosenfeld MG: Molecular determinants of nuclear receptor-corepressor interaction. Genes Dev 1999;13:3198–3208.

48 Xu HE, Stanley TB, Montana VG, Lambert MH, Shearer BG, Cobb JE, McKee DD, Galardi CM, Plunket KD, Nolte RT, Parks DJ, Moore JT, Kliewer SA, Willson TM, Stimmel JB: Structural basis for antagonist-mediated recruitment of nuclear co-repressors by PPARα. Nature 2002; 415:813–817.

49 Tagami T, Lutz WH, Kumar R, Jameson JL: The interaction of the vitamin D receptor with nuclear receptor corepressors and coactivators. Biochem Biophys Res Commun 1998;253:358–363.

50 Polly P, Herdick M, Moehren U, Baniahmad A, Heinzel T, Carlberg C: VDR-Alien: a novel, DNA-selective vitamin D_3 receptor corepressor partnership. FASEB J 2000;14:1455–1463.

51 Renaud JP, Rochel N, Ruff M, Vivat V, Chambon P, Gronemeyer H, Moras D: Crystal structure of the RAR-γ ligand-binding domain bound to all-*trans* retinoic acid. Nature 1995;378: 681–689.

52 Bourguet W, Vivat V, Wurtz J-M, Chambon P, Gronemeyer H, Moras D: Crystal structure of a heterodimeric complex of RAR and RXR ligand-binding domain. Mol Cell 2000;5:289–298.

53 Gampe RT, Montana VG, Lambert MH, Miller AB, Bledsoe RK, Milburn MV, Kliewer SA, Willson TM, Xu HE: Asymmetry in the PPARγ/RXRα crystal structure reveals the molecular basis of heterodimerization among nuclear receptors. Mol Cell 2000;5:545–555.

54 Malloy PJ, Pike JW, Feldman D: The vitamin D receptor and the syndrome of hereditary 1,25-dihydroxyvitamin D-resistant rickets. Endocrine Rev 1999;20:156–188.

55 Choi M, Yamamoto K, Masuno H, Nakashima K, Taga T, Yamada S: Ligand recognition by the vitamin D receptor. Bioorg Med Chem 2001;9:1721–1730.

56 Jurutka PW, Hsieh J-C, Remus LS, Whitfield GK, Thompson PD, Haussler CA, Blanco JCG, Ozato K, Haussler MR: Mutation in the 1,25-dihydroxyvitamin D_3 receptor identifying C-terminal amino acids required for transcriptional activation that are functionally dissociated from hormone binding, heterodimeric DNA binding, and interaction with basal transcription factor IIB, in vitro. J Biol Chem 1997;272:14592–14599.

57 Yoshizawa T, Handa Y, Uematsu Y, Takeda S, Sekine K, Yoshihara Y, Kawakami T, Arioka K, Sato H, Uchiyama Y, Masushige S, Fukamizu A, Matsumoto T, Kato S: Mice lacking the vitamin D receptor exhibit impaired bone formation, uterine hypoplasia and growth retardation after weaning. Nature Gene 1997;16:391–396.

58 Perrot-Applanat M, Logeat F, Groyer-Picard MT, Milgrom E: Immunocytochemical study of mammalian progesterone receptor using monoclonal antibodies. Endocrinology 1985;116: 1473–1484.

59 King WJ, Greene GL: Monoclonal antibodies localize estrogen receptor in the nuclei of target cell. Nature 1984;307:745–749.

60 Wilkström AC, Bakke O, Okret S, Brönnegard M, Gustafsson JA: Intracellular localization of the glucocorticoid receptor: Evidence for cytoplasmic and nuclear localization. Endocrinology 1987;120:1232–1242.

61 Haussler MR, Jurutka PW, Hsieh J-C, Thompson PD, Haussler CA, Selznick SH, Remus LS, Whitfield GK: Nuclear vitamin D receptor: structure-function, phosphorylation, and control of gene transcription; in Feldman D, Glorieux FH, Pike JW (eds): Vitamin D. San Diego, Academic Press, 1997, pp 149–177.

62 Chelsky D, Ralph R, Jonak G: Sequence requirements for synthetic peptide-mediated translocation to the nucleus. Mol Cell Biol 1989;9:2487–2492.

63 Luo Z, Rouvinen J, Maenpaa PH: A peptide C-terminal to the second Zn finger of human vitamin D receptor is able to specify nuclear localization. Eur J Biochem 1994;233:381–387.

64 Hsieh J-C, Shimizu Y, Minoshima S, Shimizu N, Haussler CA, Jurutka PW, Haussler MR: Novel nuclear localization signal between the two DNA-binding zinc fingers in the human vitamin D receptor. J Cell Biochem 1998;70:94–109.

65 Michigami T, Suga A, Yamazaki M, Shimizu C, Cai G, Okada S, Ozono K: Identification of amino acid sequence in the hinge region of human vitamin D receptor that transfers a cytosolic protein to the nucleus. J Biol Chem 1999;274:33531–33538.
66 Yamada S, Shimizu M, Yamamoto K: Structure-function relationships of vitamin D including ligand recognition by the vitamin D receptor. Med Res Rev 2003;23:89–115.

Sachiko Yamada, PhD
Department of Molecular Recognition
Institute of Biomaterials and Bioengineering
Tokyo Medical and Dental University
2–3–10 Kanda-Surugadai, Chiyoda-ku, Tokyo 101-0062 (Japan)
Tel. +81 3 5280 8036, Fax +81 3 5280 8039, E-Mail yamada.mr@tmd.ac.jp

Hochberg Z (ed): Vitamin D and Rickets.
Endocr Dev. Basel, Karger, 2003, vol 6, pp 69–79

The Rachitic Bone

Frank Rauch

Genetics Unit, Shriners Hospital for Children, Montréal, Québec, Canada

Contents

Outline

Rickets is caused by deficient mineralization at the level of the growth plate and is usually accompanied by osteomalacia, i.e. impaired mineralization of bone matrix. The disease manifestations at the growth plate are examined radiologically. However, precise characterization of the mineralization defect in bone tissue requires transiliac bone biopsy specimens. Biopsies are obtained after patients have received two short courses of tetracycline to label actively forming bone surfaces. Osteomalacia is said to be present when both osteoid thickness and mineralization lag time are increased. In calcipenic forms of rickets, histologic signs of hyperparathyroidism are typically found in addition to osteomalacia. Phosphopenic rickets is not usually associated with hyperparathyroidism. X-linked hypophosphatemic rickets can be distinguished from other forms of rickets by the presence of periosteocytic hypomineralized lesions. In clinical practice, histologic studies are usually not necessary for the diagnosis of rickets, but may be helpful in unclear cases.

Introduction

In the growing skeleton, mineralization occurs in two different types of tissue, growth plate cartilage and bone matrix. Rickets refers to the changes caused by deficient mineralization at the growth plate. Osteomalacia refers to impaired mineralization of the bone matrix. Rickets and osteomalacia usually occur together as long as the growth plates are open; only osteomalacia occurs after the growth plates have fused.

Rickets is usually diagnosed clinically or radiographically by evaluating signs and symptoms of the typical growth plate defects. Osteomalacia is also associated with clinical, radiological and biochemical abnormalities, but is more precisely evaluated in iliac bone specimens.

The physiological process of mineralization represents the incorporation of mineral (Ca, P and others) into organic bone matrix, after it has been synthesized and deposited by osteoblasts. Discussing mineralization disorders has become somewhat complicated in recent years by the widespread misuse of the term 'mineralization' in the field of bone densitometry. 'Decreased bone mineralization' is often said to be present when low bone mineral density is found. However, mineralization of bones can only occur at locations where bone matrix has been deposited before. Most cases of low bone density are not caused by a problem with incorporating enough minerals into the bone matrix, but rather reflect insufficient matrix production or increased matrix removal. The present chapter exclusively deals with disturbances of mineralization in the original sense, i.e. disordered incorporation of mineral into organic bone matrix.

Bone Biopsy: Procedure and Sample Processing

Most of what we know about the histologic features of human bone diseases is based on the analysis of iliac bone biopsy samples. This is also true for mineralization disorders. A brief description of how bone biopsies are obtained on how they are analyzed may therefore be helpful.

There are basically two ways to analyze bone tissue. The first is simply to look at a bone sample under the microscope and to qualitatively describe the observations. This corresponds to a histologic evaluation, similar to what is done in pathology. The second approach is to measure the amount of the various structures and cell types that are visible under the microscope. The aim is to convert the picture into numbers. This technique called histomorphometry.

Bone specimen for standard histologic and histomorphometric evaluation are horizontal full-thickness (transfixing) biopsies of the ilium from a site 2 cm posterior of the anterior superior iliac spine. This bone is easily accessible, does not require extensive surgery, and is associated with few postoperative complications. In principle, histomorphometric analysis can be performed in any bone. In clinical pediatrics, however, only ilium samples can be used for quantitative analysis, because this is the only site where reference data are available.

It is also important to note that horizontal transiliac samples are required for histomorphometric evaluation. Vertical samples (from the iliac crest downwards) can not be used. The transiliac sample must be obtained at a site well below the iliac crest growth plate. Specimens containing growth cartilage do not allow for a reliable quantitative analysis, because turnover is very high and cortical thickness is very low in the bone adjacent to the growth plate.

The usual bone biopsy instrument is the Bordier trephine. The inner diameter of the biopsy needle must be at least 5 mm and should preferably be 6 or 7 mm. Most children below 14 years of age will require general anesthesia for the procedure. Local anesthesia can be sufficient for older adolescents. This procedure does not have side effects other than transient local discomfort. Patients are allowed to get out of bed after 3 h and can usually be discharged on the same day.

Another prerequisite for histomorphometric evaluation is bone labeling with tetracycline. Tetracycline labeling is especially important for the evaluation of mineralization disorders. Dynamic parameters of bone cell function can only be measured when the patient has received two courses of tetracycline label prior to biopsy. The tetracycline trapped at formation sites can then be visualized under fluorescent light.

Once the sample is obtained, it should be placed into a fixative as soon as possible. Then it can be sent to the laboratory. There the sample is dehydrated, embedded in plastic, cut on a special microtome and stained. The actual histomorphometric analysis requires a high-quality microscope and is done with a semi-automatic computerized system. Despite computerization, histomorphometric analysis is still time-consuming, because even the most advanced systems rely on the operator's judgement to correctly identify the individual components of the bone tissue.

Basic Concepts of Bone Metabolism

Bone histology and histomorphometry provide information on two aspects of bone metabolism, bone remodeling (fig. 1) and bone modeling (fig. 2).

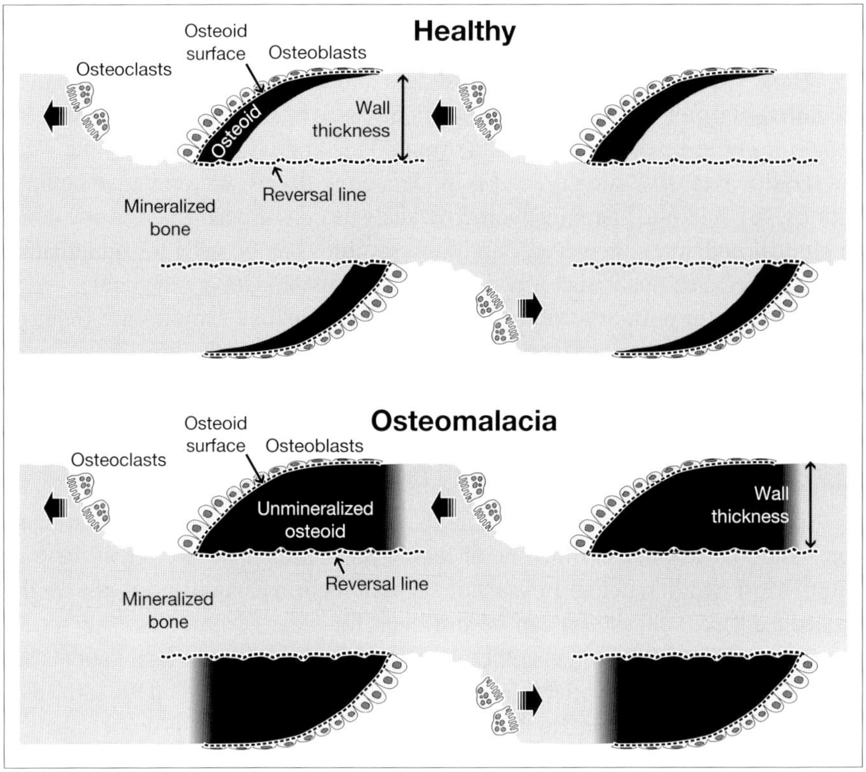

Fig. 1. Remodeling of trabecular bone. Upper panel: Normal remodeling. Bone tissue is continuously turned over by remodeling units. These consist of a team of osteoclasts followed by a team of osteoblasts which are successively active on the same surface of the trabecula. The units move parallel to the surface, as indicated by the arrows. Lower panel: Remodeling in severe mineralization disorders. The osteoid that is deposited by osteoblasts fails to mineralize. The net effect of a remodeling cycle in this situation is to remove normally mineralized bone (that was created before the disease process started) and to replace it with unmineralized bone matrix.

Remodeling is a maintenance process which has a relatively small effect on the amount of bone. In remodeling, a group of osteoclasts removes a small quantity of bone tissue, which then is put back by a team of osteoblasts (fig. 1). In contrast, bone modeling is the mechanism whereby fast and large changes in bone shape and mass can occur (fig. 2). Bone modeling involves the same cell types as bone remodeling. However, in modeling osteoblast and osteoclasts act on different surfaces, whereas the two cell types are sequentially active on the same bone surface in remodeling. A typical example for modeling is the growth of long-bone shafts in width (fig. 2). Typically osteoblasts are located on the

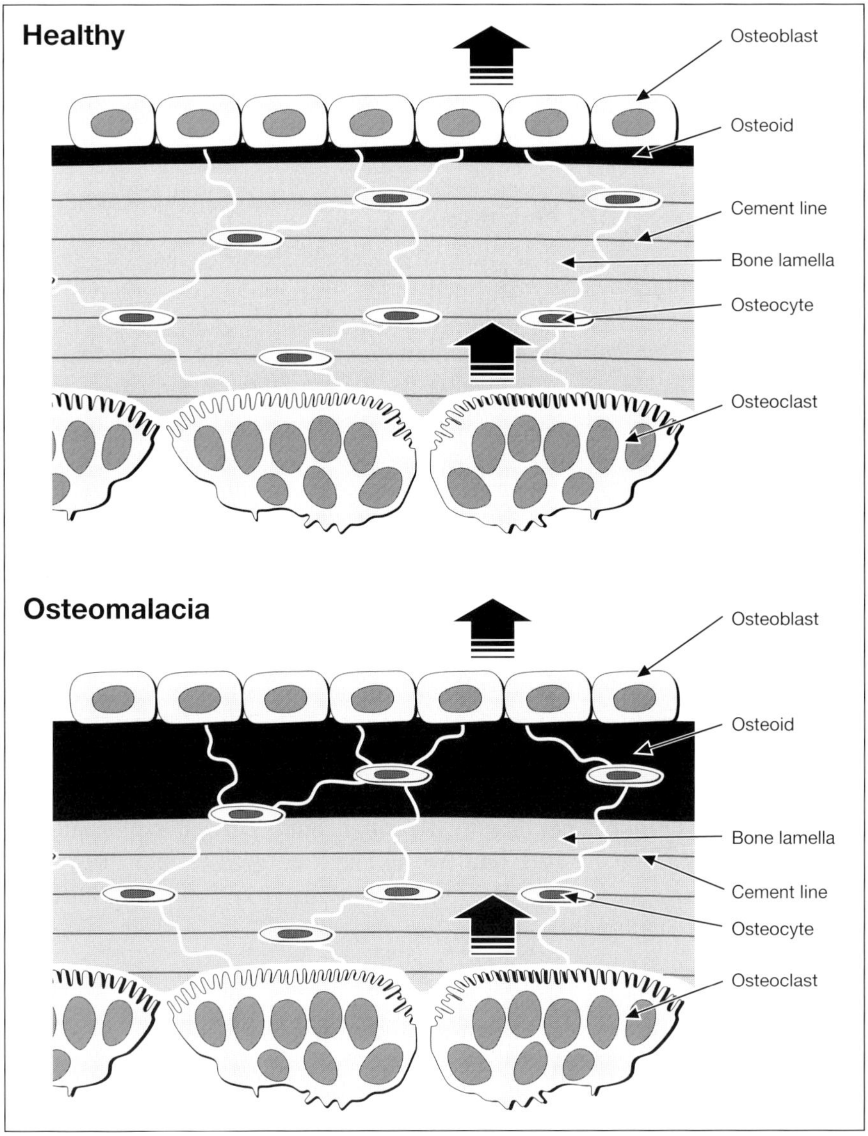

Fig. 2. Modeling of cortical bone. Upper panel: Normal modeling. Osteoblasts and osteoclasts are located on opposite sides of the bone cortex. As indicated by the arrows, osteoblasts add bone to the outer (periosteal) surface, whereas osteoclasts remove bone from the inner (endocortical) surface. Thus, the piece of bone in this example is moving upwards. The thickness of the cortex will increase, if osteoblasts add more bone than the osteoclasts remove. Lower panel: Modeling in osteomalacia. The bone matrix that is deposited by osteoblasts is not mineralized. As osteoclasts continue to resorb bone from the other side of the bone, the mineralized part of the cortex is becoming thinner.

outer surface of the bone cortex, where they secrete bone matrix and later mineralize it. Thereby, the outer bone size is increased. At the same time, osteoclasts located on the inner surface of the cortex resorb bone, thus increasing the size of the marrow cavity.

Histomorphometric Measures

Histomorphometric analyses quantify the most important aspects of bone structure and bone metabolism within a biopsy sample. The most important measures of bone structure are the amount of trabecular bone and the thickness of the bone cortex. Measures reflecting the activity of bone formation are the amount of unmineralized bone tissue, the amount of osteoblasts, the length of the tetracycline labels and the distance between the labels. The last two items on this list are the most accurate markers of bone formation, which however can only be obtained when the patient has received two courses of tetracycline prior to biopsy. Regarding bone resorption, the most important measure is the number of osteoclasts in a tissue section.

Osteoid thickness and mineralization lag time are the key parameters for the evaluation of mineralization disorders. The thickness of osteoid seams can be directly measured in histologic bone sections. Mineralization lag time is the interval between the secretion of organic bone matrix and the start of mineralization in this newly secreted matrix. This parameter can only be determined when the patient has received two courses of tetracycline prior to biopsy. Mineralization lag time is not directly measured, but is derived mathematically from the time interval between the two tetracycline courses and three basic histomorphometric measures – the length of tetracycline labels, the distance between double labels and osteoid thickness.

Skeletal Histology and Histomorphometry in Rickets

Rickets is characterized by thickening of growth plates. Growth plate thickness is determined by two opposing processes. On the epiphyseal two thirds of a typical growth plate, cartilage tissue is created through chondrocyte proliferation and hypertrophy. On the metaphyseal side of the growth plate, cartilage tissue is removed by vascular invasion followed by conversion into primary bone spongiosa.

Four layers can be distinguished in a growth plate. These are the resting zone, the proliferative zone, the hypertrophic zone and the zone of provisional calcification. In rickets, the resting and proliferative zones are not significantly altered from the normal pattern. However, the hypertrophic zone is grossly abnormal, with a disorganized increase in the number of cells and a loss of normal columnar pattern. At the same time, the mineralization of cartilage in the zone of provisional calcification is perturbed.

Cartilage mineralization is a prerequisite for the invasion of growth plate cartilage by metaphyseal blood vessels. Thus, when cartilage mineralization is prevented by a deficiency of calcium or phosphorus, vascular invasion and subsequent removal of cartilage become inefficient and growth plate tissue accumulates. This is reflected radiologically by widening of the growth plates and loss of a clear border between growth plate and metaphysis. In addition, the primary spongiosa that does form is inadequately mineralized and haversian systems are not properly formed in cortical bone. Unmineralized osteoid accumulates at all locations where new bone formation occurs.

These abnormalities decrease the biomechanical resistance of the involved skeletal sites, leading to a secondary increase in the diameters of the growth plate and metaphysis. These changes may be regarded as an attempt to compensate for decreased bone strength by increased bone size. Nonetheless, bone stability is compromised, and if the underlying condition does not improve, bowing occurs.

The histological abnormalities of the growth plate cannot be directly examined in clinical samples, because transiliac biopsy specimens do not include growth plate tissue. Therefore, the histological and histomorphometrical characterization of mineralization defects focuses on events that occur in mature bone tissue, i.e. osteomalacia.

As mentioned before, osteomalacia is caused by disturbed incorporation of mineral into organic bone matrix. This leads to an accumulation of unmineralized bone matrix, because osteoblasts continue to secrete osteoid for some time (fig. 1–3). The aspect of tetracycline labels reflects the severity of the mineralization defect. In a mild mineralization disorder, the proportion of tetracycline-labeled osteoid is decreased and the distance between labels is decreased. In severe cases, the tetracycline labels may be blurred (fig. 4) and can even be absent.

In quantitative histomorphometric terms, osteomalacia is defined as the simultaneous occurrence of increased osteoid thickness and increased mineralization lag time. The criteria for abnormality in these parameters depend on the source of reference data. The cutoffs used in adults are 12.5 μm for osteoid thickness and 100 days for mineralization lag time. These values are probably not appropriate for children, because bone turnover is faster during growth. Following a widely used approach to separate 'normal' from 'abnormal', a value higher than 2 standard deviations above the mean in healthy subjects might be used to define an 'increased result'. On the basis of reference data for

a

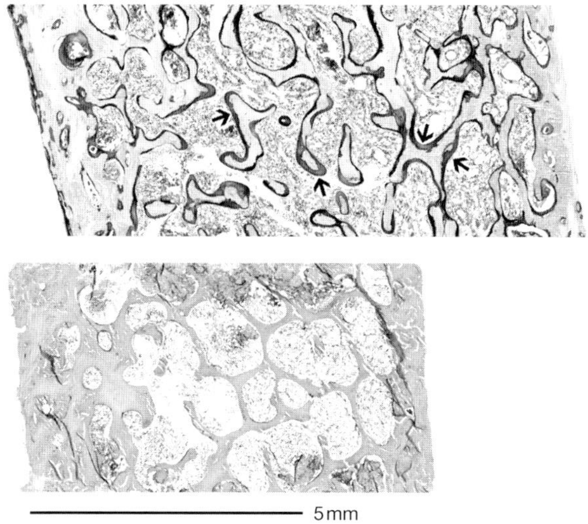

b

Fig. 3. Full thickness iliac biopsy samples. Mineralized bone is shown in light grey, unmineralized osteoid is shown in dark grey. ***a*** Sample from a 14-year-old girl with untreated X-linked hypophosphatemic rickets. Accumulation of osteoid is obvious. ***b*** Specimen from age-matched control.

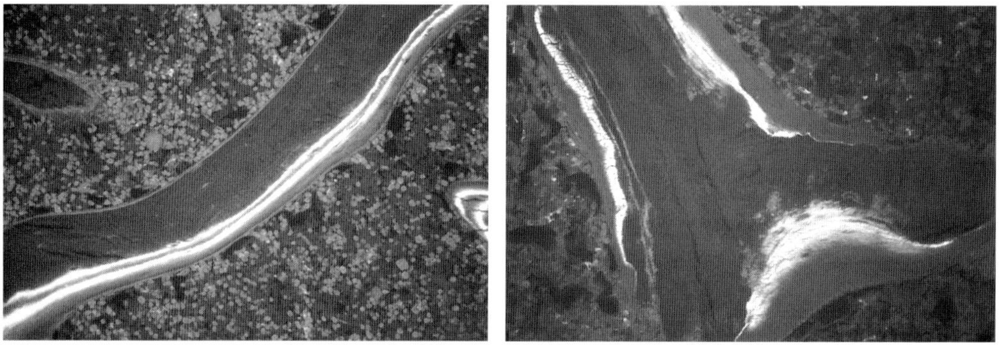

a *b*

Fig. 4. ***a*** Normal tetracycline double labels. ***b*** Labels are blurred, indicating a mineralization defect. Original magnification ×200.

pediatric histomorphometry, the cutoff values for osteoid thickness and mineralization lag time would be 9 μm and 25 days, respectively.

It is important to realize that the diagnosis of osteomalacia can only be confirmed when both osteoid thickness and mineralization lag time are abnormally high. An isolated increase in osteoid thickness can be due to an increased osteoid production rate, while an isolated increase in mineralization lag time can be due to slow bone turnover. Osteomalacia is not only characterized by abnormally high osteoid thickness and mineralization lag time, but also by reduced mineral apposition rate. However reduced mineral apposition rate is not specific, because it cannot only be caused by a defect in mineralization. Low mineral apposition rate may also result from a reduction in matrix deposition rate, as occurs in osteogenesis imperfecta and other osteopenic disorders.

Calcipenic Disorders of Bone Mineralization

In calcipenic forms of rickets and osteomalacia, hyperparathyroidism occurs in addition to the mineralization defect. This secondary hyperparathyroidism leads to increased bone turnover and deep osteoclastic resorption cavities during the earlier stages of the disease. As osteomalacia progresses, the mineralized bone surface is increasingly covered with thick osteoid seams and thus becomes inaccessible to osteoclasts. Paratrabecular fibrosis can be seen in severe forms of hyperparathyroid bone disease.

Vitamin D Deficiency

Although vitamin D deficiency rickets/osteomalacia is very frequent in many parts of the world, histomorphometric data from children with this condition have not been published. This is probably because the diagnosis can be confirmed with less invasive methods, treatment is straightforward and leads to rapid improvement.

Calcium Deficiency

Calcium deficiency can cause histologic and histomorphometric abnormalities that follow the usual pattern of a calcipenic mineralization defect, as outlined earlier. In younger children osteomalacia appears to predominate, whereas in teenagers histologic signs of hyperparathyroidism, overt osteomalacia or a mixture of both can be found. As described earlier, hyperparathyroid bone disease and frank osteomalacia may reflect different stages of the mineralization defect. Alternatively, variations in phosphorus intake may be responsible for the development of the two different histological defects. In fact, baboons fed a diet with low calcium and low phosphorus develop osteomalacia, whereas baboons on a low calcium, high phosphorus diet have features of hyperparathyroid bone disease.

The effects of low calcium intake can be exacerbated by concomitant fluorosis, as has been reported from South Africa and India. In fluorosis, high cancellous bone volume is usually found in addition to osteomalacia.

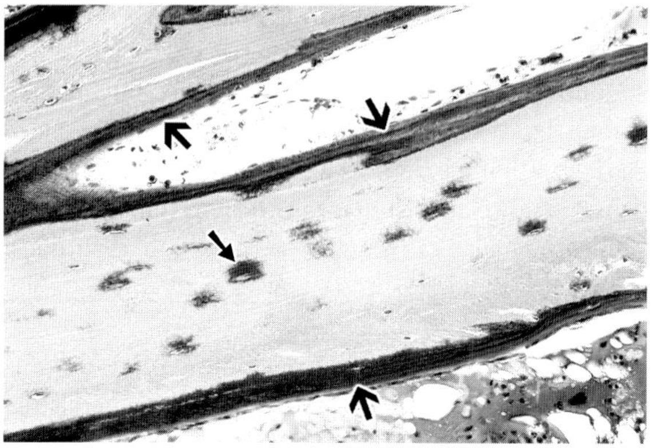

Fig. 5. Periosteocytic hypomineralized lesions. In X-linked hypophosphatemic rickets osteoid is not only accumulating on bone surfaces (large arrows), but also around osteocytes (small arrow).

Phosphopenic Disorders of Bone Mineralization

Secondary hyperparathyroidism is typically absent in phosphopenic forms of osteomalacia. Consequently, increased bone turnover and deep erosion cavities are not usually seen in these disorders.

X-Linked Hypophosphatemic Rickets

Children and adults with classical X-linked hypophosphatemic rickets show the typical features of osteomalacia (fig. 3). There are very thick osteoid seams and a grossly increased mineralization lag time, both in trabecular and in cortical bone. Despite low bone turnover rates, a large proportion of the bone surface is covered by osteoid, because mineralization proceeds slowly at individual remodeling sites.

The amount of trabecular bone is high in most patients, but a large proportion of this is unmineralized matrix. X-linked hypophosphatemic rickets can be distinguished histologically from other causes of osteomalacia, because osteocytes are surrounded by a halo of unmineralized bone (fig. 5).

Upon current standard treatment with phosphate and calcitriol, osteoid thickness and mineralization lag time decrease markedly. However, in many patients these parameters do not normalize completely. Also, the periosteocytic lesions persist to a large extent despite adequate therapy.

Other Forms of Hypophosphatemic Rickets

The histological features of non-X-linked hypophosphatemic rickets/osteomalacia have been studied in less detail than those of the X-linked disease.

Hypomineralized periosteocytic lesions do not occur in these disorders. Apart from that, histomorphometric findings in hereditary hypophosphatemic rickets with hypercalciuria resemble those of the X-linked form.

Only case reports are available on the bone tissue features of tumor induced osteomalacia. Trabecular bone surfaces are almost completely covered with thick layers of osteoid and osteoblast activity is low. These findings quickly normalize once the underlying tumor is removed.

Conclusions

Bone histology and histomorphometry are not usually needed to diagnose mineralization disorders in children, because in most cases the diagnosis can be established with less invasive methods. However, rickets can take an unusual appearance in adolescents and a bone biopsy may be helpful for diagnosis in this context. Bone biopsies also can be useful to distinguish X-linked hypophosphatemic rickets from other forms of phosphopenic disorders.

References

1 Pitt MJ: Rickets and osteomalacia are still around. Radiol Clin N Am 1991;29:97–118.

2 Parfitt AM: The physiologic and pathogenetic significance of bone histomophometric data; in Coe FL, Favus MJ (eds): Disorders of Bone and Mineral Metabolism. New York, Raven Press, 1992, pp 475–489.

3 Monier-Faugere MC, Langub MC, Malluche HH: Bone biopsies: A modern approach; in Avioli LV, Krane SM (eds): Metabolic Bone Disease and Clinically Related Disorders, ed 3. San Diego, Academic Press, 1998, pp 237–273.

4 Parfitt AM: Vitamin D and the pathogenesis of rickets and osteomalacia; in Feldman D, Glorieux FH, Pike JW (eds): Vitamin D. San Diego, Academic Press, 1997, pp 645–662.

5 Glorieux FH, Travers R, Taylor A, Bowen JR, Rauch F, Norman M, Parfitt AM: Normative data for iliac bone histomorphometry in growing children. Bone 2000;26:103–109.

Frank Rauch, MD
Genetics Unit, Shriners Hospital for Children
1529 Cedar Avenue, Montréal, Québec H3G 1A6 (Canada)
Tel. +1 514 842 5964, Fax +1 514 842 5581, E-Mail: frauch@shriners.mcgill.ca

Hochberg Z (ed): Vitamin D and Rickets.
Endocr Dev. Basel, Karger, 2003, vol 6, pp 80–92

Imaging of Rachitic Bone

Lisa J. States

The Children's Hospital of Radiology, Department of Radiology,
Philadelphia, Pa., USA

The skeleton is the one of the largest organ systems in the body. Though they may seem static, the bones are dynamic structures and sites of physiologic activity. The bones are major repositories for calcium and phosphorus, and play a key role in calcium metabolism. This chapter will review the imaging findings of rachitic bone.

Rickets is a form of metabolic bone disease characterized by inadequate mineralization of growing bones caused by diseases that alter vitamin D metabolism. Bone development requires appropriate amounts of a variety of vitamins, minerals, and hormones, in particular, calcium, phosphorus, and vitamin D. Calcium and phosphorus are needed for the formation of crystals of hydroxyapatite, which are the mineral building blocks of bone. Vitamin D is crucial as it stimulates the active absorption of calcium from the intestines and resorption in the proximal tubules of the kidney and thus helps to maintain adequate levels of both calcium and phosphorus in the body. Deficiency of vitamin D can result from inadequate exposure to the sun and disorders affecting the liver or kidney and has a profound effect on bone mineralization. Similarly, the lack of adequate calcium intake and diseases of the gastrointestinal tract and kidneys which effect calcium metabolism also cause abnormalities in bone mineralization.

Bone mineralization occurs by both intramembranous and enchondral ossification. In intramembranous ossification, bone is formed directly from bone cells. The skull and facial bones form by intramembranous ossification. In enchondral ossification a calcified cartilage matrix is remodeled into bone. Enchondral ossification results in longitudinal growth of the bones and occurs at the epiphyseal cartilaginous growth plate, the physis. Bones formed by enchondral ossification include the tubular bones, flat bones and cuboidal bones. The mandible and clavicle form by both mechanisms [1].

The physis is composed of columns of cartilage cells that are organized in four parallel zones; resting, proliferating, hypertrophic, and calcifying. The resting zone is a site of little activity. The proliferating and hypertrophic zones are sites of active cartilage cell division and maturation, respectively. Adjacent to the metaphysis is the calcifying zone, also known as the zone of provisional calcification. This is where osteoid matrix is formed and mineralized. Bone remodeling with absorption of osteoid and calcium by osteoclasts occurs in the adjacent metaphyseal region called the primary spongiosa.

On radiographs of the normal child, the first three zones of the physis are lucent and the zone of provisional calcification is similar in density to the mature mineralized bone. Abnormalities of mineralization affect the appearance of the zone of provisional calcification. As a result, radiographs of the physis of the growing child play a crucial role in the diagnosis and management of rickets.

Plain radiograph is the primary imaging tool for the evaluation of suspected metabolic bone disease due to rickets. Currently, there is no role for computed tomography or nuclear bone scintigraphy in the evaluation of rachitic bone. Magnetic resonance imaging (MRI) is an ideal imaging modality for evaluating cartilaginous structures; however, subtle mineralization is not well seen, therefore MRI has limited usefulness in the evaluation of rickets. In addition, sedation is necessary in most children younger than 6 years of age. Ultrasound can be used to identify a metaphyseal fracture in the setting of rickets [2].

When assessing radiographs, the degree of mineralization, the morphology of the bone and the appearance of the physis should be noted. Hypomineralization of the skeleton, referred to as osteopenia, is a key feature of rickets but is not specific for rickets. Both osteoporosis and osteomalacia appear radiographically as osteopenia. Osteoporosis is characterized by normal mineralization of diminished bone mass, whereas osteomalacia is characterized by diminished mineralization of normal bone mass. The morphology or shape of the bone should also be noted since bowing deformity due to bone softening often occurs. The most specific abnormality occurs at the metaphyseal-physeal region, thus evaluation of this site is essential for the diagnosis of rickets.

Choosing the part of the body to image depends on the age of the child. The rate of longitudinal growth and physiologic activity differs in bones throughout the skeleton. Therefore, the evaluation of a child with suspected rickets begins with radiographs of the areas with the most rapidly growing bones, which will vary depending on the age of the child.

A chest radiograph is very useful in detecting abnormal mineralization in the neonate, infant and young child. Abnormalities of the metaphyseal-physeal region can be seen in the proximal humeri and anterior rib ends. In most children, the wrists and knees are regions of rapid growth and show the most change and, therefore, a typical metabolic bone series includes views of the hands and the knees. Bilateral views of these regions are recommended to help determine if abnormal findings are due to generalized metabolic disease or a unilateral process such as infection or trauma.

Accelerated or delayed bone age are also common manifestations of metabolic bone disease. Therefore, the radiograph of the left hand can be most useful as it not only provides a view of the physeal region of the distal radius and ulna, but can also be used to determine the patient's skeletal age. Similarly, in children less than 1 year of age the knee radiograph allows evaluation of the distal femoral and proximal tibial and fibular physes, and can also be used to determine skeletal age.

The primary metabolic abnormality in rickets occurs at the zone of provisional calcification of the physis. Diminished calcification of cartilage cell columns, continued osteoid production by osteoblasts and diminished resorption of osteoid and calcium due to impaired osteoclast function results in a widened, irregularly calcified physis. The contiguous metaphysis is also affected and manifests as enlargement of the wrists, knees and rib ends (rachitic rosary). Metaphyseal broadening or 'cupping' is thought to result from changes related to stress at sites of ligament attachment, splaying of cartilage cells peripherally and microfracturing of the primary spongiosa by herniation of cartilage into this area [3].

The increasing number of viable, premature (<32 weeks' gestation), low birth weight (<1,500 g) infants has led to an increase in neonatal rickets [4–7]. The term osteopenia of prematurity has been used to categorize these patients since a hypomineralized skeleton is often the only finding of rickets. An early finding of rachitic change is rarefaction or lucency of the metaphyses and metadiaphyseal regions [6] (fig. 1). The typical metaphyseal findings of irregularity and broadening are not present since these neonates are not weight-bearing and are not growing at a normal rate. After 8 weeks of age, the humeri, knees, wrists and proximal femurs may show metaphyseal irregularity and growth plate widening (fig. 2). Findings may be seen earlier in a very small or early gestational age premature infant. Ongoing rickets will manifest as acute and healing fractures, most commonly seen at the ribs and forearms [7] (fig. 3).

Beyond the neonatal period, the classic rachitic changes are present. Radiographs of the long bones reveal widening and irregularity of all the physes, as well as 'fraying' and broadening of the metaphyses. The fraying may resemble the appearance of a paintbrush (fig. 4) or be disordered and irregular. In addition, the bones are demineralized and the cortical outlines of the epiphyseal ossification centers become blurred or nonapparent. A chest radiograph shows irregularity of the proximal humeral metaphyses and enlargement and irregularity of the anterior rib ends (fig. 5). In the long bones there is loss of the metaphyseal collar, a straight-edged segment of 1–3 mm in length representing the newly ossified metaphysis [8].

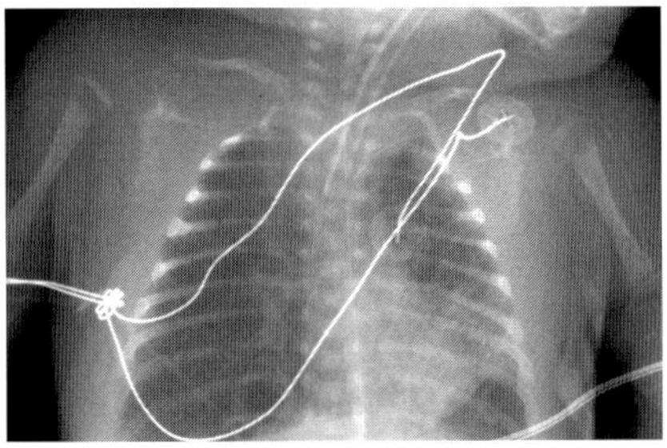

Fig. 1. Chest radiograph of an ex-25 weeks' gestation, premature infant with respiratory distress syndrome shows signs of early rickets. At 3 weeks of age there is diffuse osteopenia and a wide band of lucency in the humeral metaphyses.

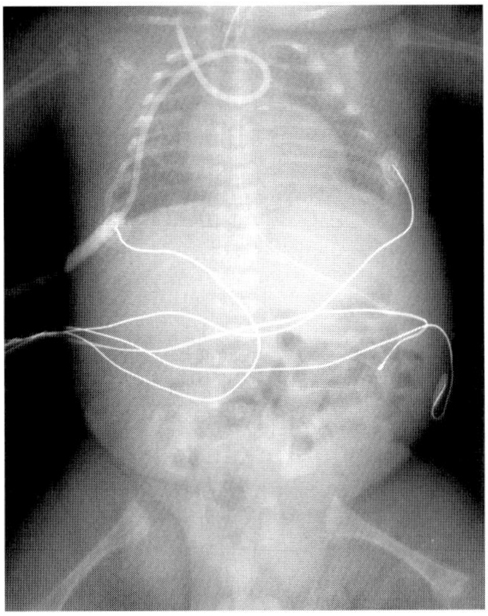

Fig. 2. Chest and abdomen radiograph of a 12-week-old infant with multiple medical problems related to low birth weight and prematurity shows classic rachitic changes. The skeleton is diffusely demineralized. Note the irregularity, cupping and widening of the metaphyses of all the long bones characteristic of rickets.

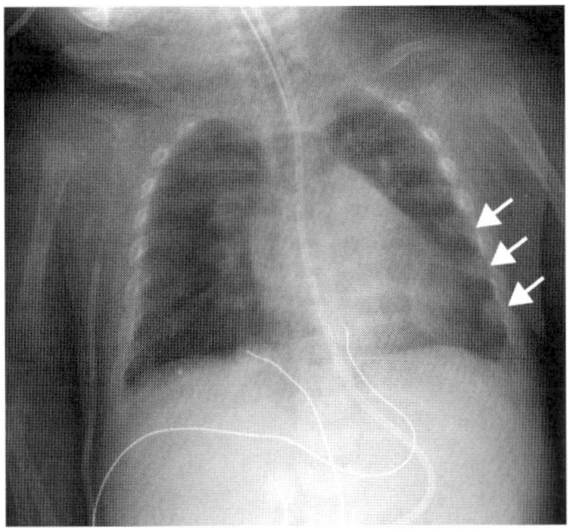

Fig. 3. Chest radiograph of a 9-month-old with chronic lung disease, on diuretic therapy, shows untreated rickets. Note the osteopenia, irregularity of the humeral metaphyses and the multiple healing fractures (arrows).

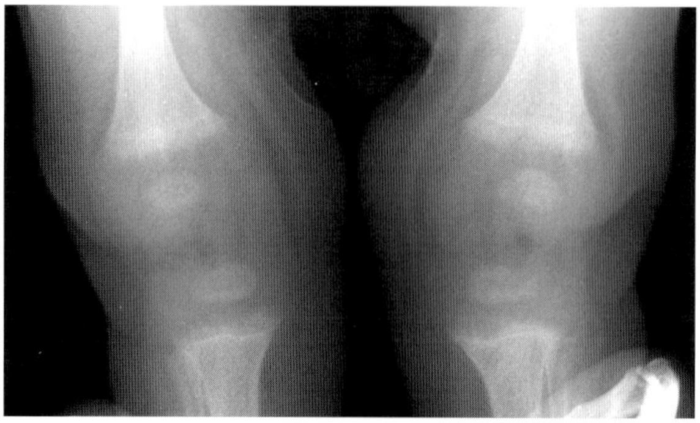

Fig. 4. Knee radiograph of a 7-month-old African-American boy with nutritional rickets show classic findings of metaphyseal fraying in a paintbrush pattern. Blurring of the trabeculae and cortical outlines is due to severe demineralization.

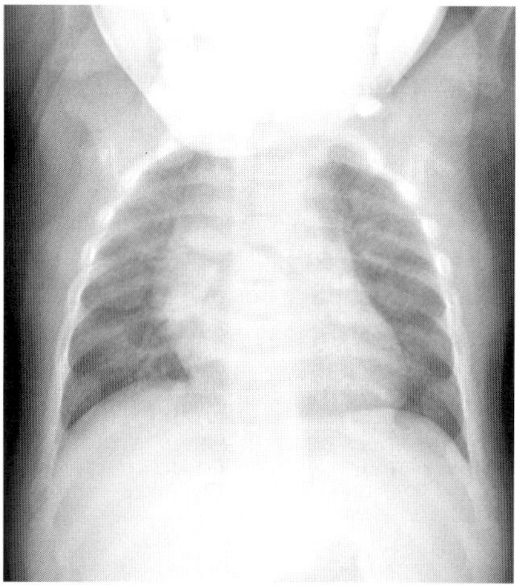

Fig. 5. Chest radiograph of an 8-month-old with nutritional rickets, enlarged joints and palpable rachitic rosary shows enlargement of the anterior rib ends is most prominent in middle ribs. In the proximal humeri, metaphyseal changes of lucency, irregularity, and broadening are well seen.

In cases of ongoing, untreated rickets, deformities due to softening of bone occur in the face of normal stress on the skeleton. Femoral and tibial bowing is most common and is typically seen in the newly crawling or walking child. Children with poor muscle tone may develop genu valgum (knock knees). Findings in the pelvis include coxa vara and protrusio acetabuli. The thorax may develop an hourglass shape. In the skull, postural molding and frontal bossing occur [3].

Radiographs are extremely useful in detecting response to therapy. With vitamin D therapy, calcium is laid down in the zone of provisional calcification.

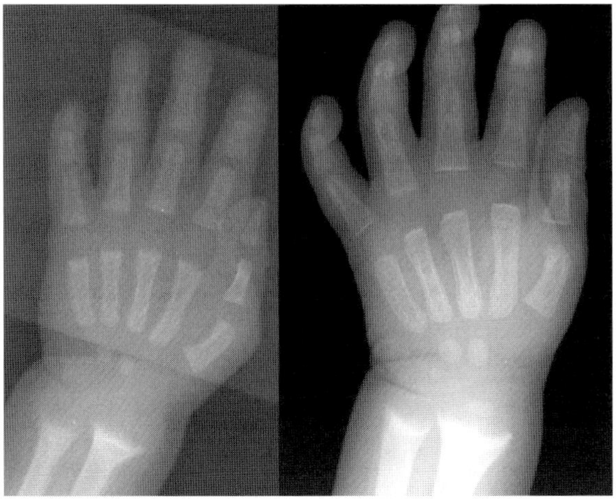

Fig. 6. Hand radiographs in a 7-month-old before treatment and 6 months after treatment. The pretreatment radiograph reveals significant blurring of the cortical outlines of all the bones. The metaphyses are widened and frayed. After treatment, a dense band is seen in the metaphysis of the radius and ulna at the zone of provisional calcification. The cortical outlines have become sharp and the trabeculae are easier to idenitify.

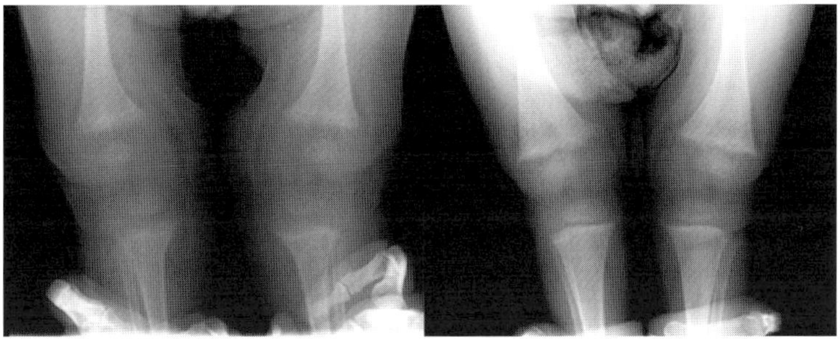

Fig. 7. Knee radiographs of the same patient as above, before and after treatment, show dense bands at the zone of provisional calcification after treatment. Also note the residual deformity of femoral bowing and flaring of the metaphyses. Residual metaphyseal irregularity suggests that healing is not complete.

On radiographs, the newly repaired zone of provisional calcification will appear as a dense metaphyseal band (fig. 6). These findings are seen as early as 2–3 weeks after the initiation of therapy in children with nutritional rickets and after 2–3 months in children with renal rickets [9]. Deformities due to bone softening, however, may persist after successful treatment (fig. 7).

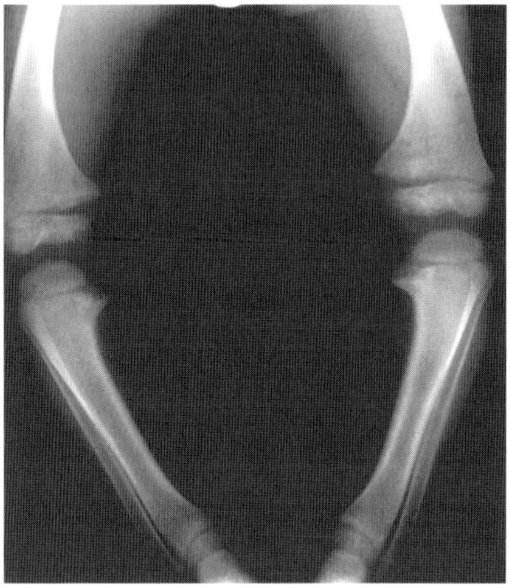

Fig. 8. Lower extremity radiographs of a 4-year-old boy with x-linked hypophosphatemic rickets show broadening of the bones and coarsened trabeculae. Irregularity at the metaphyses is mild. Note the bowing deformity of the femurs and tibias.

The imaging findings of most causes of rickets, whether due to nutritional deficiency, medication, or disease in the liver, kidneys or gastrointestinal tract, are usually indistinguishable. Age at presentation and maternal medical history are often helpful in the search for the etiology of rickets.

When rickets develops in a full-term infant less than 6 months of age a wide variety of maternal problems during pregnancy should be considered. Maternal vitamin D deficiency [10, 11], poorly controlled hyperparathyroidism, or renal insufficiency [12, 13], or administration of phosphate enemas during pregnancy [14] have all been found to cause congenital rickets. Alternatively, early presentation of rickets may occur in those with proximal renal tubular acidosis, or neonatal obstructive jaundice [6]. In addition, primary hyperparathyroidism [15] or hypophosphatasia [16] can be confused with rickets in this age group. Nutritional rickets in an otherwise normal infant will not usually become clinically apparent before 6 months of age due to prenatal stores of vitamin D imparted by the mother.

There are some interesting distinguishing features of some of the renal causes of rickets. Vitamin D-resistant rickets, also known as familial hypophosphatemic rickets or X-linked hypophosphatemic rickets, is most commonly brought to medical attention in the setting of progressive femoral bowing in a child over 18 months of age. According to Swischuk and Hayden [17] two different radiographic patterns, referred to as type A and type B, can be seen in this disorder. In type A, rachitic changes in the knees out of proportion to the wrists were common, a finding not described in any other type of rickets. In type B, a modeling defect with short, squat long bones and coarse bone trabeculation of the axial skeleton was found. This finding was seen predominantly in males, thought to be a reflection of the X-linked inheritance (fig. 8).

Vitamin D-dependent rickets, also known as pseudodeficiency rickets, is a hereditary form of rickets caused by impaired 1α hydroxylation in the renal proximal tubule. An additional form of vitamin D-dependent rickets, referred to as type II, is characterized by end-organ resistance to active vitamin D [18]. Symptoms of hypocalcemia manifest during the first few months of life. In both these disorders, radiographic findings are indistinguishable from other forms of rickets. Another cause of rickets is renal tubular insufficiency characteristic of Fanconi syndrome with its various subtypes of hypophosphatemic vitamin D-refractory rickets. Hypophosphatemic rickets may also occur as a result of nephrotoxicity due to ifosfamide therapy [19, 20]. Rickets may also develop as a paraneoplastic syndrome with phosphate loss in the urine and is referred to as oncogenic rickets [21].

Renal osteodystrophy is a combination of osteomalacia, rickets (osteomalacia of growing bone), and secondary hyperparathyroidism that develops in children with chronic renal disease. Both glomerular and tubular dysfunction, contribute to the development of this metabolic bone disease. Impaired glomerular function causes phosphorus retention, which results in hypocalcemia. Tubular dysfunction also causes hypocalcemia due to impaired synthesis of 1,25-hydroxyvitamin D. Hyperparathyroidism then develops as the body's response to diminished serum calcium levels and causes a variety of manifestations, including demineralization of the bones. This results in osteomalacia, the development of which may be exacerbated by the presence of chronic acidosis, aluminum toxicity due to dialysis, or total parenteral nutrition [22, 23].

Bone changes due to secondary hyperparathyroidism are well described. The classic features are subperiosteal resorption, endosteal resorption and osteopenia [24]. Subperiosteal resorption is best seen in the middle phalanges of the hands, upper medial proximal tibias, medial femoral neck, distal clavicles, distal radius and ulna (fig. 4), and lamina dura of teeth. The outer cortex has a hazy, ill-defined appearance. Endosteal resorption results in a lacy pattern of the inner cortex and is referred to as *cortical tunneling*. Acro-osteolysis may also occur. Osteomalacia can appear as diminished density, or coarsening of the residual mineralized matrix and trabeculae. An additional feature of hyperparathyriodism is the development of cysts and brown tumors due to hemorrhage in fibrous tissue that has replaced the resorbed bone matrix (fig. 9). Children with renal osteodystrophy are particularly at risk for developing slipped capital femoral epiphysis (fig. 10). The age at presentation is younger than the general population [25].

An interesting association is the presence of rickets in the infant or child with osteopetrosis [28, 29]. This has been referred to as osteopetrorickets. Osteopetrosis is a rare, autosomal-recessive disorder characterized by abnormal osteoclast function resulting in failure of resorption of bone. As a result, the bones throughout the skeleton are extremely dense. In some of these patients,

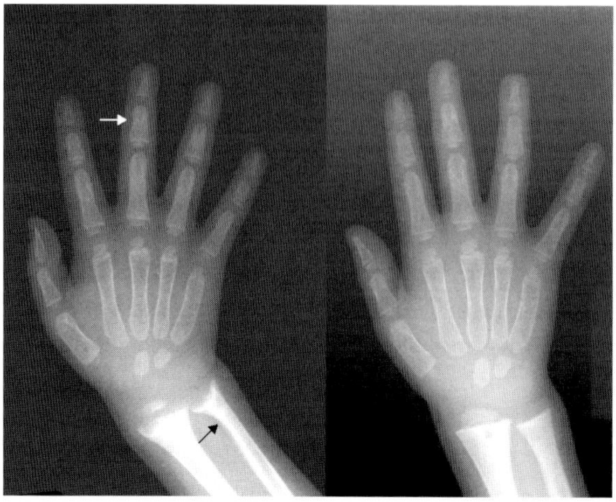

Fig. 9. Hand radiographs of a 3-year-old boy with pseudodeficiency rickets show changes of renal osteodystrophy before treatment and 6 months after treatment. Before treatment the trabeculae are coarsened due to osteomalacia. Typical rachitic changes are seen in the metaphyses of the distal radius and ulna. Subperiosteal resorption is seen along the inner border of the distal ulna (arrows) and middle phalanges. The tufts of the distal phalanges are poorly seen due to acro-osteolysis. After treatment, the zone of provisional calcification appears sharp and normal. The trabeculae are seen better. A new finding is a round lucency in the metaphysis likely representing a brown tumor.

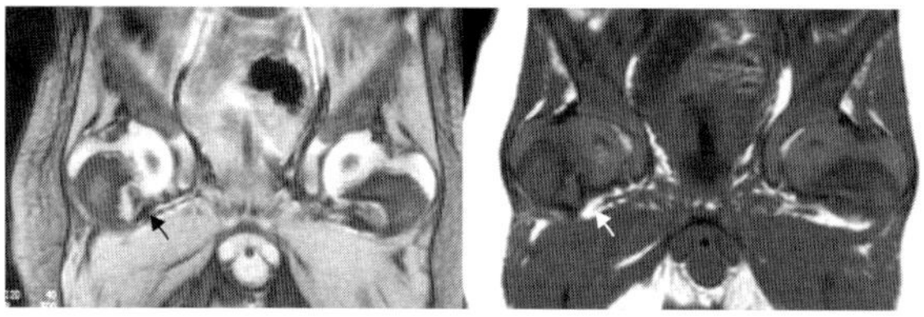

Fig. 10. Coronal magnetic resonance images of a 3-year-old with renal osteodystrophy due to prune belly syndrome show irregularity of the metaphyses. The gradient echo (left) and T1-weighted (right) images show the epiphyseal cartilage distinct from the metaphysics. Irregularity of the metaphyses is due to unossified tongues of cartilage alternating with ossified cartilage. A fracture fragment is seen along the medial aspect of the right femoral metaphysis (arrow).

despite a positive calcium balance, the calcium phosphorus product in the extracellular fluid is insufficient and rickets develops. Widening of the physes, osteopenia and pseudofractures occur (fig. 11). Widening and cupping of the metaphyses can also be seen.

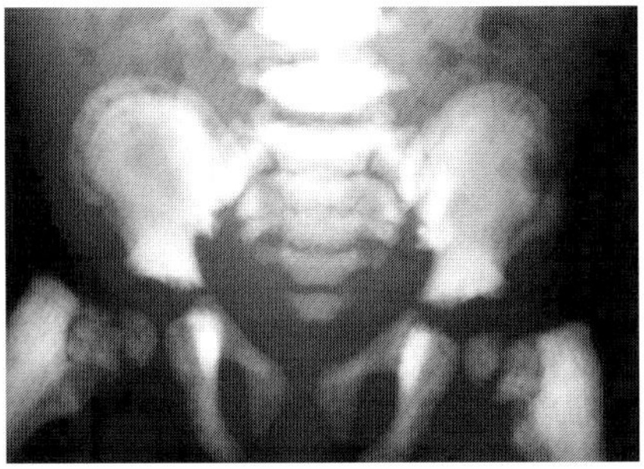

Fig. 11. Pelvic radiograph in a child with osteopetrorickets shows diffusely sclerotic bones characteristic of osteopetrosis. Changes of rickets include osteopenia of the widening of the physes. Pseudofractures are seen at the base of the femoral neck. In addition, the right femoral head is displaced due to a slipped capital femoral epiphysis. Lucency of the peripheral iliac wings represents metaphyseal lucency.

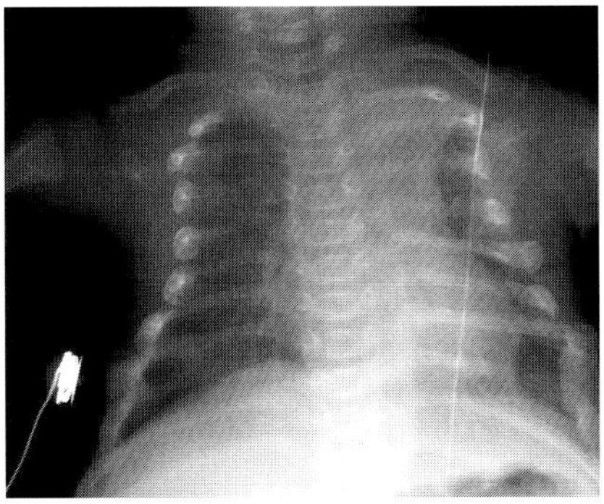

Fig. 12. Chest radiograph of a neonate with primary hyperparathyroidism shows diffuse osteopenia, wavy, deformed ribs and clavicles and healing fractures. The humeral metaphyses are normal.

There are several disorders that can be confused with rickets but close attention to the radiographic findings can be helpful. These disorders include primary hyperparathyroidism, hypophosphatasia, osteogenesis imperfecta, nonaccidental trauma and some of the metaphyseal dysplasias [8].

Primary hyperparathyroidism, a rare disorder, is usually diagnosed within the first three months of life [27]. Radiographs demonstrate osteopenia, subperiosteal bone resorption, and pathologic fractures (fig. 12). Focal lytic lesions may be present. Metaphyseal changes are not a feature of this disorder.

Hypophosphatasia, an uncommon inherited disorder, is characterized by deficiency of the enzyme alkaline phosphatase and accumulation of inorganic pyrophosphate. Excess inorganic pyrophosphate results in undermineralized bone with incomplete ossification of cartilage and metaphyseal regions. Soft tissue calcification and nephrocalcinosis may develop due to hypercalcemia. Radiographs reveal short, irregular, long bones with poor ossification. Bowed long bones and fractures are often present. Focal, round, lytic areas in the metaphyses due to clusters of unmineralized osteoid distinguish this disorder from rickets [14, 26] (fig. 13).

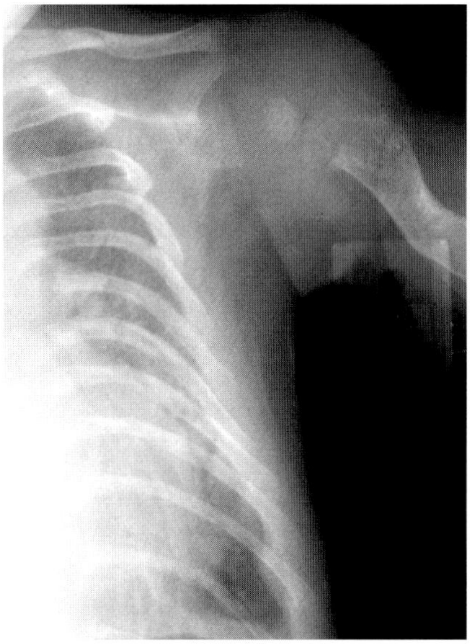

13

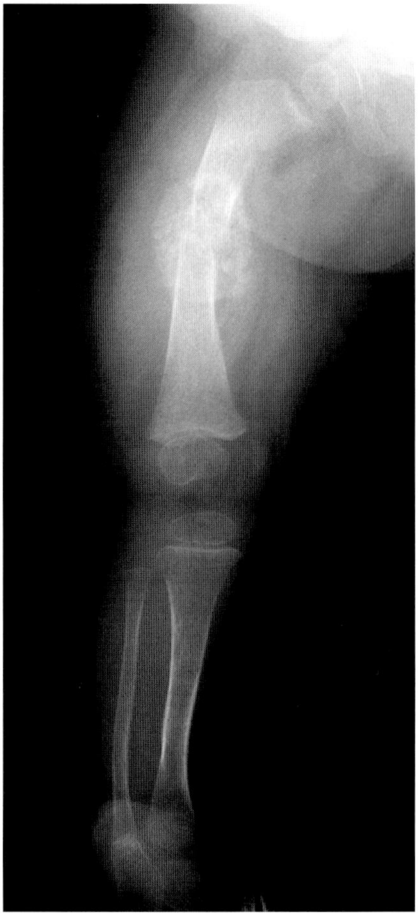

14

Fig. 13. Shoulder radiograph of a newborn with hypophosphatasia shows a focal lucency in the humeral metaphysis. The broad, bowed humerus, excludes rickets.

Fig. 14. Lower extremity radiograph of a 6-month-old with osteogenesis imperfecta shows diffusely demineralized bones. A healing fracture of the femur and bowing of the femur and fibula suggest the diagnosis in this nonambulating infant. Note the normal metaphyses.

Osteogenesis imperfecta (OI) can manifest with bowing and fractures (fig. 14). Bones are demineralized but have normal metaphyses. Broad or gracile long bones and wormian bones in the skull, features of OI, are features not seen in rickets.

The metaphyseal chondrodysplasias are forms of short-limbed dwarfism with varying degrees of dysmorphism. The metaphyseal findings of irregularity, and flaring with widening of the growth plates resemble rickets. The metaphyseal collar is intact distinguishing this from rickets [8]. A full skeletal survey in these patients may show additional findings not seen in rickets.

In conclusion, radiographs remain the imaging study of choice in evaluation of the child with metabolic bone disease due to rickets. A variety of disorders cause rickets and most of these are radiographically indistinguishable. The age of the patient is an important factor to be considered in the evaluation of the infant or child with suspected rickets. A chest radiograph is adequate in the neonate and infant, whereas radiographs of the knees and wrists are appropriate in children. Furthermore, radiographs are a valuable tool to assess the response to therapy.

References

1 Greenfield GB: Analytical approach to bone radiology. Radiology of Bone Diseases, ed 5. Philadelphia, Lippincott, 1990, pp 1–5.

2 Markowitz RI, Hubbard AM, Harty MP, Bellah RD, Kessler A, Meyer JS: Sonography of the knee in normal and abused infants. Pediatr Radiol 1993;23:264–267.

3 Schneider R: Radiologic methods of evaluating generalized osteopenia. Symposium on Metabolic Bone Diseases. Orthop Clin N Am 1984;15:631–651.

4 Roberts L, Badger V: Osteomalacia of very-low-birth-weight infants. J Pediatr Orthop 1984;4: 593–598.

5 Lyon AJ, McIntosh N, Wheeler K, William JE: Radiological rickets in extremely low birthweight infants. Pediatr Radiol 1987;17:56–58.

6 Wong HB: Rickets in Singapore infants and children. J Singapore Paediatr Soc 1986;28:12–19.

7 Koo WWK, Sherman R, Succop P, Krug-Wispe S, Tsang RC, Steichen JJ, Crawford, AH, Oestreich AE: Fractures and rickets in very low birth weight infants: Conservation management and outcome. J Pediatr Orthop 1989;9:326–330.

8 Oestreich AE, Ahmad BS: The periphysis and its effect on the metaphysis. Sketal Radiol 1993;22: 115–119.

9 Reade TM, Scriva CR, Glorieux FH, et al: Response to crystalline 1α-hydroxy vitamin D_3 in vitamin D dependency. Pediatr Res 1975;9:593–599.

10 Moncrieff H, Fadahunsi T: Congenital rickets due to maternal vitamin D deficiency. Arch Dis Child 1974;49:810–811.

11 Begum R, Continho ML, Dormandy TL: Maternal malabsorption presenting congenital rickets. Lancet 1968;i:1048–1052.

12 Al-Senan K, Al-Alaiyan S, Al-Abbad A, LeQuesne G: Imaging casebook: Congenital rickets secondary to untreated maternal renal failure. J Perinatol 2001;21:473–475.

13 Levin TL, States L, Greig A, Goldman H: Maternal renal insufficiency: A cause of congenital rickets and secondary hyperparathyroidism. Pediatr Radiol 1992;22:315–316.

14 Rimensberger P, Scubiger G, Willi U: Connatal rickets following repeated administration of phosphate enemas in pregnancy: A case report. Eur J Pediatr 1992;151:54–56.

15 Landing BH, Kamoshita S: Congenital hyperparathyroidism secondary to maternal hypoparathyroidism. J Pediatr 1970;77:842–847.

16 Currarino GD, Neuhauser EBD, Reyersbach GC, et al: Hypophosphatasia. Am J Roentgenol 1957; 78:392–419.

17 Swischuk LE, Hayden CK Jr: Rickets: A roentgenographic scheme for diagnosis. Pediatr Radiol 1970;8:203–208.

18 Demay M: Inherited defects of vitamin D metabolism; in Adrianne Bendich A (series ed): Nutrition and Health; in Holick MF (ed): Vitamin D Physiology, Molecular Biology, and Clinical Applications. Totowa, Humana Press, 1999, chap 18.

19 Silberzweig E, Haller JO, Miller S: Case report. Ifosfamide: A new case of rickets. AJR 1992;159: 823–824.

20 Sweeney LE: Hypophosphataemic rickets after ifosfamide treatment in children. Clin Radiol 1993;45:345–347.

21 Nuovo MA, Dorfman HD, Sun CC, Chalew SA: Tumor-induced osteomalacia and rickets. Am J Surg Path 1989;13:588–599.

22 Burtis WJ, Lang R: Chemical abnormalities. Orthop Clin N Am 1984;15:653–669.

23 Norman ME: Vitamin D in bone disease. Pediatr Clins N Am 1982;229:947–971.
24 Steinbach HL, Noetzli M: Roentgen appearance of the skeleton in osteomalacia and rickets. AJR 1964;91:955–972.
25 Goldman HB, Lane JM, Salvata E: Slipped capital femoral epiphyses complicating renal dystrophy: A report of three cases. Radiology 1978;126:333–339.
26 Currarino GD: Hypophastasia; in Kaufmann HJ (ed): Intrinsic Diseases of Bones. Progr Pediatr Radiol. Karger, Basel, 1973, pp 469–494.
27 Ross AJ, Cooper A, Attie MF: Primary hyperparathyroidism in infancy. Presented at 54th Annual Meeting, Surgical Section. San Antonio, American Academy of Pediatrics, 1985.
28 Di Rocco M, Buoncompagni A, Loy A, Dellacqua A: Osteopetrorickets: Case report. Eur J Pediatr 2000;159:579–581.
29 Donnelly LF, Johnson JF, Benzing G: Infantile osteopetrosis complicated by rickets. AJR 1995; 164:968–970.

Lisa J. States, MD
Alfred I. duPont Hospital for Children
Department of Medical Imaging
PO Box 269
Wilmington, DE 19899 (USA)
Tel. +1 302 651 4643, Fax +1 302 651 4626, E-Mail ljstates@comcast.net

Hochberg Z (ed): Vitamin D and Rickets.
Endocr Dev. Basel, Karger, 2003, vol 6, pp 93–104

Vitamin D Deficiency Rickets

Nicholas J. Shaw

Birmingham Children's Hospital, Birmingham, UK

Contents

Historical Perspective

Although traditionally associated with the process of industrialisation in developed countries in the 19th century there are much earlier descriptions of rickets (Homer 900 BC, Soranus Ephesius AD 130). A detailed description of the clinical features of rickets was published by the anatomist Francis Glisson in 1651. In the late 19th and early 20th centuries rickets was prevalent in cities in Northern Europe and the United States. In 1898, 80% of infants under the age of 2 years at the Infants Hospital in Boston had signs of rickets with a similar prevalence seen in Glasgow associated with children living in the dark crowded tenements that had sprung up with the Industrial Revolution. The importance of sunlight and diet in the aetiology of vitamin D deficiency became clarified in the early part of the 20th century. Mellanby [1] demonstrated the healing of rickets in dogs by adding cod liver oil to their diet and the presence of a vitamin was assumed and designated vitamin D. At around the same time in a classic experiment Hess and Unger [2] showed healing of rickets in children in New York by exposing them to sunlight on the roof of the hospital. Similarly, radiation from a mercury arc lamp was found to be effective (fig. 1). It was only after many years of research that in 1960 it was

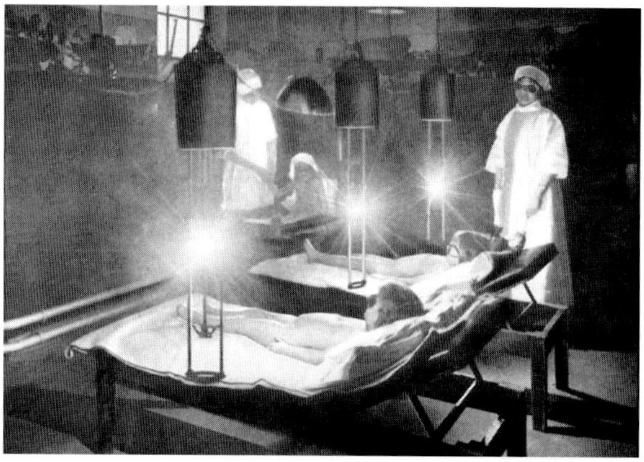

Fig. 1. Ultraviolet light treatment with a mercury arc lamp – Birmingham Children's Hospital 1930s.

clear that the effects ascribed to 'vitamin D' were due to the synthesis of a hormone which was dependent on the action of ultraviolet light on an endogenous steroid precursor from irradiated ergosterol in plants and 7-dehydrocholesterol in skin. The identification of ergocalciferol provided an effective and easily administered source of vitamin D. This led to the supplementation of cow's milk formulas and the provision of vitamin D supplements to breast-fed infants in the 1930s in the United States with the subsequent virtual disappearance of rickets in the mid-20th century. Similar food fortification introduced during the Second World War in the United Kingdom led to a rapid reduction in the prevalence of rickets. Unfortunately, this was followed by a rise in the incidence of idiopathic hypercalcaemia in infants which was attributed to uncontrolled vitamin D fortification. As a consequence, food fortification and the use of vitamin D supplements was significantly reduced in the United Kingdom.

A significant resurgence in the prevalence of vitamin D deficiency rickets occurred in the United Kingdom in the 1970s in children of South-East Asian immigrants. This was particularly seen in northern cities with a high Asian population such as Bradford and Glasgow [3]. This was followed by a nationwide public health initiative (the Stop Rickets campaign) which introduced measures such as ensuring that pregnant women and breast-fed infants received vitamin D supplements which are still official Department of Health guidelines [4]. A significant reduction in prevalence was then seen throughout the United Kingdom, which was well documented in one study from Glasgow [5]. However, in the final years of the 20th century a further significant resurgence of rickets and hypocalcaemia secondary to vitamin D deficiency has been seen in the United Kingdom particularly again in children of South-East Asian

Table 1. Aetiological factors for vitamin D deficiency

Vitamin D synthesis
Latitude
Atmospheric pollution
Clothing
Melanin pigmentation
Sunlight exposure
Vitamin D intake
Breast-feeding
Maternal vitamin D deficiency
Unusual diets
Vitamin D metabolism
Low calcium intake
Intestinal calcium absorption
Genetic variation

ethnic origin [6]. A high prevalence of asymptomatic vitamin D deficiency has also been reported in Asian 2-year-old children [7] and pregnant Asian women [8]. A survey undertaken of paediatricians in the West Midlands region identified 24 cases of symptomatic vitamin D deficiency in children under the age of 5 years in 1 year (incidence 6.8 per 100,000) the majority of these occurring in South-East Asian children [9]. At the same time a resurgence has been documented in the United States particularly seen in black breast-fed infants who were not receiving vitamin D supplements [10]. In addition, there continues to be reports from around the world of vitamin D deficiency rickets.

Aetiology and Epidemiology

The aetiology of vitamin D deficiency rickets is usually due to one or more of the factors listed in table 1 with different factors being more significant in different situations. It is now rare to see it occurring in Caucasian children in the absence of gastrointestinal or liver disease or extreme restriction of sunlight exposure. An example is a report of a white infant in Toronto with rickets which appeared to be entirely due to the use of a potent sunscreen. The majority of reports worldwide occur in dark-skinned infants and children. It is well known that increased melanin pigmentation reduces cutaneous vitamin D synthesis [11] but this factor alone is unlikely to explain the occurrence of rickets in such children particularly in countries with plenty of sunlight. The absence of any significant cutaneous vitamin D synthesis during the winter months in countries with latitudes above and below 35° is a contributory factor with dark skinned children being more susceptible. This will account for the resurgence of rickets being seen in South-East Asian children in the United Kingdom and Norway and black children in the United States. This is particularly so in breast-fed infants who are not receiving oral vitamin D to supplement the minimal vitamin D content of breast milk (approximately 12–60 IU/l). An additional factor in many of these populations will be maternal vitamin D deficiency which has been demonstrated in pregnant and breast feeding women. Thus the infants will be born with depleted vitamin D stores which are not subsequently replenished because of inadequate cutaneous vitamin D synthesis and the absence of vitamin D in breast milk and no oral vitamin D supplementation.

Less commonly diets of abnormal composition for infants are responsible which include prolonged exclusive breast feeding, macrobiotic and vegan diets without any vitamin D supplements. Again, these are more often reported in dark skinned infants in countries where cutaneous vitamin D synthesis is compromised for a significant part of the year.

As previously commented there are many reports of rickets occurring in countries with plenty of sunlight throughout the year such as Saudi Arabia, India and Australia. Here limited sunlight exposure may be due to cultural practices such as clothing and veiling in Muslim women and spending a lot of time indoors at home. Certainly, reports of rickets from Australia are almost exclusively from ethnic minority groups with such cultural practices. In addition, overcrowding may limit sunlight exposure in some countries. The effect of atmospheric pollution in countries undergoing rapid industrialisation may also limit vitamin D synthesis. A recent report from Delhi showed a clear difference in vitamin D status between children in rural areas and those living in the polluted urban areas of the city [12].

The role of calcium intake influencing vitamin D metabolism has also attracted attention in the past decade. Animal studies have shown that a low calcium intake enhances the catabolism of 25-hydroxyvitamin D. This is due to the effect of increased 1,25-dihydroxyvitamin D synthesis as a consequence of increased parathyroid hormone secretion. The elevated 1,25-dihydroxy-vitamin D then acts on the liver to enhance the metabolic destruction of 25-hydroxyvitamin D [13]. This effect is seen in humans in other situations where 1,25-dihydroxyvitamin D concentrations are raised such as primary hyperparathyroidism and chronic gastrointestinal disease. Thus, the same populations who are more susceptible to the impact of vitamin D deficiency often have a diet that is low in calcium. Alternatively, intestinal calcium absorption may be impaired as was speculated to contribute to vitamin D deficiency in South-East Asians in the United Kingdom due to the phytate content of chapati flour.

Finally a potential contributory factor may be genetic factors influencing Vitamin D metabolism. One study has suggested that Asian subjects living in the United States have enhanced catabolism of 25-hydroxyvitamin D due to

Table 2. Clinical presentation of vitamin D deficiency

Convulsions
Stridor
Tetany
Cardiomyopathy
Bowed legs
Delayed walking
Fracture
Coincidental X-ray findings
Hypercalcaemia due to 3° hyperparathyroidism

increased 25(OH)D, 24-hydroxylase activity [14]. As yet, this work has not been confirmed by other studies.

Although historically the presence of rickets has been linked to poverty this is not a consistent association as rickets is also seen in affluent well educated populations. In addition to symptomatic vitamin D deficiency there is considerable evidence of subclinical vitamin D deficiency in a variety of populations. Thus, there are reports of South-East Asian 2-year-olds in the United Kingdom [7] and French adolescent boys during winter [15] with a high prevalence of biochemical vitamin D deficiency. This may be of relevance in relation to the risk of adult disease such as osteoporosis, diabetes and ischaemic heart disease where such epidemiological associations have been described.

Clinical Presentation

The presenting features of symptomatic vitamin D deficiency vary depending on the age of the affected child. In the survey undertaken in the West Midlands region in the United Kingdom of children presenting under the age of 5 years there were three different modes of presentation [9]. One group presented under the age of 6 months with symptomatic hypocalcaemia, usually convulsions, another group presented with signs of rickets particularly bowed legs from the age of 1 year and the third group presented with delayed walking with evidence of hypotonia and a proximal myopathy beyond the age of 18 months. This latter group were all black children of African-Caribbean ethnic origin who had received prolonged breast-feeding. Cardiomyopathy or stridor as a consequence of hypocalcaemia are other recognised modes of presentation in infancy (table 2).

Some infants may present in the neonatal period with hypocalcaemia and evidence of rickets due to severe maternal vitamin D deficiency which has been termed ‘congenital rickets’. On occasions, rickets may be identified as a coincidental finding on an X-ray taken in a child presenting with another illness.

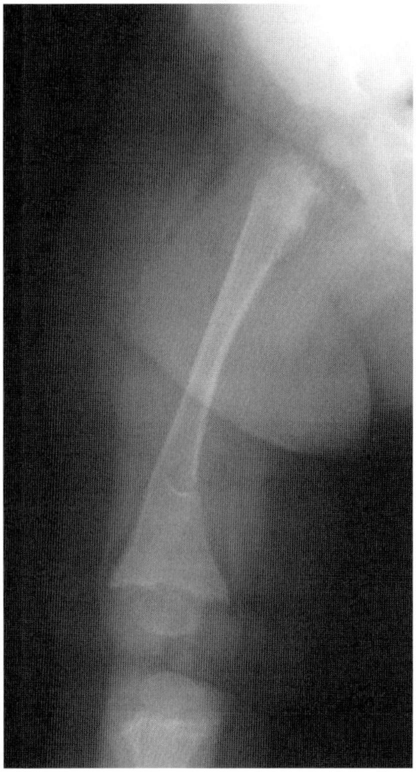

2

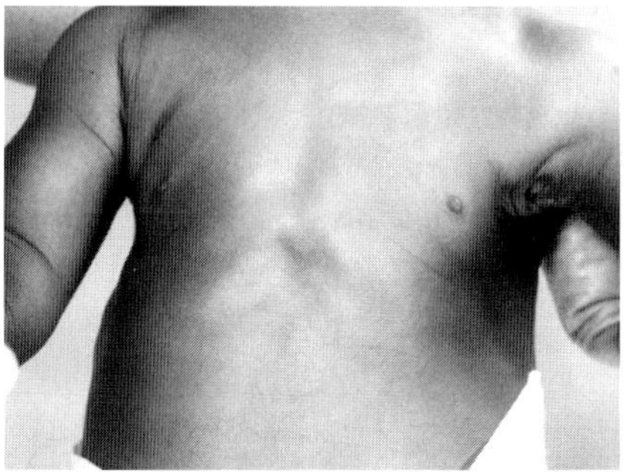

3

Fig. 2. Femoral shaft fracture in a child with rickets.

Fig. 3. Appearance of Harrison's sulci in a child with severe rickets.

The occurrence of a fracture in the osteopenic bones of a child with rickets is another potential mode of presentation (fig. 2).

In the first year of life the predominant clinical signs are palpable and visible enlargement of the extremities of the long bones, particularly wrists and ankles and costochondral junctions in the thorax ('rachitic rosary'). There may be a Harrison's sulcus (fig. 3) due to the inward pull of the diaphragm on softened lower ribs. Examination of the skull will often show signs of poor mineralisation with softening of the occipital area ('craniotabes') enlarged sutures and delayed closure of the fontanelles.

After the first year of life the effects of weight bearing become evident in the legs resulting in genu varum (bow legs) or genu valgum (knock knees). Development of the teeth is frequently impaired in vitamin D deficiency with delayed eruption and enamel hypoplasia. This is a useful distinguishing feature from hypophosphataemic rickets where early tooth development is normal. Older children may complain of bone pain and fatigue. Evidence of an associated iron deficiency anaemia is often seen in infants. Rarely a more severe haematological disorder is seen (the von Jacksch-Luzet syndrome) which causes a severe anaemia with leucocytosis, thrombocytopenia and hepatosplenomegaly. It resembles chronic myeloid leukaemia but is rapidly cured with vitamin D therapy. There is a recognised association between coincidental illness particularly gastrointestinal and symptomatic hypocalcaemia in infants with Vitamin D deficiency. There is also evidence of an increased risk of pneumonia in children with vitamin D deficiency [16].

The other age group where symptomatic Vitamin D deficiency presents is during adolescence. In one study from Saudi Arabia its prevalence is reported as 68/100,000 children aged 10–15 years [17]. Such individuals who are often in early or mid puberty usually present with hypocalcaemia either as convulsions or tetany. Other reported symptoms include diffuse limb pains and generalised weakness. There are often no clinical or radiological features of rickets in this age group. There is a striking female predominance when presenting at this age and they are often consuming a diet low in calcium and vitamin D and have limited sunlight exposure. A rare presentation in this age group is with hypercalcaemia due to tertiary hyperparathyroidism secondary to prolonged parathyroid gland stimulation from severe vitamin D deficiency.

Biochemical Features

As a consequence of vitamin D deficiency there is reduced intestinal calcium absorption, decreased extracellular calcium leading to defective mineralisation and secondary hyperparathyroidism (fig. 4). Biochemical findings are usually low or normal serum calcium levels and high serum parathyroid hormone levels leading to decreased tubular reabsorption of phosphate, aminoaciduria and low serum phosphate. There is evidence of increased bone turnover with high levels of alkaline phosphatase which are much higher than seen in hypophosphataemic rickets. Defective tubular reabsorption of bicarbonate may also be seen leading to a mild hyperchloraemic acidosis. Serum levels of 25-hydroxyvitamin D are usually low (<8 ng/ml) but may be within the normal range if there has been recent exposure to vitamin D. Levels of 1,25-dihydroxyvitamin D are usually within normal or low normal range but have also been reported to be elevated but considered to be inappropriately low for the degree of hyperparathyroidism. Occasionally, elevated levels of serum phosphate can be seen in the face of secondary hyperparathyroidism giving a biochemical profile similar to that seen in pseudohypoparathyroidism. This entity which appears to occur more often in infants and adolescents who

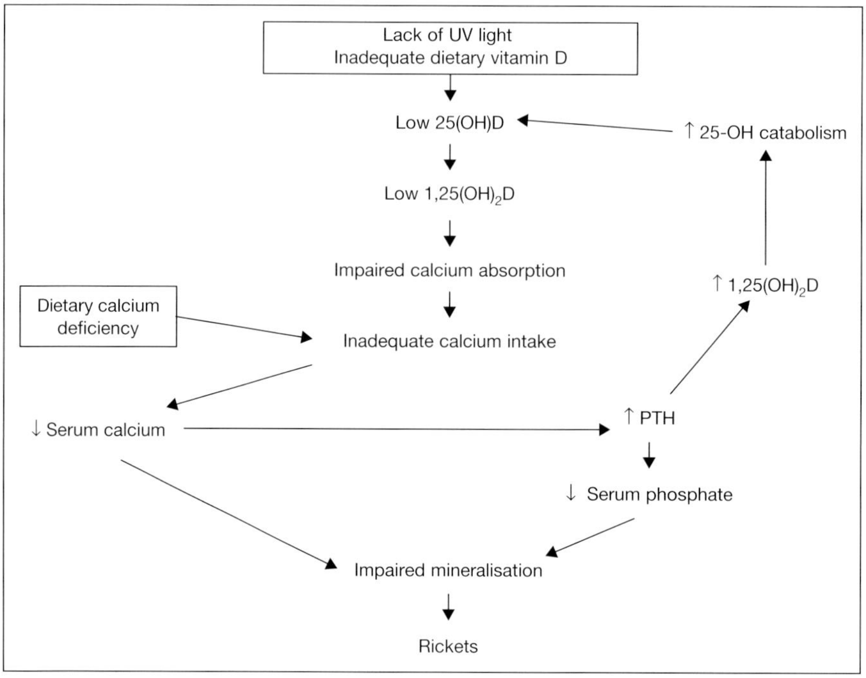

Fig. 4. Factors involved in the development of vitamin D deficiency rickets.

present with hypocalcaemia has also been termed 'partial hypoparathyroidism' and has been interpreted as a defective renal responsiveness to PTH [18]. Markers of bone turnover are usually elevated in vitamin D deficiency rickets other than osteocalcin which have been reported to be low or normal and rise rapidly when treatment is initiated. However, the monitoring of other bone markers in addition to alkaline phosphatase does not usually aid clinical management.

Three stages of vitamin D deficiency rickets can be identified.

Stage I arises from impaired intestinal calcium absorption and calcium resorption from bone leading to hypocalcaemia. Although this stage is felt to only last a few days before stage II, it may be prolonged leading to symptomatic hypocalcaemia in infants between the ages of 2 and 9 months.

In stage II, serum calcium is normal, but a low serum phosphate appears as a consequence of secondary hyperparathyroidism. In stage III, hypocalcaemia recurs as a consequence of insufficient mobilisation of calcium from bone and at this point the bone disease is severe. In clinical practice, it is often difficult to distinguish between these three stages.

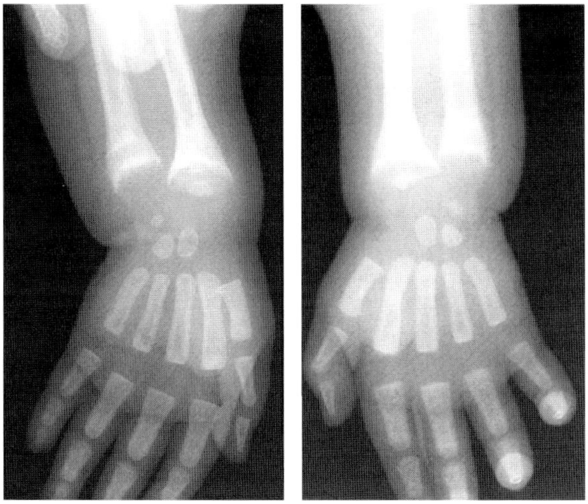

Fig. 5. X-ray changes of florid vitamin D deficiency rickets.

Radiological Features

Radiological features predominantly appear at the growth plate and usually X-rays of the knee or wrist are the most useful for detecting early changes. The distal ulna is the best site to show early changes of rickets particularly in young children. In older children, the metaphyses above and below the knees are more useful. There is widening of the radiolucent space between the metaphyses and epiphyses as a consequence of the accumulation of uncalcified cartilage. With increasing severity of rickets the metaphyses show fraying and cupping or lateral spreading forming cortical spurs (fig. 5). The centres of ossification may be pale and irregular and their appearance may be delayed. The shafts of the long bones usually show reduced density with thin cortices and may show deformity, particularly bowing of the tibiae and femurs. In addition pathological fractures may be noted particularly unrecognised fractures of the ribs and fibula. On a chest X-ray similar cupping at the costochondral junctions is seen corresponding to the palpable rachitic rosary. When rickets occurs during adolescence typical changes may not be seen at the wrists and knees due to the narrowing and fusion of the epiphyseal growth plates. Here radiographs of the pelvis may be useful as the centres of secondary ossification in the ischium and ilium may be abnormally wide. The appearance at the knees in an infant with rickets in conjunction with disproportionate short stature has on occasion been thought to be that of a metaphyseal dysplasia. However these changes rapidly resolve with vitamin D treatment. The first sign of healing rickets is the appearance of a zone of provisional calcification at the ends of the metaphyses. This is usually seen within 3–4 weeks. There is a gradual improvement in the coarse trabecular pattern which may take up to 6 months to resolve. Periosteal new bone formation may also be seen which is gradually incorporated into the cortices of the long bones.

Treatment

The most effective and physiological treatment for an infant with symptomatic hypocalcaemia, or rickets due to vitamin D deficiency, is either ergocalciferol (D_2) or cholecalciferol (D_3). This is the fastest means to replenish the depleted 25(OH)D levels, improve intestinal calcium absorption and suppress the effect of secondary hyperparathyroidism. Alfacalcidol or calcitriol are not appropriate treatments and children treated with these preparations initially are often resistant to their effect. Currently, in the United Kingdom preparations of ergocalciferol or cholecalciferol are not readily available and a liquid preparation suitable for infants is not listed in the British National Formulary. A calciferol solution containing 3,000 units per ml is available from Martindale Pharmaceuticals (Bampton Road, Harold Hill, Romford, Essex, RM3 8UG). A dose of 3,000 units daily for infants less than six months and 6,000 units daily for those older than 6 months for 6 weeks – 4 months is usually adequate to replenish depleted vitamin D stores, correct biochemical abnormalities and heal rickets. Normalisation of calcium and phosphate levels will occur within 3 weeks although alkaline phosphatase may remain elevated for several months. Measurement of serum PTH on treatment is also useful as it should normalise when the vitamin D deficiency has resolved. $1,25(OH)_2D$ concentrations rise rapidly with treatment and remain elevated for up to 10 weeks. Oral calcium supplements are also usually required initially if the child is hypocalcaemic and/or dietary intake is poor. One study from Nigeria in children with rickets and a low calcium intake indicated more rapid healing when calcium supplements were given alone or in combination with vitamin D than vitamin D alone [19]. Although they primarily had calcium deficiency as the cause of the rickets one third had additional evidence of vitamin D deficiency raising the suggestion that calcium supplements should be routinely used in the treatment of vitamin D deficiency rickets. It is not necessary to continue treatment until any leg deformity resolves which may take several years for which orthopaedic correction is rarely required. For the occasional adolescent presenting with symptomatic hypocalcaemia, a tablet preparation containing 10,000 units of cholecalciferol is available and is the most appropriate for this age group.

Following successful healing of rickets it is important to continue vitamin D in a prophylactic dose of 400 IU per day. Spontaneous healing of rickets may occur during the summer months as a consequence of increased ultraviolet light exposure. Where there are concerns about compliance single large oral or intramuscular doses of 200–600,000 IU have been used without inducing vitamin D toxicity [20].

References

1 Mellanby E: An experimental investigation on rickets. Lancet 1919;i:407–412.

2 Hess AF, Unger LJ: Cure of infantile rickets by sunlight. JAMA 1921;77:39–43.

3 Ford JA, McIntosh WV, Butterfield R, Preece MA, Pietrek J, Arrowsmith WA, Arthurton MW, Turner W, O'Riordan JL, Dunnigan MG: Clinical and subclinical vitamin D deficiency in Bradford children. Arch Dis Child 1976;51:939–943.

4 Department of Health: Dietary Reference Values for Food Energy and Nutrients for the United Kingdom. London, HMSO, 1991. (Report on health and social subjects 41.)

5 Dunnigan MG, Glekin BM, Henderson JB, McIntosh WB, Sumner D, Sutherland GR: Prevention of rickets in Asian children: Assessment of the Glasgow Campaign. BMJ 1985;291: 239–242.

6 Shaw NJ, Pal BR: Vitamin D deficiency in UK Asian families: Activating a new concern. Arch Dis Child 2002;86:147–149.

7 Lawson M, Thomas M: Vitamin D concentrations in Asian children aged 2 years living in England: Population survey. BMJ 1999;318:28.

8 Alfaham M, Woodhead S, Pask G, Davies D: Vitamin D deficiency: A concern in pregnant Asian women. Br J Nutr 1995;73:881–887.

9 Callaghan A, Booth IW, Moy RGD, Shaw NJ, Debelle G: Rickets returns. Arch Dis Child 2002;86(suppl 1):A35.

10 Kreiter SR, Schwartz RP, Kirkman HN Jr, Charlton PA, Calikoglu AS, Davenport ML: Nutritional rickets in African-American breast-fed infants. J Pediatr 2000;137:153–157.

11 Holick MF: Vitamin D: The underappreciated D-lightful hormone that is important for skeletal and cellular health. Curr Opin Endocrinol Diab 2002;8:87–98.

12 Agarwal KS, Mughal MZ, Upadhyay P, Berry JL, Mawer EB, Puliyel JM: The impact of atmospheric pollution on vitamin D status of infants and toddlers in Delhi, India. Arch Dis Child 2002;87:111–113.

13 Clements MR, Johnson L, Fraser DR: A new mechanism for induced vitamin D deficiency in calcium deprivation. Nature 1987;324:62–65.

14 Awumey EMK, Mitra DA, Hollis BW, Kumar R, Bell NH: Vitamin D metabolism is altered in Asian Indians in the Southern United States: A clinical research center study. J Clin Endocrinol Metab 1998;83:169–173.

15 Guillemant J, Le HT, Maria A, Allemandou A, Peres G, Guillemant S: Wintertime vitamin D deficiency in male adolescents: Effect on parathyroid function and response to vitamin D_3 supplements. Osteoporos Int 2001;12:875–879.

16 Muhe L, Lulseged S, Mason KE, Simoes EA: Case-control study of the role of nutritional rickets in the risk of developing pneumonia in Ethiopian children. Lancet 1997;349:1801–1804.

17 Narchi H, Jamil ME, Kulaylat N: Symptomatic rickets in adolescence. Arch Dis Child 2001;84: 501–503.

18 Rao S, Parfitt AM, Kleerekoper M, Pumo BS, Frame B: Disassociation between the effects of endogenous parathyroid hormone on adenosine 3′,5′-monophosphate generation and phosphate reabsorption in hypocalcaemia due to vitamin D depletion: An acquired disorder resembling pseudohypoparathyroidism type II. J Clin Endocrinol Metab 1985;61:285–290.

19 Thacher TD, Fischer PR, Pettifor JM, Lawson JO, Isichei BM, Reading JC, Chan GM: A Comparison of calcium, vitamin D, or both for nutritional rickets in Nigerian children. N Engl J Med 1999;341:563–568.
20 Shah BR, Finberg L: Single day therapy for vitamin D deficiency rickets: A preferred method. J Pediatr 1994;125:487–490.

Dr. Nicholas J. Shaw
Department of Endocrinology, Birmingham Children's Hospital
Steelhouse Lane, Birmingham, B4 6NH (UK)
Tel. +44 121 333 8189, Fax +44 121 333 8191, E-Mail nick.shaw@bch.nhs.uk

Hochberg Z (ed): Vitamin D and Rickets.
Endocr Dev. Basel, Karger, 2003, vol 6, pp 105–125

Calcium-Deficiency Rickets

Tom D. Thacher

Department of Family Medicine, Jos University Teaching Hospital, Jos, Nigeria

Contents

Calcium, present within bone as crystals of hydroxyapatite ($Ca_{10}(PO_4)_6(OH)_2$), comprises about 40% of bone mass. During bone growth in infancy and childhood, endochondral ossification occurs at the growth plates resulting in lengthening of bone. Successful mineralization of the matrix formed by chondrocytes of the growth plate requires sufficient calcium and phosphate to permit crystal formation. An inadequate supply of calcium restricts mineralization of the growing bone, leading to the clinical features of nutritional rickets.

Epidemiology

Far from being eradicated, nutritional rickets has been described in over 20 countries in the last 10 years. Many of these countries are in the tropics where sunlight is abundant. Vitamin D-deficiency rickets still occurs in sunny locales if mothers remain indoors during pregnancy and lactation along with their young infants. Because of their dependency on breast milk and limited mobility, infants typically present with vitamin D-deficiency rickets in the first year of life.

Despite adequate sunlight exposure, nutritional rickets develops in some children beyond the first year of life, and the apparent oxymoron 'sunshine rickets' has been used to describe this observation. Evidence from several tropical countries indicates that many children with nutritional rickets have adequate vitamin D status, based on the normal serum 25-hydroxyvitamin D values found in the majority of children [1–3]. Reports of calcium deficiency as a cause of rickets in these children have originated from South Africa [1], Nigeria [2, 3], and Bangladesh [4]. Though most reports are limited to these three countries, calcium-deficiency rickets likely occurs in many tropical countries, but may be misdiagnosed as vitamin D deficiency in the absence of laboratory measurement of 25-hydroxyvitamin D. Calcium-deficiency rickets was first reported and is still occasionally described among American and European children whose milk intake is restricted [5–7].

Inadequate data are available to determine the true prevalence of nutritional rickets in most countries. Some surveys have been done relying solely on selected clinical or biochemical features for the diagnosis of rickets, but these overestimate the true prevalence [8]. Only 38% of Nigerian children who presented with clinical features consistent with rickets (primarily leg deformities) had active rickets radiologically [9]. The remainder presumably had residual leg deformity from rickets in the past or had physiologic bow leg or knock knee deformity. In Ethiopian children under 5 years of age with pneumonia, 38% had radiographic evidence of rickets [10]. Most of these were young infants with presumed vitamin D deficiency, but 25-hydroxyvitamin D values were not reported. In some regions of India one quarter of the children had clinical signs of rickets, but among 600 children examined radiographically only 6.3% had rickets [11]. Epidemiological surveys in Bangladesh indicate that clinical signs of rickets may be found in 6–9% of children; however, the prevalence of radiologically confirmed rickets was about 1% [12]. In northeastern Nigeria, clinically overt rickets was found in 2.4% and abnormalities suggestive of rickets in 15% of 461 households [13]. Similarly, 9% of urban children between the ages of 6 months and 3 years in a community survey in central Nigeria had clinical signs of rickets [14]. In both Nigerian studies radiographs were not done. However, in another community survey in central Nigeria, radiologically active rickets was found in 1.2% of children between the ages of 12 and 18 months [unpubl. data].

Few studies report serum 25-hydroxyvitamin D values that would discriminate between calcium and vitamin D deficiency and permit determination of the relative proportion of each. Nearly all studies have been carried out in selected populations rather than in randomly sampled communities. Varying definitions of rickets have used inconsistent combinations of clinical, biochemical, and radiologic data. Rigorous population studies are needed to accurately determine the prevalence and incidence of calcium-deficiency rickets in various populations and the burden of disability it causes.

Pathophysiology

In either vitamin D-deficiency or calcium-deficiency rickets, calcium is the limiting nutrient for growth plate mineralization. Lack of calcium for bone mineralization could theoretically arise from reduced intake or absorption of calcium, impaired utilization of calcium at the growth plate, or increased calcium loss from the body. Vitamin D deficiency impairs intestinal calcium absorption, because 1,25-dihydroxyvitamin D concentrations are inadequate to stimulate vitamin D receptors in the gut. Exposure to sunlight can easily provide children with sufficient vitamin D. Adequate sunlight exposure has not been clearly defined, but at a latitude of 39°N (Cincinnati) even a fully clothed infant without a hat has been estimated to require only 2 h of sunlight per week to maintain 25-hydroxyvitamin D values in the normal range [15]. For an infant clothed only in a diaper, 20 min of sunshine per week should be sufficient. Dark skin pigmentation may triple the amount of time required, but it does not limit the quantity of 25-hydroxyvitamin D produced. Melanin absorbs ultraviolet photons and reduces the energy available for vitamin D synthesis; however, melanin also limits the photodegradation of synthesized vitamin D to inactive sterols resulting from prolonged sunlight exposure.

Even if sun exposure is adequate, and vitamin D status is sufficient, low dietary calcium intake can result in nutritional rickets. In response to a fall in serum ionized calcium concentration, parathyroid hormone (PTH) secretion stimulates renal 1,25-dihydroxyvitamin D synthesis. Though PTH concentrations are inconsistently elevated, 1,25-dihydroxyvitamin D values are invariably elevated in calcium-deficiency rickets. The primary effect of raised 1,25-dihydroxyvitamin D concentrations is to maximize intestinal absorption of ingested calcium.

Breast milk is the primary source of calcium during infancy, particularly for children in developing countries who typically breast-feed well into the second year of life. With increasing duration of lactation, the concentration of calcium in breast milk declines, while the volume of breast milk intake increases. In addition, nearly twofold variation in the concentration of calcium in breast milk has been observed between African mothers at the same stage of lactation [16]. Concentrations of calcium in breast milk of African women were 15–20% lower than those of British women. However, calcium supplementation in the mother does not alter the calcium content of breast milk. Breast milk calcium apparently derives from mobilization of bone and renal conservation of calcium, rather than from dietary intake.

Depending on the stage of lactation and individual variation, one liter of breast milk contains between 120 and 360 mg of calcium. The infant's daily intake of calcium from breast milk has been estimated to be about 210 mg. In contrast, cow's milk contains nearly 1,200 mg of calcium per liter, but the fractional absorption of calcium in cow's milk is less than human milk. Consequently, in countries where children are weaned from breast milk to vitamin D-fortified cow's milk or breast milk substitutes, prolonged breast-feeding may be a risk factor for nutritional rickets. However, in countries where dairy product intake is minimal, prolonged breast-feeding may supply sufficient calcium to prevent rickets from developing. Whether the breast milk calcium concentrations of mothers of children who develop calcium-deficiency rickets differ from those of mothers whose children do not develop rickets has not been determined.

Dietary calcium intakes in developing countries are generally very low, because dairy product consumption is low. Calcium requirements are difficult to satisfy apart from dairy product intake. However, not all children with low calcium intake develop rickets. In a case-control study of 123 Nigerian children with rickets, there was no difference in calcium intake between children with rickets and age- and sex-matched control children [17]. Both groups had a very low mean daily calcium intake of about 220 mg. However, a South African study reported lower intakes of calcium in children with rickets than in control children [18]. Limitations of dietary recall techniques and disparity between the actual calcium content of foods and values in food composition tables make it difficult to detect small differences in calcium intake between groups [19].

Other nutritional and dietary factors may further limit available calcium. Dietary components that inhibit intestinal absorption of calcium include oxalate (present in spinach, sweet potatoes, and beans) and phytate (a phosphorus-rich component of grains, seeds, and nuts). The predominantly vegetarian diet found in many developing countries, high in oxalates and phytates, may compound the effect of restricted dairy product intake to exacerbate dietary calcium insufficiency. The age an infant is introduced to complementary foods that interact with breast milk calcium may also relate to the risk of rickets. In one Nigerian study, nutritional rickets was associated with late introduction of cereals (after age 7 months) [13], suggesting that the additional calcium provided by cereals, though minimal, may offset any inhibition of calcium absorption.

The effect of dietary protein on intestinal calcium absorption is unclear, but some data indicate that calcium absorption is reduced on a restricted protein intake. Furthermore, meat protein may protect against rickets, possibly by selectively increasing the oxidation of vitamin D to 25-hydroxyvitamin D [20]. However, compared with matched controls, Nigerian children with rickets did not have greater wasting [17] or lower serum albumin or prealbumin values [21] that would indicate greater protein malnutrition. Both high protein and high sodium intakes increase calcium excretion by the kidney, but there is no evidence of increased urinary calcium or sodium excretion (directly reflecting sodium intake) in children with calcium-deficiency rickets. Other nutrient factors that have been reported to affect calcium balance or bone mineralization include vitamins A and C, zinc, magnesium, phosphorus, and saturated fat. However, the contribution of any of these nutrients in calcium-deficiency rickets is undefined.

Wide individual variation exists in the amount of calcium absorbed from the diet. Given a diet uniformly low in calcium, children who more poorly absorb calcium should be predisposed to develop rickets. Genetic polymorphisms of the vitamin D receptor (VDR) have been related to calcium absorption, and it is likely that there are many genetic determinants of calcium absorption efficiency. However, in Nigerian children with rickets, we have been unable to detect a difference in calcium absorption compared with that of matched control children [Graff, unpubl. data]. Children with rickets absorbed 61% (SD 19%) of an orally administered stable isotope of calcium as compared with 63% (SD 13%) in control children. These values of fractional calcium absorption greatly exceed the 25–40% fractional absorption found in Western populations accustomed to greater dietary calcium intakes.

Several children from the same family frequently develop calcium-deficiency rickets (fig. 1). Fifteen percent of Nigerian children with rickets had a first-degree relative with a history of rickets [17]. This familial association could reflect either an underlying genetic risk or shared environmental factors. In a study of VDR alleles in Nigerian children, only polymorphism of the *Fok*I cleavage site was associated with calcium-deficiency rickets [22]. The cleavage site was more frequently absent (F allele) among children with rickets than in controls. Studies in American children have suggested that the VDR encoded by the F allele has greater functional activity than that encoded by the f allele. Children with the FF genotype have increased calcium absorption and greater bone density than those with either the Ff or ff genotypes. Why a better functioning VDR variant (F allele) is associated with calcium-deficiency rickets is unclear. Such children could be destined for greater bone size and density, but could also be more prone to develop rickets when deprived of calcium. This hypothesis remains to be tested.

Increased urinary calcium excretion (hypercalciuria) possibly due to PTH resistance could be postulated to lead to calcium-deficiency rickets. However, calcium excretion is universally extremely low in African children with nutritional rickets, and calcium wasting does not appear to contribute to the disease.

Impaired utilization of calcium at the growth plate has not been investigated in the pathogenesis of calcium-deficiency rickets. Theoretically, an environmental endocrine disrupter, a substance in the environment that perturbs the

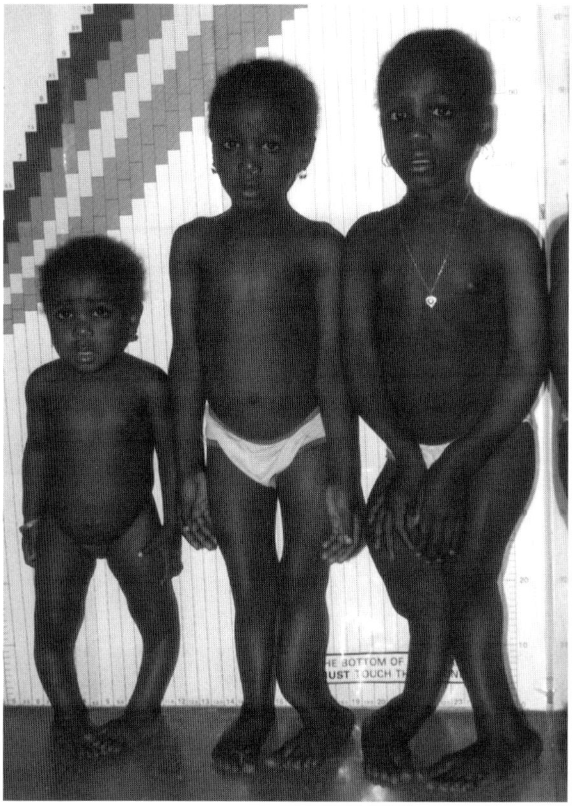

Fig. 1. Familial clustering of calcium-deficiency rickets. The three sisters all had calcium-deficiency rickets.

calcium-vitamin D axis, could impair adaptation to a low calcium diet. Dietary calcium deficiency increases the absorption of ingested lead, and toxic lead levels are found in many Nigerian children. However, elevated lead concentrations do not appear to be associated with calcium-deficiency rickets [unpubl. data]. Whether other environmental factors interfere with effective incorporation of calcium into bone requires further investigation. Aluminum, fluoride, strontium, and manganese have all been reported to impair bone mineralization.

Bone histology of children with calcium-deficiency rickets displays severe osteomalacia, characterized by increased osteoid volume, surface, and thickness, a reduced calcification front, and a prolonged mineralization lag time [23]. These findings indicate that the rate of synthesis of bone matrix exceeds the rate of bone mineralization. Treatment with calcium alone resulted in marked histologic improvement and successful bone mineralization.

That inadequate dietary calcium plays a central role in the pathogenesis of nutritional rickets in African children has been established by the response to calcium supplementation. In a randomized, controlled trial comparing treatment of nutritional rickets in Nigerian children with calcium, vitamin D, or both drugs combined, the groups that received calcium healed more rapidly than the group that received vitamin D alone [24]. After 6 months, 61% of the calcium alone group, 58% of the vitamin D and calcium group, and 19% of the vitamin D alone group demonstrated both radiologic and biochemical healing. Other studies have also demonstrated healing of nutritional rickets with calcium alone [1–3, 21].

It may be useful to avoid categorizing nutritional rickets as either purely due to calcium deficiency or to vitamin D deficiency, but rather consider these as two extremes of a continuum over which varying degrees of vitamin D and calcium insufficiency interact [20]. Both calcium- and vitamin D-deficiency rickets share a final common causal pathway of inadequate calcium for bone mineralization. Vitamin D requirements are probably greater in those with reduced availability of dietary calcium. When calcium intake is restricted, parathyroid hormone secretion increases 1,25-dihydroxyvitamin D concentrations. Elevation of 1,25-dihydroxyvitamin D increases the catabolism of 25-hydroxyvitamin D, resulting in a reduction in circulating 25-hydroxyvitamin D [25]. Likewise, calcium requirements would be greater in those with limited sunlight exposure and dietary vitamin D intake. Combined interaction of a low calcium intake with suboptimal vitamin D status may be a more common cause of nutritional rickets than either factor alone. Though not in the vitamin D-deficient range, 25-hydroxyvitamin D values are consistently lower in Nigerian children with rickets than in age-matched controls [3, 17]. A study in baboons demonstrated that addition of maize to the diet markedly exacerbated vitamin D deficiency, resulting in more rapid development of rickets [26]. Populations with predominantly cereal diets may thus be at greater risk of rickets due to combined calcium and vitamin D deficiency. Rickets could be initiated by vitamin D deficiency in early infancy and subsequently sustained by dietary calcium deficiency. If such were the case, subclinical vitamin D deficiency in young infants should be common in populations with a high prevalence of nutritional rickets. However, a community survey of 218 Nigerian children under 3 years of age failed to identify any with 25-hydroxyvitamin D values less than 25 nmol/l [14].

Diagnosis

Clinical Features

Many of the clinical features of calcium-deficiency rickets are identical to those found in vitamin D-deficiency rickets (fig. 2). Possibly because calcium

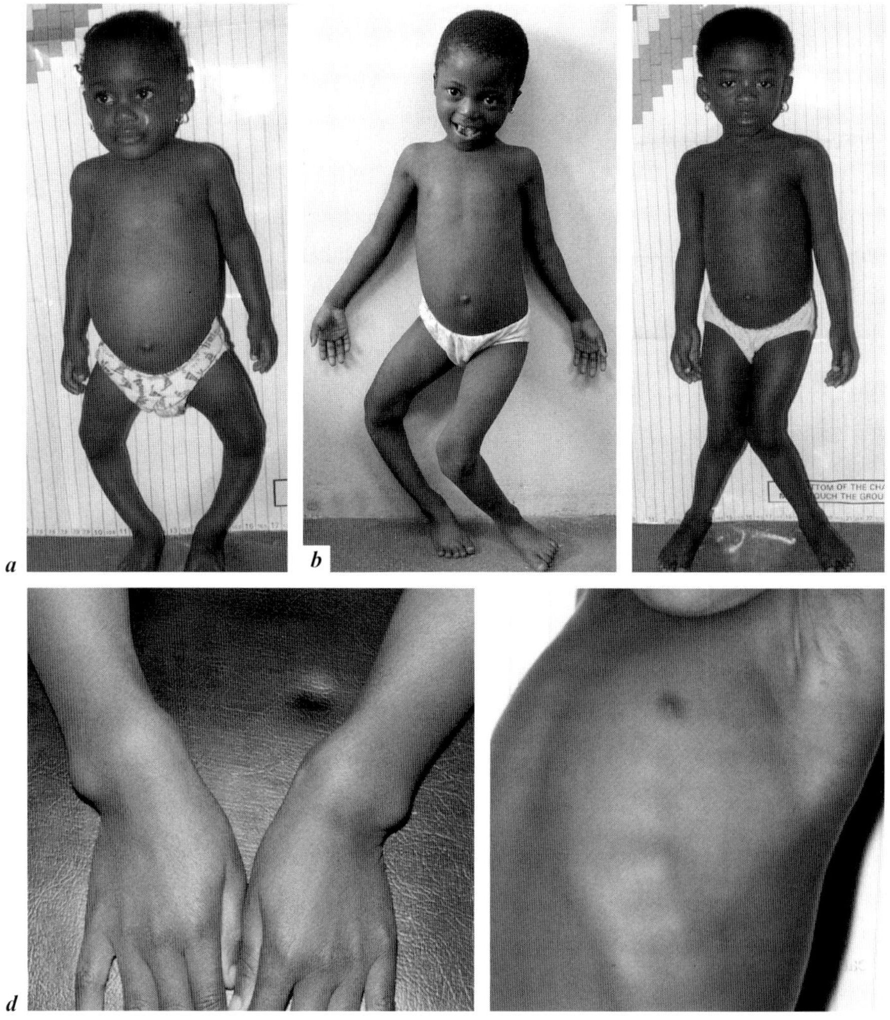

Fig. 2. Clinical signs of calcium-deficiency rickets. ***a*** Genu varum. ***b*** Windswept deformity. ***c*** Genu valgum. ***d*** Wrist enlargement. ***e*** Rib beading.

deficiency tends to occur in older children, features that are more frequent in young infants with vitamin D deficiency (e.g. craniotabes, hypotonia, tetany) are typically absent in children with calcium-deficiency rickets. Rickets due to vitamin D deficiency typically manifests within the first year of life, whereas most children with calcium deficiency generally present after the age of 18 months. In Nigeria, calcium-deficiency rickets has peak prevalence between

Table 1. Clinical features and their utility in predicting radiologically active rickets in Nigerian children over age 18 months [9] with leg deformities or inability to walk (% values)

Characteristic	Sensitivity[1]	Specificity[2]	PPV[3]
Symptoms			
Weakness	65	52	45
Leg pain during walking	60	55	42
Excessive falling	58	55	41
Leg pain at rest	22	87	50
Unable to walk	11	98	75
Previous fracture	9	92	43
Signs			
Enlarged costochondral junctions (beading)	77	64	56
Enlarged wrists	75	81	71
Genu varum (bow leg deformity)	48	47	35
Enlarged ankles	38	83	57
Genu valgum (knock knee deformity)	32	68	38
Rib cage deformities	15	96	67
Windswept deformity of legs	14	88	41
Open anterior fontanel	12	94	55
Dental enamel defects	11	90	39
Harrison's sulcus	7	96	50

[1]Sensitivity is the proportion of children with active rickets who have the clinical feature.

[2]Specificity is the proportion of children without active rickets who do not have the clinical feature.

[3]Positive predictive value is the proportion of children with the clinical feature who have active rickets.

2 and 4 years of age, and it may even present or persist into adolescence. A familial predisposition is also noted.

The symptoms and signs of calcium-deficiency rickets and their diagnostic utility are shown in table 1. Not all children with clinical signs of rickets have active disease radiologically or biochemically. Muscle weakness often manifests as fatigue after walking a short distance or as difficulty in rising from a squatting position. Leg pain and delay in walking are frequently reported. Children with calcium-deficiency rickets most frequently present for medical attention because of leg deformities. Because resolution of bony deformity after treatment is very gradual, it is important to document the degree of deformity at presentation. The intermalleolar distance in genu valgum or the intercondylar distance in genu varum should be measured in the supine position, because ligamentous laxity may exaggerate these measures while a child is standing. A goniometer can be used to measure the femoral-tibial angle.

The type of leg deformity is related to the age of onset of rickets. Children with an onset of rickets younger than age 2 years, when there is normally a varus femoral-tibial angle, tend to develop bow leg deformity. Children with an onset of rickets after the age of 2 years tend to develop knock-knee deformity, exaggerating the normal valgus femoral-tibial angle. Bow leg deformity is less specific for active rickets than knock-knee or windswept deformity, possibly because of the frequent occurrence of physiologic bow leg. Children may have severe residual leg deformities from rickets without radiologically active rickets at the growth plates. Because of leg deformities and impaired bone growth, height for age less than two standard deviations below the mean (z-score <-2) is associated with active rickets.

Wrist enlargement and costochondral enlargement (also called rib beading or rachitic rosary) are the most sensitive clinical signs in predicting radiologically active rickets in children with leg deformities. The presence of either wrist or costochondral enlargement had a sensitivity of about 90% in detecting active rickets in children with leg deformities. Defining wrist and costochondral enlargement objectively is difficult, and the ability of clinical signs to predict active rickets may vary among different examiners. Rib cage deformities and Harrison's sulcus (indentation of the lower rib cage by tension from the diaphragm) were specific for rickets, but lacked sensitivity. The clinical features that were independently predictive of radiologically active rickets were an age less than 5 years, height for age z-score <-2, leg pain with walking, wrist enlargement, and costochondral enlargement. The presence of any 3 of these predicted active rickets with a sensitivity of 87% and specificity of 76%. Reliance on clinical findings for the diagnosis of active rickets may be essential in developing countries or in nutritional surveys where access to radiographic facilities are limited.

Biochemical Features

Apart from the values of vitamin D metabolites, the biochemical features of calcium-deficiency rickets are quite similar to those of vitamin D-deficiency rickets (table 2). Hypocalcemia is generally, but not invariably, a feature of calcium-deficiency rickets. About 40–50% of the calcium in blood exists in ionized form at normal albumin concentrations and pH. PTH and vitamin D regulate only the ionized form. Most of the non-ionized serum calcium is bound to blood proteins. When serum albumin is reduced, the total serum calcium is

Table 2. Comparison of biochemical features of calcium-deficiency with vitamin D-deficiency rickets

Biochemical test	Calcium-deficiency rickets	Vitamin D-deficiency rickets
Calcium	↓ or N	↓ or N
Phosphorus	↓ or N	↓
Alkaline phosphatase	↑	↑
PTH	N or ↑	↑
25-Hydroxyvitamin D	N or ↓	↓↓
1,25-Dihydroxyvitamin D	↑↑	↓ or N

N = Normal; ↑ = increased; ↑↑ = markedly increased; ↓ = decreased; ↓↓ = markedly decreased.

reduced without affecting the concentration of ionized calcium (normal values 1.12–1.23 mmol/l). Because malnutrition is frequent in populations with calcium deficiency, serum calcium concentrations should be corrected for the albumin concentration to determine if hypocalcemia is metabolically important. The following formula may be used to standardize serum calcium to an albumin value of 4 g/l:

$$\text{Corrected calcium (mmol/l)} = \text{Total calcium} + 0.03\ [40 - \text{albumin (g/l)}]$$

Hypophosphatemia is also a usual feature, but a markedly depressed serum phosphorus value may suggest severe renal phosphate wasting as in X-linked hypophosphatemic rickets. The most constant biochemical feature is raised serum alkaline phosphatase. Normal alkaline phosphatase values are greater in children than in adults, but values more than 3 times the upper limit of adult norms are characteristic of calcium-deficiency rickets. The magnitude of elevation of alkaline phosphatase values parallels the severity of bone disease as assessed radiologically [27]. Alkaline phosphatase produced by osteoblasts is believed to promote hydroxyapatite crystal formation in the bone. If liver disease is suspected, bone specific alkaline phosphatase may be used to characterize the specific contribution from bone. Urinary calcium excretion in calcium-deficiency rickets is extremely low ($<$40 mg/g creatinine or $<$10 mg/24 h).

Measurement of vitamin D metabolites assists to differentiate calcium-deficiency from vitamin D-deficiency rickets. Serum concentrations of 25-hydroxyvitamin D measure the adequacy of vitamin D status. Vitamin D produced in the skin is converted to 25-hydroxyvitamin D within a few hours, and 25-hydroxyvitamin D has a half-life of about 3 weeks. There have been varying attempts to define the lower limit of normal 25-hydroxyvitamin D concentrations. The typical laboratory lower limit is two standard deviations below the population mean. However, others advocate using a value of 25-hydroxyvitamin D (~50 nmol/l) above which PTH no longer continues to decline. Others use values of 25-hydroxyvitamin D (25–40 nmol/l), above which 1,25-dihydroxyvitamin D fails to rise in response to physiologic doses of vitamin D. However, in the case of vitamin D deficiency severe enough to cause rickets, concentrations of 25-hydroxyvitamin D are generally below 12 nmol/l. The concentration of 25-hydroxyvitamin D in calcium-deficiency rickets is usually well above this value, with mean values typically reported in the range of 32–50 nmol/l. However, compared with control children 25-hydroxyvitamin D values are lower in children with calcium-deficiency rickets. These values rise with calcium supplementation alone, lending support to the contention that calcium deficiency reduces serum 25-hydroxyvitamin D by increasing its catabolism [25].

In contrast to the low or normal values usually found in vitamin D-deficiency rickets, concentrations of 1,25-dihydroxyvitamin D are markedly elevated in calcium deficiency. This is consistent with an attempt to maximize calcium absorption from the diet. As healing of rickets occurs with calcium supplementation, the elevated 1,25-dihydroxyvitamin D values decline. Some evidence indicates that 1,25-dihydroxyvitamin D concentrations are greater and 25-hydroxyvitamin D values are lower in black than in white races [28]. Serum values of 1,25-dihydroxyvitamin D increase markedly in children with vitamin D-deficiency rickets who receive vitamin D, causing possible confusion with the biochemical features of calcium-deficiency rickets.

Given that hypocalcemia typically accompanies calcium-deficiency rickets, PTH should be markedly elevated. However, there seems to be wide variability of PTH concentrations in children with calcium-deficiency rickets. In some cases PTH concentrations are low normal and increase in response to calcium supplementation, suggesting loss of parathyroid responsiveness in chronic calcium-deficiency rickets [21]. PTH increases the renal production of 1,25-dihydroxyvitamin D, and yet 1,25-dihydroxyvitamin D values bear no relationship to PTH concentrations in children with calcium-deficiency rickets. Just how much the variability of PTH concentrations in reported studies may be due to prolonged storage prior to assay is unclear. Further research of the PTH response during treatment of calcium-deficiency rickets and the regulation of 1,25-dihydroxyvitamin D by PTH in calcium-deficiency rickets is needed.

Collagen metabolites have also been examined in calcium-deficiency rickets. Interpretation of serum values of these metabolites must take into account the change in the range of normal values with age. Urinary deoxypyridinoline excretion, which reflects bone resorption, is increased in calcium-deficiency rickets.

Deoxypyridinoline excretion correlates closely with serum alkaline phosphatase and declines with calcium supplementation. Another marker of bone resorption, the C-terminal telopeptide of type I collagen, is similarly increased. Markers of bone formation, including the C-terminal propeptide cleaved from type I procollagen and the N-terminal propeptides of collagen types I and III, are also increased in children with calcium-deficiency rickets. However, osteocalcin, another marker of bone formation, does not appear to be consistently increased, despite elevated 1,25-dihydroxyvitamin D values.

As in vitamin D-deficiency rickets, generalized aminoaciduria also occurs in calcium-deficiency rickets [29]. Serum amino acids are also increased in calcium deficiency. Amino acids derived from collagen (hydroxyproline, hydroxylysine) and muscle (3-methylhistidine) are significantly increased in the serum and decline to normal values with calcium supplementation.

Radiographic Assessment

Rickets is principally a radiographic diagnosis. Both vitamin D- and calcium-deficiency rickets share characteristic cupping and fraying of the metaphyses and longitudinal widening of the growth plates. Radiographs of the wrists and knees can be scored to assess the severity of rickets and monitor the response to treatment [27], particularly in clinical trials (fig. 3). After 12 months of age, appendicular growth is greater than axial growth, thus making the long bones of the arms and legs most likely to show the radiographic changes of rickets. Radiographs are essential to distinguish rickets from other causes of leg deformities, particularly Blount's disease, epiphyseal and metaphyseal dysplasias, and physiologic varus and valgus deformities. The femoral-tibial angle can be measured on radiographs to follow changes with treatment.

Bone densitometry is not generally indicated in the clinical management of patients with rickets. Volumetric bone density changes very little during growth, but because bone density is typically measured by X-ray attenuation within the projected bone area, areal bone density measurements increase during growth. Calcium supplementation dramatically increases areal bone density of children with rickets. How much of this increase is of permanent benefit is not clear. An increase in bone density can result simply from the bone-remodeling transient, through inhibition of activation of new remodeling units by calcium [30]. Studies of short-term (up to 18 months) calcium supplementation in healthy children indicate that the incremental increase in bone density is not maintained after the withdrawal of calcium supplementation [31]. Some decline in bone density is observed when calcium treatment is stopped in calcium-deficiency rickets after radiographic healing is complete, but radiographs rarely show any recurrence of rachitic changes [unpubl. data].

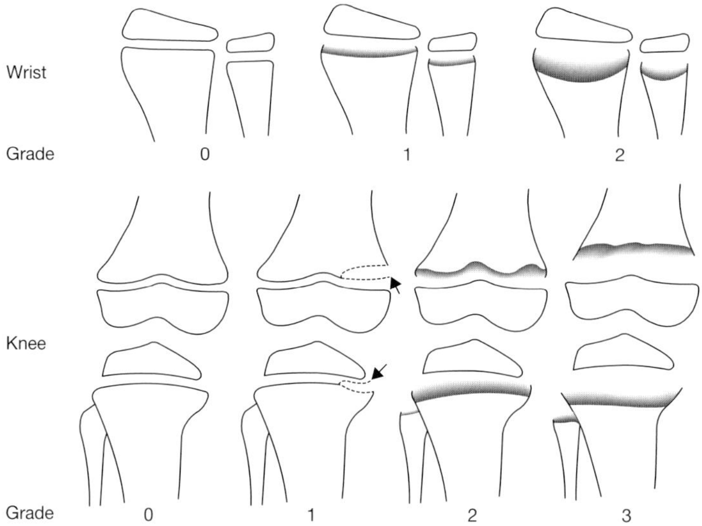

Wrist* Radius and ulna scored separately

Grade	Radiographic features
1	Widened growth plate, irregularity or fraying of metaphyseal margin, but without concave cupping
2	Metaphyseal concavity with fraying of margin

2 bones × 2 grade points = 4 points possible

Knee* Femur and tibia scored separately
Multiply the grade in part A by the multiplier in part B for each bone, then add femur and tibia scores together

A Grade	Degree of lucency and widening of zone of provisional calcification
1	Partial lucency, smooth margin of metaphysis visible
2	Partial lucency, smooth margin of metaphysis not visible
3	Complete lucency, epiphysis appears widely separated from distal metaphysis

B Multiplier	Portion of growth plate affected
0.5	≤ Half of the growth plate affected (as shown for grade 1 in figure)
1	> Half of the growth plate affected

2 bones × 1 multiplier point × 3 grade points = 6 points possible

Total: 10 points possible

*Score the worst knee and the worst wrist.

Fig. 3. Ten-point radiographic scoring method of the severity of rickets [27].

Treatment

Calcium is the most essential component of treatment for calcium-deficiency rickets, and it has a clear advantage over vitamin D alone [24]. The dosage of calcium required for healing of rickets has not been precisely defined. Most studies demonstrate healing with daily dosages of 1,000 mg elemental

Table 3. Calcium content of various oral calcium salts

Calcium salt	Calcium content mg/1,000 mg salt
Calcium carbonate	400
Calcium citrate	211
Calcium glubionate	65
Calcium gluconate	90
Calcium lactate	130
Calcium phosphate dibasic	230
Calcium phosphate tribasic	400

calcium given for 6 months. Whether lower doses are sufficient to heal an equal proportion of children with calcium-deficiency rickets, or whether higher doses would result in more rapid healing remains to be tested. Giving calcium supplements at bedtime or with food and dividing the dose into 2–3 times daily may further improve utilization and absorption of ingested calcium.

In calculating the calcium dose, a common error is to base the dose on the calcium salt rather than on the elemental calcium content (table 3). For instance, calcium lactate, commonly available in African countries, contains only 39 mg of calcium in a 300-mg tablet. Instead of providing 900 mg of calcium a day, three tablets of calcium lactate 300 mg provide only 117 mg of elemental calcium. Over 20 tablets of calcium lactate are required to provide a treatment dose of 1,000 mg of elemental calcium. The solubility differences of various calcium salts are probably not clinically important, as all forms appear to be adequately absorbed.

Rather than provide supplements, increasing the dietary intake of calcium-containing foods may be a better means of establishing improved dietary habits. Dairy products are the richest sources of food calcium. A cup of milk (~250 ml) contains nearly 300 mg of elemental calcium, so 3 cups a day should prove sufficient to heal calcium-deficiency rickets. However, many families in developing countries cannot afford this quantity of milk over the course of 6 months of treatment, let alone throughout childhood. Therefore, less expensive, indigenous forms of calcium are essential. Small dried fish are a component of the diet in many countries where calcium-deficiency rickets occurs, and if ground into fishmeal, the bones can be a good source of calcium [32]. Limestone (predominantly calcium carbonate) is an inexpensive source of calcium and is abundant in almost all parts of the globe. Limestone has been used in food processing, and in powdered form it can easily be mixed with a child's food. The baobab leaf, commonly used in some African diets, is also rich in calcium. Supplementation of the diet with fishmeal or limestone leads to

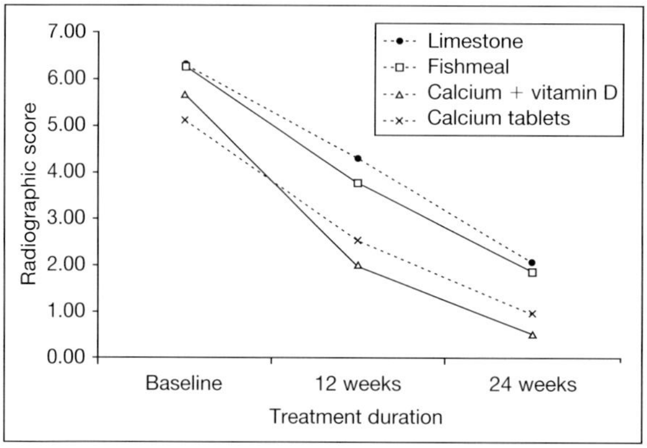

Fig. 4. Comparison of the radiographic response to various calcium supplements in Nigerian children with calcium-deficiency rickets.

healing of calcium-deficiency rickets at a rate similar to supplementation with calcium tablets (fig. 4) [unpubl. data].

Vitamin D does not clearly provide added benefit to calcium alone in the treatment of calcium-deficiency rickets. On a low calcium diet, vitamin D-dependent mechanisms of absorption are already nearly saturated, and the major benefit of additional calcium appears to result from calcium absorption through a vitamin D-independent mechanism (i.e. passive transfer across electrochemical gradients) [33]. However, inadequate calcium intake does increase the requirement for vitamin D. Regular sunlight exposure for as little as 15 min daily in tropical latitudes should provide for adequate vitamin D synthesis in the skin. However, if consistent sunlight exposure cannot be ensured, vitamin D supplementation may be prudent.

Symptomatic response to treatment occurs fairly rapidly. Within the first month, leg pain reduces, and children become stronger and more active. Radiologic healing of the growth plate usually requires 3–6 months of calcium supplementation, but some children may require additional calcium for complete healing. Radiographs every 3 months are sufficient to document healing. Monitoring serum calcium, phosphorus, and alkaline phosphatase assists to objectively confirm response to treatment, particularly within the first month.

Clinical signs of rickets require a longer time to resolve than do radiologic or biochemical abnormalities. Even after the growth plates have healed radiologically, bony deformities require many more months, even years, to remodel. The child's growth should be monitored. The intermalleolar or intercondylar distance and the femoral-tibial angle should be measured at 6-monthly intervals to verify resolution of leg deformities.

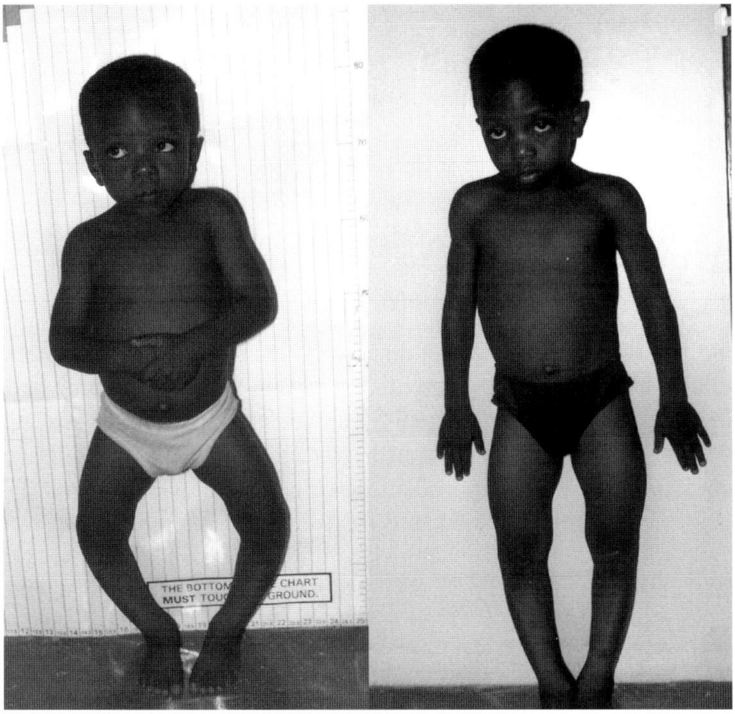

Fig. 5. Child with calcium-deficiency rickets before treatment and 2 years following treatment with 6 months of calcium.

Orthopedic treatment of deformities associated with calcium-deficiency rickets is usually unnecessary in children with mild deformities in early childhood. Serial wedging of plaster casts has been advocated to bring about more rapid correction of leg deformities, but there is no good evidence of benefit. Even without such intervention, satisfactory remodeling occurs over 2–4 years (fig. 5). Surgical management, including femoral and tibial osteotomies or unilateral stapling of the growth plate, should be reserved for older children with marked deformities. Surgical correction should only be undertaken after demonstrated radiographic healing of the growth plates, in order to avoid recurrent deformity after the procedure.

Prevention

Provision of adequate dietary calcium should prevent calcium-deficiency rickets. Many children in developing countries have average daily calcium intakes

Age	Adequate intake mg/day
0–6 months	210
7–12 months	270
1–3 years	500
4–8 years	800
9–18 years	1,300

Table 4. Dietary reference intake of calcium in children [34]

of only 200 mg, yet the majority of them do not develop rickets, and no adverse effect on adult bone mineral content has been clearly documented. Recommended daily allowances of calcium for a population refer to intakes sufficient to meet the nutrient requirement of nearly all individuals. In countries where calcium-deficiency rickets is prevalent, determination of the recommended daily allowance of calcium should be based on data establishing the amount of calcium that prevents calcium-deficiency rickets in those at risk. However, data on prevention of calcium-deficiency rickets in susceptible populations is lacking.

Recently, a standing committee of the Institute of Medicine (US) formulated adequate intake values for calcium (table 4) [34]. Adequate intakes were based on calcium balance studies and formulated to provide desirable calcium retention in healthy North Americans. They were neither intended for international use nor designed with calcium-deficiency rickets in mind. Adequate intake was used rather than recommended daily allowance, because the data considered by the committee were inadequate to establish a recommended daily allowance. Adequate intakes were judged to be intakes sufficient to reduce the risk of osteoporosis and fractures, but the intake required to avoid these outcomes in 98% of the population was not known with sufficient certainty to establish a recommended daily allowance. Osteoporosis is distinctly uncommon in African populations, so the dietary reference intake for calcium may not apply to African children.

Lacking other data to the contrary, the adequate intake values for North American children are probably sufficient to prevent calcium-deficiency rickets. Given the rapid healing of calcium-deficiency rickets with 1,000 mg of daily calcium supplementation, it is not unreasonable to conclude that the adequate intake values of 500–800 mg of calcium would be sufficient to prevent calcium-deficiency rickets in children from 1 to 8 years of age. However, intakes of this magnitude are very unusual in developing countries, and calcium-deficiency rickets has not been seen where daily calcium intakes exceed 400 mg. It is possible that deprivation of calcium in early life may program the body for better retention and utilization of calcium, thus reducing the calcium requirement to maintain a healthy adult skeleton. This could explain the lower risk of osteoporosis in African populations, but this hypothesis remains to be tested. The consequence of calcium-deficiency rickets in childhood for the adult skeleton has also not been examined.

The relative intake of other nutritional factors can influence the calcium requirement. Despite the same intake of calcium, nutrient interactions may result in differing bioavailability of calcium in individuals on different diets. Furthermore, the amount of calcium required to prevent calcium-deficiency rickets depends on the adequacy of vitamin D in the diet or from sunlight. Mothers should be encouraged to expose their infants and children to sunlight for an average of 15–30 min a day. Pregnant and breast-feeding mothers should also regularly expose themselves to sunshine to ensure optimal vitamin D status in young infants. In areas where sunlight is not available year-round, supplementation of infants with single large doses of vitamin D (stosstherapy) at times of immunization may be indicated.

Increasing the calcium intake of children can be attained in one of three ways: through dietary supplements, through food fortification, or through change of dietary habits. In developing countries, where most calcium-deficiency rickets occurs, dietary supplementation would be prohibitively expensive and pose difficulties in distribution and compliance. Fortification of staple foods, such as maize or wheat flour, with calcium or limestone might be reasonable in regions with a high prevalence of calcium deficiency. However, most staple foods in developing countries are locally produced, making fortification difficult to implement. The most reasonable option to effect an increased calcium intake for children in most developing countries is to promote dietary habits that include calcium-rich foods.

Milk and other dairy products are not only a rich source of calcium, but provide other important nutrients for children in developing countries who may be prone to other nutrient deficiencies. Measures to make milk products more affordable for those in developing countries can make this option accessible to a greater number of people. Milk can be added to the diet beginning at one year of age, while continuing to promote breast-feeding. Lactose intolerance is probably not an important deterrent to milk intake for African and Asian children, as it is infrequent in the pediatric age group. Other potentially less expensive sources of calcium for prevention of rickets in developing countries could include fishmeal, baobab leaf, or limestone. Indigenous food items that are rich in calcium should be identified within the diets of individual ethnic groups.

Public enlightenment campaigns can educate populations about calcium-rich foods, but changing entrenched dietary habits is not easy. However, as awareness that calcium-deficiency rickets can be treated, and most likely prevented, with calcium-rich foods, adoption of a healthy diet should gain greater acceptance. The message that calcium is important for bone health should be conveyed in all populations, not only for prevention of osteoporosis, but also for prevention of calcium-deficiency rickets.

Acknowledgments

I am grateful to John M. Pettifor and Philip R. Fischer for their helpful comments on this chapter.

References

1 Pettifor JM, Ross P, Wang J, Moodley G, Couper-Smith J: Rickets in children of rural origin in South Africa: Is low dietary calcium a factor? J Pediatr 1978;92:320–324.
2 Okonofua F, Gill DS, Alabi ZO, Thomas M, Bell JL, Dandona P: Rickets in Nigerian children: A consequence of calcium malnutrition. Metabolism 1991;40:209–213.
3 Oginni LM, Worsfold M, Oyelami OA, Sharp CA, Powell DE, Davie MWJ: Etiology of rickets in Nigerian children. J Pediatr 1996;128:692–694.
4 Fischer PR, Rahman A, Cimma JP, Kyaw-Myint TO, Kabir ARML, Talukder K, et al: Nutritional rickets without vitamin D deficiency in Bangladesh. J Trop Pediatr 1999;45:291–293.
5 Maltz HE, Fish MB, Holliday MA: Calcium deficiency rickets and the renal response to calcium infusion. Pediatrics 1970;46:865–870.
6 Kooh SW, Fraser D, Reilly BJ, Hamilton JR, Gall DG, Bell L: Rickets due to calcium deficiency. N Engl J Med 1977;297:1264–1266.
7 Legius E, Proesmans W, Eggermont E, Vandamme-Lonbaerts R, Bouillon R, Smet M: Rickets due to dietary calcium deficiency. Eur J Pediatr 1989;148:784–785.
8 Bishop N: The global burden of rickets; in Combs GF Jr (ed): Improving Health and Economic Development: Approaches to Preventing Diet-Related Rickets – An International Symposium. Ithaca, Cornell University, 2001, pp 18–22.
9 Thacher TD, Fischer PR, Pettifor JM: The utility of clinical features to identify active rickets. Ann Trop Paediatr 2002;22:229–237.
10 Muhe L, Lulseged S, Mason KE, Simoes EAF: Case-control study of the role of nutritional rickets in the risk of developing pneumonia in Ethiopian children. Lancet 1997;349:1801–1804.
11 Bhattacharyya AK: Nutritional rickets in the tropics; in Simopoulos AP (ed): Nutritional Triggers for Health and in Disease. World Rev Nutr Diet. Basel, Karger, 1992, vol 67, pp 140–197.
12 Kabir LA, Mannan MA: Rickets in Chakaria, Bangladesh; in Combs GF Jr (ed): Improving Health and Economic Development: Approaches to Preventing Diet-Related Rickets – An International Symposium. Ithaca, Cornell University, 2001, pp 34–38.
13 Akpede GO, Omotara BA, Ambe JP: Rickets and deprivation: A Nigerian Study. J R Soc Hlth 1999;119:216–222.
14 Pfitzner MA, Thacher TD, Pettifor JM, Zoakah AI, Lawson JO, Isichei CO, Fischer PR: Absence of vitamin D deficiency in young Nigerian children. J Pediatr 1998;133:740–744.
15 Specker BL, Valanis B, Hertzberg V, Edwards N, Tsang RC: Sunshine exposure and serum 25-hydroxyvitamin D concentrations in exclusively breast-fed infants. J Pediatr 1985;107:372–376.
16 Prentice A, Barclay DV: Breast-milk calcium and phosphorus concentrations of mothers in rural Zaire. Eur J Clin Nutr 1991;45:611–617.
17 Thacher TD, Fischer PR, Pettifor JM, Lawson JO, Isichei CO, Chan GM: Case-control study of factors associated with nutritional rickets in Nigerian children. J Pediatr 2000;137:367–373.
18 Eyberg C, Pettifor JM, Moodley G: Dietary calcium intake in rural black South African children: The relationship between calcium intake and calcium nutritional status. Hum Nutr Clin Nutr 1986;40C:69–74.

19 Heaney RP: Nutrient effects: Discrepancy between data from controlled trials and observational studies. Bone 1997;21:469–471.
20 Dunnigan MG, Henderson JB: An epidemiological model of privational rickets and osteomalacia. Proc Nutr Soc 1997;56:939–956.
21 Thacher TD, Glew RH, Isichei CO, Lawson JO, Scariano JK, Hollis BW, VanderJagt DJ: Rickets in Nigerian children: Response to calcium supplementation. J Trop Pediatr 1999;45:202–207. [Erratum: J Trop Pediatr 2000;46:62.]
22 Fischer PR, Thacher TD, Pettifor JM, Jorde LB, Eccleshall R, Feldman D: A vitamin D receptor polymorphism relates to calcium deficiency rickets in Nigerian children. J Bone Miner Res 2000;15:2206–2210.
23 Marie PJ, Pettifor JM, Ross FP, Glorieux FH: Histological osteomalacia due to dietary calcium deficiency in children. N Engl J Med 1982;307:584–588.
24 Thacher TD, Fischer PR, Pettifor JM, et al: A comparison of calcium, vitamin D, or both for nutritional rickets in Nigerian children. N Engl J Med 1999;341:563–568.
25 Clements MR, Johnson L, Fraser DR: A new mechanism for induced vitamin D deficiency in calcium deprivation. Nature 1987;325:62–65.
26 Sly MR, van der Walt WH, Du Bruyn DB, Pettifor JM, Marie PJ: Exacerbation of rickets and osteomalacia by maize: A study of bone histomorphometry and composition in young baboons. Calcif Tissue Int 1984;36:370–379.
27 Thacher TD, Fischer PR, Pettifor JM, Lawson JO, Manaster BJ, Reading JC: Radiographic scoring method for the assessment of the severity of rickets. J Trop Pediatr 2000;46:132–139.
28 Bell NH, Greene A, Epstein S, Oexmann MJ, Shaw S, Shary J: Evidence for alteration of the vitamin D-endocrine system in blacks. J Clin Invest 1985;76:470–473.
29 VanderJagt DJ, Peery B, Thacher TD, Pastuszyn A, Glew RH: Aminoaciduria in calcium deficiency rickets in northern Nigeria. J Trop Pediatr 1999;45:258–264.
30 Heaney RP: The bone-remodeling transient: implications for interpretation of clinical studies of bone mass change. J Bone Miner Res 1994;9:1515–1523.
31 Lee WT, Leung SS, Leung DM, Cheng JC: A follow-up study on the effects of calcium-supplement withdrawal and puberty on bone acquisition of children. Am J Clin Nutr 1996;64:71–77.
32 Larsen T, Thilsted SH, Kongsbak K, Hansen M: Whole small fish as a rich calcium source. Br J Nutr 2000;83:191–196.
33 Sheikh MS, Ramirez A, Emmett M, Santa Ana C, Schiller LR, Fordtran JS: Role of vitamin D-dependent and vitamin D-independent mechanisms in absorption of food calcium. J Clin Invest 1988;81:126–132.
34 Standing Committee on the Scientific Evaluation of Dietary Reference Intakes, Food and Nutrition Board, Institute of Medicine: Dietary Reference Intakes for Calcium, Phosphorus, Magnesium, Vitamin D, and Fluoride. Washington, National Academy Press, 1999.

Tom D. Thacher, MD
Department of Family Medicine, Jos University Teaching Hospital
PMB 2076, Jos (Nigeria)
Tel. +1 234 73 452 355, E-Mail tom@thachers.org

Hochberg Z (ed): Vitamin D and Rickets.
Endocr Dev. Basel, Karger, 2003, vol 6, pp 126–155

Hypophosphatemic Rickets

Marc K. Drezner

William F. Middleton Memorial Veterans Administration Hospital and Department of Medicine, University of Wisconsin, Madison, Wisc., USA

Contents

Osteomalacia and rickets are disorders of calcification characterized by defects of bone and cartilage mineralization, respectively. In osteomalacia, there is a failure to normally mineralize the newly formed organic matrix (osteoid) of bone. In rickets, there is defective cartilage growth plate calcification, as well as delayed maturation of the cellular sequence and disorganization of the cartilage cell arrangement, resulting in thickening of the epiphyeal plates. Although each of these disorders is phenotypically similar, the pathogenesis of the mineralization defect, the biochemical alterations and the therapeutic approaches differ in these conditions.

Hypophosphatemia is the characteristic biochemical abnormality in many of these disorders. Such phosphopenic diseases usually develop from an abnormality of transepithelial phosphate transport in the nephron, resulting in phosphate wasting. Often the underlying abnormality is due to a genetic defect, which directly or indirectly influences renal phosphate handling. As a rule, patients with these disorders maintain a normal serum calcium concentration and parathyroid hormone level, as well as normal bone turnover.

The remainder of this chapter concentrates on summarizing information regarding the pathophysiology of the hypophosphatemic rachitic and osteomalacic disorders, which affect children throughout the world today, as well as a systematic approach to the diagnosis and management of these diseases. The focus will include those clinical states that are primary disorders of phosphate homeostasis such as: X-linked hypophosphatemic rickets/osteomalacia (XLH), tumor-induced osteomalacia (TIO), autosomal-dominant hypophosphatemic rickets, X-linked recessive hypophosphatemic rickets, and hereditary hypophosphatemic rickets with hypercalciuria (HHRH).

Histopathology

Calcification of bone is a complex process in which a calcium-phosphate mineral phase is deposited in a highly ordered fashion within the organic matrix [1]. Abnormal mineralization in the hypophosphatemic disorders is due most likely to phosphopenia at calcification sites and, in some cases, paracrine inhibitory factors, resulting in accumulation of unmineralized osteoid, a sine qua non for the diagnosis of osteomalacia. However, establishing the diagnosis of phosphopenic osteomalacia histopathologically requires demonstration that the abundant osteoid results from abnormal mineralization, and not increased osteoid production [2, 3]. Thus, histopathological detection of an increase in the bone-forming surface covered by incompletely mineralized osteoid, an increase in osteoid volume and thickness and a decrease in the mineralization front (the percentage of osteoid-covered bone-forming surface undergoing calcification) or the mineral apposition rate is requisite (fig. 1).

Inadequate cartilage mineralization in hypophosphatemic rickets is confined to the maturation zone of cartilage, wherein the height of the cell columns is increased, the cells are closely packed and irregularly aligned, and calcification in the interstitial regions of this hypertrophic zone is defective. These changes result in increased thickness of the epiphyseal plates, accompanied by an increase in transverse diameter that often extends beyond the ends of the bone and causes cupping or flaring.

Radiographic Abnormalities

Although reduced bone density is the most common radiographic abnormality associated with phosphopenic osteomalacia [4], coarsening of the trabeculae and Looser's zone or pseudofractures in long bones occurs infrequently as does a trefoil (or triangular) pelvis and/or concave (or 'codfish') vertebrae in advanced disease. The radiographic defects of the trabeculae are due to inadequate mineralization of osteoid and loss of secondary trabeculae. Looser's zones most often occur symmetrically and are generally present at the medial aspect of the femurs, in the metatarsals or in the pelvis. They manifest as ribbon-like zones of rarefaction, a few millimeters to several centimeters in length, oriented perpendicular to the bone surface.

The rachitic abnormalities in children with phosphopenic disease produce a variety of pathopneumonic radiographic findings in the skeleton, some of which may persist into adulthood. Most commonly, the growth plates of long bones are cupped and display increased thickness and an irregular hazy appearance at the diaphyseal line, secondary to irregular invasion of recently calcified cartilage by bone tissue (fig. 2, 3). Since these abnormalities occur at sites of rapid growth, widening of the forearm at the wrist and thickening of the costochondral junctions frequently occur. The costochondral abnormality, rachitic rosary, often remains evident in adults. Indentation of the lower ribs, at the sites of diaphragmatic attachment, an abnormality known as Harrison's groove, may also develop. Rapid growth of the long bones also results in bowing of the lower extremities (fig. 4) and that of the skull (in neonates) in parietal flattening, frontal bossing and widened sutures.

Laboratory Abnormalities

Abnormal transepithelial phosphate transport in the nephron, resulting in renal phosphate wasting, underlies the majority of the hypophosphatemic rachitic disorders. In general, patients with these disorders maintain a normal serum calcium concentration, while the serum phosphorus is characteristically low. In contrast, the serum 25(OH)D and parathyroid hormone levels are normal, but the serum $1,25(OH)_2D$ level is usually normal or mildly decreased, in spite of the prevailing hypophosphatemia, which should increase the circulating concentration of this active vitamin D metabolite. However, an elevated serum 1,25$(OH)_2$D concentration was recently reported in two rare genetic phosphopenic disorders, Hereditary hypophosphatemic rickets with hypercalciuria and Fanconi syndrome, type 2. While the elevated calcitriol level underlies enhanced gastrointestinal absorption of calcium and hypercalciuria in these diseases, the impact of abnormal vitamin D metabolism on the phenotypic manifestations of the more common phosphopenic disorders is less certain.

A marker of the bone disease in all forms of hypophosphatemic rickets is increased plasma alkaline phosphatase activity. Physicians often overlook this abnormality in children, since normal levels are high, particularly during growth spurts. Surprisingly, however, in some affected patients normal enzyme activity is manifest. Moreover, in adults, the alkaline phosphatase levels are often inexplicably normal.

Clinical Presentation

The primary clinical symptoms of hypophosphatemic rickets are skeletal pain and deformity, bone fractures, slipped epiphyses and abnormalities of growth [5]. In infants and young children, additional signs of disease include listlessness and irritability. By 6 months of age, classic skeletal deformities may appear, such as frontal bossing with flattening at the back of the head. Later a lateral collapse of both chest walls (Harrison's sulcus) and rachitic rosary may become evident. If untreated, progressive bone deformities often result in bowing of the long bones, particularly the tibia, femur, radius and ulna, and fractures. In addition, dental eruption may be delayed and teeth may exhibit inadequate dentine calcification, which predisposes to dental abscesses.

In contrast, the clinical signs of phosphopenic osteomalacia are nondescript and often overlooked. When present, they often include diffuse skeletal pain and muscle weakness. The weakness primarily involves proximal muscles and often occurs with wasting, hypotonia and a waddling gait. Such a myopathy is seen in almost all forms of hypophosphatemic rickets and osteomalacia, X-linked hypophosphatemia notably excepted. Phosphate supplementation to counteract the renal phosphate wasting often markedly improves the myopathy. The aching pain, associated with the hypophosphatemic disorders, frequently worsens with activity and occasionally results in an antalgic gait secondary to localization about the hips. Fractures may occur in the long bones, as well as the ribs and vertebral bodies, and lead to progressive deformities in addition to tenderness.

Hypophosphatemic Rachitic/Osteomalacic Diseases

Rachitic disorders are a part of a variety of diseases in which phosphate depletion is manifest. Most typically, these diseases have in common abnormal renal proximal tubular function, which results in an increased clearance of inorganic phosphorus (phosphate wasting) and consequent hypophosphatemia. However, the biochemical abnormalities and phenotypic presentations characteristic of these disorders are remarkably diverse (table 1). Indeed, a complete history, including ascertainment of familial disease, as well as an extensive biochemical evaluation is essential to appropriately diagnose the prevailing disorder. With continued progress in our understanding the pathophysiology of these disorders, genotypic evaluation may become central to establishing the disease subtype. In the remainder of this chapter, I will review the most common phosphopenic rachitic diseases.

X-Linked Hypophosphatemic Rickets/Osteomalacia

XLH represents the prototypic phosphate wasting disorder and is the most common 'vitamin D-resistant' disease in man. X-linked dominant inheritance,

Fig. 1. Bone biopsy from an untreated patient with X-Linked Hypophosphatemia. ***a*** Vilanueva-stained iliac trabecular bone (×100) showing abundance of osteoid (arrows) distributed over the mineralized surfaces. ***b*** Same microscopic field viewed with UV illumination. The majority of the osteoid (arrows) is unlabeled and only a paucity of single tetracycline labels is evident, consistent with impaired mineralization, characteristic of phosphopenic osteomalacia.

Fig. 2. Radiographic image of the lower extremities in a child with X-Linked hypophosphatemia. The growth plates of the femurs are cupped and display increased thickness and an irregular hazy appearance at the diaphyseal line. In addition, the femurs display characteristic bowing.

Fig. 3. Radiographic image of the forearms and hands in a child with X-linked hypophosphatemia. The growth plates of the radius and ulna are cupped and exhibit widening as well as hazy appearance – both characteristic of rickets.

Fig. 4. Lower extremities of a 18-month-old infant with untreated X-linked hypophosphatemia. Severe bowing of the femurs and tibiae are evident.

Fig. 5. Bone biopsy from a patient with X-linked hypophosphatemia after successful treatment with calcitriol and phosphorus. ***a*** Villanueva-stained iliac trabecular bone (×100) no longer exhibits excessive osteoid. Rather, thin osteoid seams (arrows) cover less than 30% of the bone surface. ***b*** The same microscopic field viewed under UV light displays increased tetracycline uptake. Indeed, an abundance of crisp appearing double labels (arrows) is evident, indicative of normal mineralization is evident.

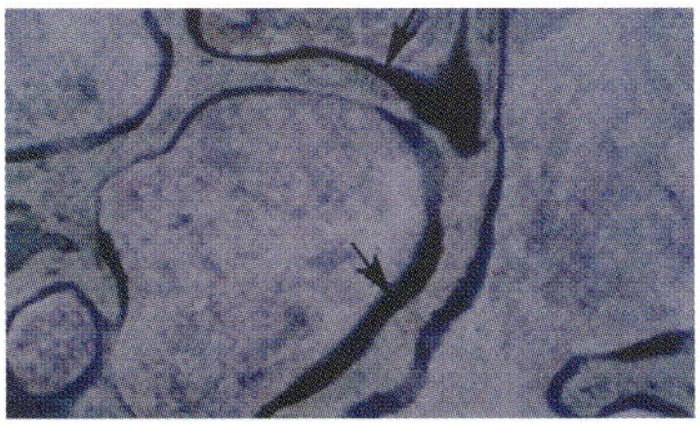

1a

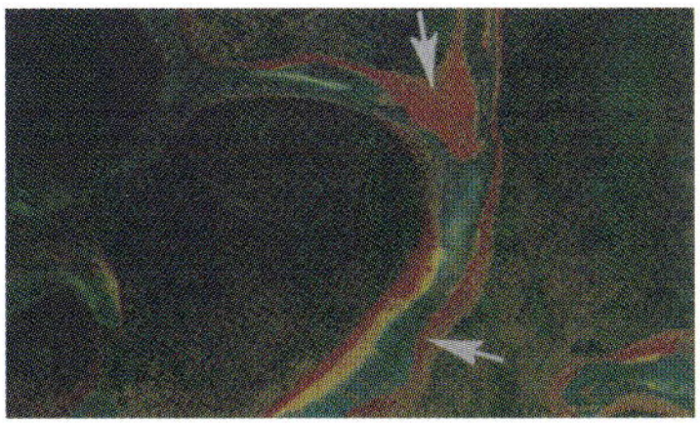

1b

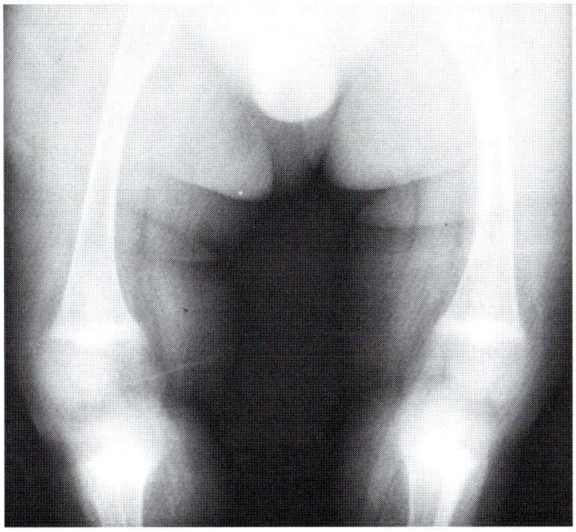

2

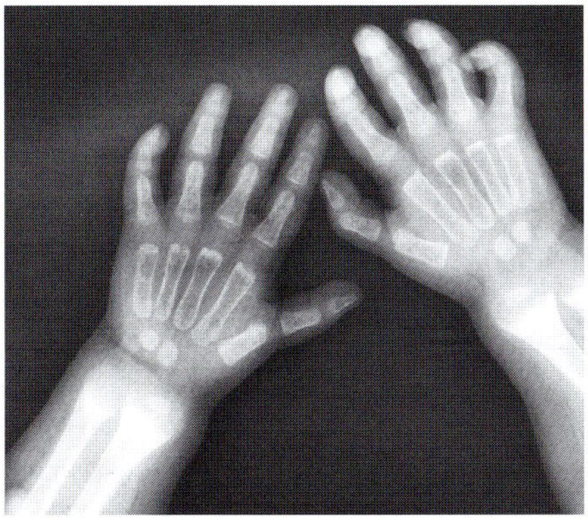

3

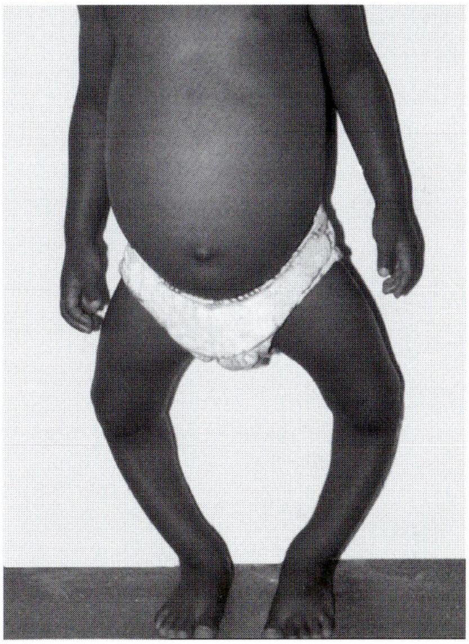

4

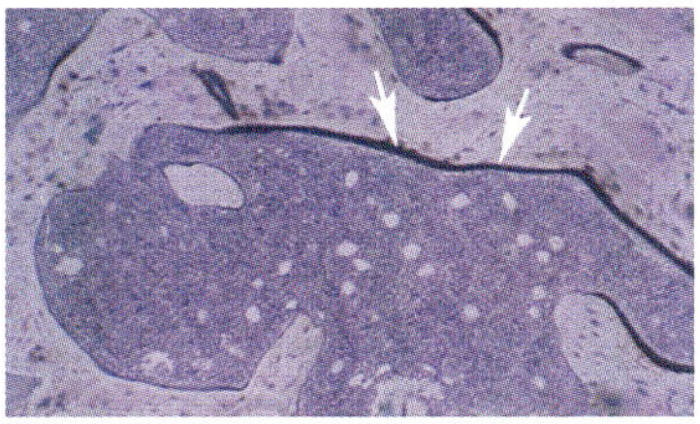

5a

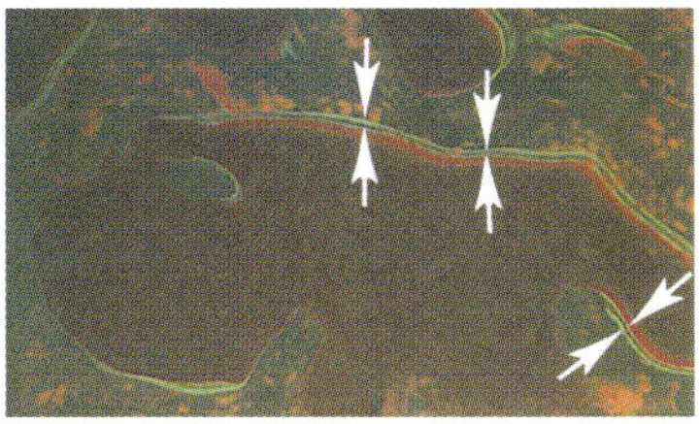

5b

Table 1. Characteristics of the phosphopenic rachitic/osteomalacic disorders in man

	XLH	TIO	ADHR	ARHR	HHRH	Fanconi's syndrome	
						type I	type II
Phosphate homeostasis							
Serum P	↓	↓	↓	↓	↓	↓	↓
Renal TmP/GFR	↓	↓	↓	↓	↓	↓	↓
GI P absorption	↓	↓	↓	↑	↑	↓	↑
FGF-23	N/↑	↑	↑	?	?	?	?
Calcium homeostasis							
Serum Ca	N	N	N	N	N	N	N
Urine Ca	↓	↓	↓	↑	↑	↓	↑
Nephrolithiasis	–	–	–	+	–	–	–
GI Ca absorption	↓	↓	↓	↑	↑	↓	↑
Serum PTH	N	N	N	N	N	N	N
Vitamin D metabolism							
25(OH)D	N	N	N	N	N	N	N
$1,25(OH)_2D$	N/↓	↓	N/↓	↑	↑	N/↓	↑
Bone metabolism							
Serum alkaline phosphatase	N/↑	N/↑	N/↑	N/↑	N/↑	N/↑	N/↑
Urine pyrydionoline crosslinks	N	N	N	N	N	N	N
Genetics							
Familial	+	–	+	+	+	variable	+
Transmission	X-linked dominant		Autosomal dominant	Autosomal recessive	Autosomal recessive	variable	?
Abnormal gene	*PHEX*		*FGF-23*	*CLCN5*	?	variable	?

N/↓ = Decreased relative to the prevailing hypophosphatemia; N/↑ = normal or increased.

progressively severe skeletal abnormalites and growth retardation [6] characterize the disorder. However, the clinical expression of the disease is widely variable. The mildest abnormality is hypophosphatemia without clinically evident bone disease [7–9] and the most common clinically evident manifestation is short stature. Whereas the hypophosphatemia often is detected at birth, its presence and/or other features of the disease may not become apparent until age 6–12 months or older [10].

The majority of affected children exhibit clinical evidence of rickets, including enlargement of the wrists and knees, a lateral collapse of both chest walls (Harrison's sulcus) and/or rachitic rosary. Bowing of the lower extremities is often present. Such defects frequently result in waddling gait and, in severely affected patients, genu varum or valgum [11]. Additional signs of the disease may include late dentition, tooth abscesses, secondary to poor mineralization of the interglobular dentine [12, 13] premature cranial synostosis and frontal bossing. Strikingly absent are common features of vitamin D deficiency osteomalacia, such as muscle weakness, tetany and convulsions.

Without treatment, a small group of patients may manifest pseudofractures, coarsened trabeculation, rarified areas and/or non-union fractures. Others, independent of treatment, develop bone overgrowth at the site of muscle attachments and around joints, which causes significant limitation of motion, particularly at the hips [14, 15]. Such overgrowth may result in fusion of the sacroiliac joint [16]. Indeed, such enthesopathic changes are a primary cause of morbidity in adults.

Bone biopsies in affected children and adults (fig. 1) reveal low turnover osteomalacia, the severity of which has no relationship to sex, the extent of the biochemical abnormalities or the severity of the clinical disability. The osteomalacia is characterized by a reduced rate of bone formation, diffuse patchy hypomineralization, a decrease in mineralizing surfaces and a unique increase in perilacunar areas of absent mineralization [17].

The characteristic hypophosphatemia in XLH is secondary not only to increased urinary phosphate excretion but to mild gastrointestinal phosphate malabsorption [18–21]. The serum calcium concentration in affected subjects is normal, despite gastrointestinal malabsorption of calcium and decreased urinary calcium. Commensurately diminished bone mineralization preserves a slightly positive calcium balance [18, 19]. Such maintenance of calcium homeostasis is associated with normal serum parathyroid hormone levels. However, administration of standard therapy for the disease, oral phosphorus and calcitriol, results in development of secondary hyperparathyroidism in many affected patients and tertiary hyperparathyroidism in a few.

Several investigators have reported normal circulating levels of 25(OH)D in patients with XLH [18, 19, 22]. In addition, untreated youths and adults have normal serum $1,25(OH)_2D$ levels [23–25], despite hypophosphatemia and phosphate depletion, factors that increase calcitriol production in several animal species [26–28] and man [29, 30]. The paradoxical occurrence of hypophosphatemia and normal serum $1,25(OH)_2D$ levels is consistent with a defect in production of this active vitamin D metabolite, most likely due to diminished 25(OH)D-1α-hydroxylase activity. This is supported by recent studies that show the serum calcitriol in patients with XLH increases far less than in normals in response to pharmacological stimulation with exogenous parathyroid hormone [31]. However, the defect is not complete since administration of calcitonin results in a normal increment in the circulating concentration of $1,25(OH)_2D$ [32].

Genetic Abnormality

Studies in *hyp* mice, the murine homologue of the human disease, suggest that elaboration of a humoral factor underlies the observed inhibition of renal phosphate transport in affected patients. In this regard, the *hyp* mouse phenotype is neither transferred nor corrected by cross-transplantation of kidneys in normal and mutant mice [33]. Moreover, although in mice the defective phosphate transport is due to underexpression of the sodium dependent phosphate co-transporter, the gene for this transporter is located on chromosome 5q35 in humans and cannot underlie X-linked hypophosphatemia [34]. Thus, it is most likely that the disorder is due to overproduction of a factor that down-regulates the expression of the sodium dependent phosphate co-transporter, resulting in renal phosphate wasting.

Such recognition led to an intensive effort to clone the gene for XLH. Indeed, the collaborative efforts of the HYP consortium [35–39] resulted in the analysis of data from 13 multigenerational pedigrees and consequent refined mapping of the Xp22.1–p21 region of the X chromosome, identification of tightly linked flanking markers for the *HYP* locus, construction of a YAC contig spanning the *HYP* gene region, and eventual cloning and identification of the disease gene as PHEX, a *P*hosphate-regulating gene with *H*omologies to *E*ndopeptidases located on the *X* chromosome. The protein product of this gene belongs to the M13 family of endopeptidases that include neutral endopeptidase 24.11 (NEP), endothelin-converting enzymes 1 and 2, the Kell blood antigen group, neprilysi-like peptide (NL1) and endothelin-converting enzyme-like I.

Not unexpectedly, identification of the gene associated with XLH as *PHEX* [39] has facilitated efforts to better understand this disease. The gene, located on chromosome Xp22.1 [40], codes for a 749-amino acid protein, consisting of three domains: (1) a small amino-terminal intracellular tail; (2) a single, short transmembrane domain, and (3) a large carboxy-terminal extracellular domain, which, typical of zinc metalloproteases [41], has ten conserved cysteine residues and a HEXXH pentapeptide motif. The homology PHEX displays with metalloproteases has resulted in inclusion of this protein into the M13 family of membrane-bound metalloproteases [42–44], which degrade or activate a variety of peptide hormones [41, 43, 45–49]. Preservation in the PHEX structure of the catalytic glutamate and histidine residues (equivalent to Glu^{648} and His^{711} of NL1) argues strongly for a similar protease activity, as does the alignment of *PHEX* mutations with regions required for peptidase activity in NL1 [50]. Additionally, like other neutral endopeptidases, immunofluorescent studies have revealed a cell-surface location for PHEX in an orientation consistent with a type II integral membrane glycoprotein [50].

Identification of the *PHEX* gene led relatively rapidly to cloning the homologous murine *Phex* gene and identification of the mutations in the murine homologues of XLH, the *hyp* and *gy* mice [51–53]. Unlike 97% of known genes, neither the human or murine gene has a Kozak sequence, a purine at the –3 position before the ATG initiation sequence [51, 53, 54]. Since such genes are often post-transcriptionally regulated, this anomaly may impact studies of hormonal and metabolic *PHEX/Phex* regulation.

PHEX mutations consisting of deletions, insertions and duplications, as well as splice site, nonsense and missense mutations, have been documented in >160 patients with XLH [39, 54–61] and are scattered throughout exons 2–22, which encode the 749-amino acid extracellular protein domain. In addition, a single mutation within the 5′-untranslated region has been identified [57]. Although these mutations invariably cause loss of function, the mechanism by which such loss of activity occurs is not clear. However, preliminary data indicate that missense mutations interfere with protein trafficking, resulting in mutant protein sequestration in the endoplasmic reticulum [60]. Until recently, *PHEX* coding region mutations had not been detected in about 35% of patients. Accordingly, Christie et al. [61] explored a group of such subjects for intronic mutations that may result in mRNA splicing abnormalities. They found in 1 patient a unique mutation in intron 7 that created a novel donor splice site, which interacts with 3 naturally occurring acceptor splice sites, leading to the incorporation of 3 pseudoexons in *PHEX* transcripts. Translation of these pseudoexons results in either the inclusion of missense amino acids into the PHEX protein or a truncated protein, lacking 5 of the 10 conserved cysteine residues and the pentapeptide zinc-binding motif. These observations suggest that intron mutations may represent a substantial proportion of the gene abnormalities yet undiscovered in a subset of patients with XLH. In any case, it is likely that mutations in the PHEX gene result in an haploinsufficiency defect, in which one-half the normal gene product in females (or null amounts in males), result in the phenotype. The alternative hypothesis that the PHEX gene results in a dominant negative effect is unlikely since, inconsistent with this possibility, several mutations reported in affected humans almost certainly result in absent message production.

Pathogenesis

Although, recent data have established the presence of a humoral factor in XLH (see above), the integration of this abnormality into the pathophysiological cascade underlying the disease has remained obscure. However, with the discovery of the *PHEX/Phex* gene, several observations suggested the likely interrelated events resulting in the characteristic phenotype of the disorder. Most notably, the absence of *PHEX/Phex* in the kidney [52, 62–66] indicated that the gene mutation must indirectly regulate the expression of NPT2/Npt2 in renal tubular cells. In addition, recognition that *PHEX* is a member of the M13 family of zinc-dependent type II cell surface membrane metalloproteinases [39] suggested that PHEX/Phex most likely inactivates a novel phosphaturic hormone (provisionally referred to as phosphatonin [67]) or possibly activates a P conserving factor. Thus, the most plausible pathophysiological basis for XLH is: (1) an inactivating mutation of *PHEX* produces inadequate amounts of the PHEX endopeptidase; (2) a resultant ineffective or inadequate degradation/inactivation of phosphatonin occurs, causing elevated circulating levels of bioactive protein, and (3) a consequent repressed expression of NPT2 manifests, resulting in renal P wasting and hypophosphatemia.

Since investigation of murine tissues and cell cultures revealed that *Phex* is predominantly expressed in bones and teeth [52, 53, 62, 64–66], the possibility that diminished *PHEX/Phex* expression in osteoblasts initiates the cascade of events responsible for the pathogenesis of XLH has been entertained. In order to confirm this hypothesis, several investigators have used targeted over-expression of *Phex* in attempts to normalize osteoblast mineralization, in vitro, and rescue the *Hyp* phenotype in vivo. Surprisingly, however, these studies [68, 69] revealed that restoration of *Phex* expression and enzymatic activity to immortalized *hyp* mouse osteoblasts, by retroviral-mediated transduction, does not restore their capacity to mineralize extracellular matrix in vitro, under conditions supporting normal mineralization. Moreover, in complementary studies, Liu et al. [69] found transgenic *hyp* mice (*Osc-Phex-Hyp*), despite expressing abundant Phex mRNA and enzyme activity in mature osteoblasts and osteocytes, exhibited hypophosphatemia and, in the setting of P depletion, histological evidence of osteomalacia, similar to that in non-transgenic *hyp* mice. These observations are consistent with several possibilities. First, despite theoretical evidence to the contrary, extraosseous *Phex* expression may play an important role in the modulation of phosphatonin activity. Second, and more likely, the temporal and developmental expression of the *Osc* promoter-driven *Phex* expression may not mimic the endogenous regulation of *Phex*. Thus, restoration of *Phex* expression to the mature osteoblast may be insufficient alone to rescue the phenotype. In this regard, the very lack of *Phex* activity early in osteoblast development (preceding *Osc* expression) may result in a failure to alter an otherwise immutable osteoblast function, the continued presence of which in mature osteoblasts results in abnormal mineralization or contributes to an impairment of this process.

Further progress in understanding the pathogenesis of XLH has been similarly limited by the inability to identify PHEX/Phex substrates, which may function as phosphatonin(s). The search for candidate substrates has been influenced by the observation that related endopeptidases have substrates that are co-expressed in an organ/cell type-specific fashion [41]. Thus, physiologically relevant PHEX/Phex substrate is likely produced in osteoblasts, the site of predominant *PHEX/Phex* expression [52, 65, 70]. Indeed, genes regulating extracellular matrix production, bone mineralization and renal P transport (e.g. stanniocalcin I [71, 72]) are synthesized in the osteoblast. Moreover, several reports indicate that cultured *hyp* mouse osteoblasts secrete a factor(s), which not only inhibits renal P transport [73, 74] but impairs bone mineralization [75, 76]. Such intrinsic osteoblast abnormalities are supported by the partial rescue of the *hyp* mouse phenotype, which occurs upon normal bone marrow transplantation [77]. In addition, Miao et al. [78] observed that cells derived from *hyp* mouse bone marrow cell cultures exhibited impaired mineralization ex vivo and reduced osteocalcin, bone sialoprotein and vitronectin at both the protein and mRNA levels. These observations suggest that the *PHEX/Phex* gene may control bone mineralization indirectly by regulating the synthesis and deposition of bone matrix proteins. Regardless of the mechanism, however, a PHEX/Phex substrate(s), which is produced by osteoblasts and influences renal P transport and/or bone mineralization, has not been unequivocally identified. In this regard, investigators have reported that membranes expressing recombinant *Phex* or soluble secreted *PHEX* failed to metabolize stanniocalcin I, osteocalcin and osteogenic growth peptide [79, 80], proteins produced by osteoblasts.

More recently, in studies of additional P wasting disorders novel phosphaturic factors have been identified, which may serve as PHEX substrates. Most notably, as discussed below, mutations in fibroblast growth factor (FGF)-23 have been discovered in patients with autosomal-dominant hypophosphatemic rickets (ADHR) [81]. These mutations protect the protein from proteolysis, thereby elevating FGF-23 circulating levels, which results in the characteristic P wasting in this disease. In further studies, elevated circulating levels of FGF-23 have been found in patients with another P wasting disorder, TIO, which return to normal upon tumor resection [82]. Moreover, White et al. [83] reported that FGF-23 and PHEX are co-expressed in tumors causing TIO. Such associations raise the possibility that FGF-23 may not only function as a phosphaturic factor in ADHR and TIO, but serve as a PHEX substrate and phosphatonin in XLH. Indeed, recent data [84] reveal that transgenic mice, expressing FGF-23, exhibit retarded growth, hypophosphatemia, decreased serum $1,25(OH)_2D$ levels and rickets/osteomalacia, all features of XLH. However, while further investigations [84, 85] documented the direct phosphaturic actions of FGF-23, both in vivo and in vitro, identification of this factor as a PHEX substrate and phosphatonin remains incomplete. Whereas Bowe et al. [85] reported that PHEX degrades native FGF-23 (but not the mutant form), Guo et al. [79] found that a peptide fragment of FGF-23, including the cleavage site mutated in ADHR [81], does not serve as a PHEX substrate. The reasons for these conflicting data are not immediately evident. Measurements of circulating FGF-23 in patients with XLH are similarly inconclusive, with elevated levels present only in a subset of treated patients [82, 86]. Thus, further studies are necessary to clarify the possible role of FGF-23 in the pathophysiology of XLH. In fact, regardless of whether FGF-23 is a substrate for PHEX, documenting osteoblast production of this factor is essential to assure that FGF-23 is phosphatonin and as such provides the activity inherent in *hyp* mouse osteoblasts that inhibits mineralization [75–78] and renal P transport [73, 74, 77]. In this regard, further studies in patients with TIO have identified tumor production of yet additional novel factors, which may serve as phosphatonin(s) [84, 87–89]. Among these is 14–3-3-γ protein, which is also produced by *hyp* mouse osteoblasts [89] and frizzle-related protein 4. Thus, additional work is crucial to determine whether phosphatonin is a single protein or a family of proteins and to ascertain the precise physiological derangement underlying XLH.

Treatment

Contemporary therapy for XLH is a combination drug regimen of $1,25(OH)_2D_3$ (or $1\alpha(OH)D_3$) and phosphorus. In general, patients respond exceptionally well to this therapeutic regimen (fig. 5) [90–94]. However, healing of the rickets and osteomalacia and acceleration of growth velocity are not universal outcomes.

The treatment regimen includes a period of titration to achieve a maximum dose of rocaltrol, 40–60 ng/kg/day in divided doses, and phosphorus, 1–2 g/day in 4–5 divided doses. Unfortunately, this therapy creates a significant risk for toxicity that is often expressed as hypercalcemica, hypercalciuria and/or decreased renal function. The occurrence of hypercalcemia, nephrocalcinosis and diminished creatinine clearance necessitates appropriate restriction of therapy and in some cases discontinuation of therapy. In spite of these complications, treatment often proceeds with limited interruptions. Whereas such combined therapy often improves growth velocity, refractoriness to the growth-promoting effects of treatment is often encountered [95]. Thus, use of recombinant growth hormone, as ancillary therapy, has been advocated [96, 97].

Indications for therapy in adults with XLH are less clear. Intractable bone pain and refractory non-union fractures often respond to treatment with calcitriol and phosphorus. However, data remain unclear regarding the effects of treatment on fracture incidence (which may not be increased in untreated patients), enthesopathy and dental abscesses. Therefore, the decision to treat affected adults must be individualized.

Tumor-Induced Osteomalacia

TIO is a sporadic condition characterized by defective bone and cartilage mineralization in children and bone mineralization in adults, which resolves after resection of a co-existing tumor. Since the original description of this syndrome [98], reports of approximately 120 affected patients have appeared [99]. In 58 cases the existent tumor has unequivocally caused the osteomalacia rickets. Other reported patients had inoperable lesions, which precluded establishing the diagnosis, incomplete reported data following surgical intervention, or only partial resolution of the syndrome during observation.

Patients generally present with long-standing vague symptoms, including bone and muscle pain, muscle weakness and infrequently recurrent long bone fractures. In youths fatigue, gait disturbances, delayed growth and bowing of the lower extremities are often additional findings. While the age at diagnosis ranges from 7 to 74 years, only 20% of the patients are <20 years at presentation. The duration of symptoms ranges from 2.5 months to 19 years.

Characteristically, patients exhibit hypophosphatemia and renal phosphate wasting. Gastrointestinal malabsorption of phosphorus contributes to the hypophosphatemia and a negative phosphorus balance. The serum 25(OH)D level is normal and the $1,25(OH)_2D$ concentration decreased or inappropriately normal relative to the prevailing hypophosphatemia. Alkaline phosphatase is commonly high and aminoaciduria often present.

Bone radiographs generally exhibit diffuse osteopenia, pseudofractures, and coarsened trabeculae, as well as widened epiphyseal plates in children. Bone histology reflects the presence of low turnover osteomalacia [13, 19, 100–103], with a marked reduction in the osteoblastic calcification rate and a consequent prolongation of the mineralization lag time and increased duration of the formation period. In contrast, the few affected patients, who have tumors that secrete a nonparathyroid hormone factor(s), which activates adenylate cyclase, exhibit changes consistent with enhanced bone turnover, including an increase in osteoclast and osteoblast number [104–106].

Tumors

Tumors are commonly of mesenchymal origin. However, malignancies of epidermal and endodermal derivation, including breast carcinoma [107], prostate carcinoma [101, 108, 109], oat cell carcinoma [110], small cell carcinoma [111], multiple myeloma and chronic lymphocytic leukemia [106] have been associated with the tumor-induced osteomalacia syndrome. Moreover, the occurrence of osteomalacia in patients with widespread fibrous dysplasia of bone [107], neurobibromatosis [112] and linear nevus sebaceous syndrome [113, 114] may also be ‘tumor’ induced. Proof of a causal relationship has been precluded by the multiplicity of lesions and the consequent inability to effect surgical cure in most patients. However, in one case of fibrous dysplasia [107] and linear nevus sebaceous syndrome [114], removal of virtually all of the abnormal bone or skin lesions, respectively, resulted in appropriate biochemical and radiographic improvements.

Although the mesenchymal tumors associated with the syndrome exhibit morphological complexity, Weidner and Cruz [115] have classified the polymorphous tumors into four distinct subtypes: (1) primitive-appearing, mixed connective tissue tumors; (2) osteoblastoma-like tumors; (3) nonossifying fibroma-like tumors, and (4) ossifying fibroma-like tumors. The most common of these, the mixed connective tissue variant, occurs in soft tissue, behaves in a benign fashion and is characterized by variable numbers of primitive-appearing stromal cells growing in poorly defined sheets and punctuated by clusters of osteoclast-like giant cells. Likely the primitive stromal cells are the source of the hormonal factor(s) that causes the syndrome. However, immunohistochemical studies have shown no evidence of epithelial, neural, vascular or neuroendocrine differentiation in these cells. Indeed, these cells are organelle poor and do not have neurosecretory granules. This, of course, does not preclude them from secreting hormonally active substances.

In any case, the tumors are commonly small, slow growing difficult to locate and present in obscure areas, such as the nasopharynx or sinus. Thus, a careful and thorough examination is necessary to document or exclude the presence of such a tumor. Indeed, variable techniques, such as CT, MRI scan, a technetium-labelled blood pool and octeotride scanning, have been used to successfully locate tumors. Despite a diligent search, however, the tumor may elude localization. Thus, if suspicion is high, continued follow-up is essential, including repeated periodic attempts at identification of a tumor, since documentation of a tumor often does not happen until the disease has progressed over several years.

Pathogenesis

Recent studies have documented that TIO is due to the elaboration of factors, so-called phosphatonins, secreted by tumor cells. Indeed, in vivo studies have consistently revealed that infusion of tumor extracts to mice and rats result in increased renal phosphate excretion and hypophosphatemia. Moreover, several investigators have documented that conditioned medium collected from cultured tumor cells obtained from affected patients reproducibly inhibits phosphate uptake in opposum kidney cells [19, 96, 105, 108]. Several additional observations reaffirm that tumor-secreted phosphonin(s) underlie TIO and provide potential insight to the identity of the circulating phosphaturic factor(s). In this regard, Cai et al. [116] reported partial purification of 'phosphatonin' from a cell culture of a sclerosing hemangioma causing tumor-induced osteomalacia. These studies support that the putative phosphatonin may be a peptide with molecular weight of 8–25 kD, which does not alter glucose or alanine transport, but inhibits sodium-dependent phosphate transport. In addition, Jan de Buer et al. [88] employed serial analysis of gene expression to identify genes that were over-expressed in tumors from affected patients and compared the expression profiles of these genes to those found in histologically similar tumors, which did not cause hypophosphatemic osteomalacia. They observed uniquely abundant expression of several hundred genes in the tumors from patients with TIO. Several of these genes encoded secreted proteins while others encoded membrane-bound or intracellular proteins. Subsequent array profiling for selected candidate genes and RT-PCR analysis of RNA revealed that frizzled-related protein (FRP)-4 and FGF-23 were highly expressed. Further, other investigators have found that MEPE is similarly over-expressed in tumors causing the syndrome [83, 87]. Interestingly, each of these proteins has demonstrable renal phosphate inhibitory activity. These varied observations indicate that the tumor-induced osteomalacia syndrome may be heterogeneous and 'phosphatonin' may represent a family of hormones.

Regardless, the mechanism by which the putative phosphatonin functions in tumor-induced osteomalacia remains unknown. In fact, the related finding that PHEX, among other proteins of osteoblast origin, is upregulated in tumors from patients with the TIO syndrome adds complexity to any model of phosphatonin action [50, 83]. In any case, it is likely that the ultimate decrease in phosphate reabsorption occurs secondary to decreased transcription of the NPT2 messenger RNA and concordant diminished protein concentration. Such a mechanism would parallel that operative in XLH in which the putative phosphatonin similarly decreases NPT2 [117, 118].

In contrast to these observations, patients with tumor-induced osteomalacia secondary to hematogenous malignancy manifest abnormalities of the syndrome due to a distinctly different mechanism. In these subjects the nephropathy induced with light chain proteinuria results in the decreased renal tubular reabsorption of phosphate characteristic of the disease. To date at least 15 patients have been reported who potentially manifest this form of the disorder [118]. In many instances, however, the diagnosis of tumor-induced osteomalacia was not considered. Nevertheless, at least in some cases of this syndrome, renal tubular damage may be mediated by tissue deposition of light chains or of some other immunoglobulin derivative with similar toxic effects on the kidney. Thus, light-chain nephropathy must be considered one possible mechanism for the tumor-induced osteomalacic syndrome.

Diagnosis and Treatment

Since the TIO syndrome has all the classical biochemical and radiological characteristics of the hypophosphatemic rickets/osteomalacias, the diagnosis is dependent on exclusion and a diligent search for tumors in patients at risk for the disease. Adequate exclusion of other phosphopenic disorders requires a detailed dietary history, a complete family history (with a focus on the existence of a broad range of genetic diseases) and an assessment of potential toxin exposure. If no other cause is apparent, several observations favor the diagnosis of TIO and include: (1) a normal serum 25(OH)D level; (2) a selective deficiency of $1,25(OH)_2D$, manifest by a decreased serum concentration; (3) presence of light chain proteinuria; (4) demonstration of phosphaturic activity in tumor extracts or the conditioned medium from cultured tumor cells, and/or (5) induction of the tumor-induced osteomalacia syndrome in athymic nude mice upon heterotransplantation of tumor tissue from affected subjects. If the suspicion for the disease is strong, a search for tumors must reflect that: (1) they range from small to large and benign to malignant, and (2) they may be present for many years before the clinical appearance of bone disease or they may remain undiscovered for many years following the discovery of bone disease, thereby lessening the importance of a temporal association between the onset of bone disease and the clinical awareness of a tumor.

In the absence of tumor, sporadic onset hypophosphatemic rickets/osteomalacia must be considered. Affected youths probably are affected by a spontaneous mutation and will exhibit the characteristics of XLH or ADH. In adults the cause of the syndrome is less certain. Biochemical abnormalities are indistinguishable from those in patients with tumor-induced osteomalacia. Thus, in the absence of genetic transmission of the disorder, careful long-term follow-up for tumor occurrence must be maintained in all patients with hypophosphatemic rickets/osteomalacia.

The foremost treatment for tumor-induced osteomalacia is complete resection of the associated tumor. Such intervention, if successful, within a matter of days to weeks results in normalization of the characteristic biochemical abnormalities. Moreover, healing of the attendant rickets/osteomalacia follows and within several months is completed. Unfortunately, recurrence of mesenchymal tumors, such as giant cell tumors of bone, or inability to resect completely certain malignancies, such as prostatic carcinoma, has created the need to develop effective medical therapeutic intervention for tumor-induced osteomalacia. In this regard, administration of calcitriol and phosphorus combination therapy has proven effective treatment. Several investigators [104, 119] have noted striking improvement of the biochemical and bone abnormalities of the syndrome in response to calcitriol (1.5–3.25 μg/day) and phosphorus (2–4 g/day). In response to this regimen biochemical abnormalities normalize and the osteomalacia improves remarkably or completely heals. The doses of medicines employed, however, potentially lead to complications, such as nephrolithiasis, nephrocalcinosis and hypercalcemia. Indeed, hypercalcemia, secondary to parathyroid hyperfunction, has been documented in 5 affected subjects, representing at least 15–20% of the long-term treated patients. All of these patients had received phosphorus (as part of a combination regiment with vitamin D_2 or calcitriol), which may have stimulated parathyroid hormone secretion and ultimately led to parathyroid autonomy. Thus, careful serial assessment of parathyroid function, serum and urinary calcium and renal function are essential to ensure safe and efficacious therapy.

Autosomal-Dominant Hypophosphatemic Rickets

Several studies have documented an autosomal-dominant inheritance of a hypophosphatemic disorder similar to XLH. Indeed, the literature currently supports the existence of two autosomal-dominant disorders, ADHR and hypophosphatemic bone disease, which may be a forme fruste of ADHR. In 1977, Bianchine et al. [120] reported autosomal-dominant transmission of hypophosphatemic rickets, an observation confirmed by Econs and McEnery [121] in their study of a large disease kindred. The phenotypic manifestations of this disorder include the expected hypophosphatemia due to renal phosphate wasting, lower extremity deformities, tooth abscesses and rickets/osteomalacia. However, current investigations indicate that there is incomplete penetrance of this disorder with variable expression and age of onset. Indeed, a few of the affected female patients exhibit onset of clinically apparent disease in the second through the fourth decades and an increased tendency for bone fracture, uncommon occurrences in XLH. Moreover, a small number of affected youths seemingly escape disease expression as they age. Limited information is available regarding other aspects of the disease including regulation of vitamin D metabolism and circulating levels of parathyroid hormone.

Studies of the genetic defect underlying this disease initially revealed localization of the abnormality to chromosome 12p13 in an 18-cM interval flanked by D12S100 distally and D12D331 proximally [122]. More recently, White et al. [123] reported that mutations of FGF-23, a new member of the growing family of FGF proteins, cause this disorder. However, the biological actions of FGF-23, the mechanisms whereby mutations of FGF-23 influence renal phosphate transport and the relationship(s) between FGF-23, PHEX and phosphatonin remain uncertain. In particular, evidence has not been presented to ascertain if FGF-23 directly or indirectly regulates renal phosphate reabsorption, or is a substrate for PHEX. Eventual elucidation of these issues will provide important information regarding the multiple genetic influences that affect renal phosphate transport.

Hypophosphatemic bone disease, described by Scriver et al. [124], has many of the characteristics of XLH and ADHR, but affected children display no evidence of rachitic disease. Since this syndrome is described in only a few small kindreds and radiographically evident rickets in not universal in children with familial hypophosphatemia, these families may have ADHR. Further observations will be necessary to discriminate this possibility.

X-Linked Recessive Hypophosphatemia

The initial description of X-linked recessive hypophosphatemic rickets involved a family in which males presented with rickets or osteomalacia, hypophosphatemia, and a reduced renal threshold for phosphate reabsorption. In contrast to patients with XLH, affected subjects exhibited hypercalciuria, elevated serum $1{,}25(OH)_2D$ levels (table 1), and proteinuria of up to 3 g/day. Patients also developed nephrolithiasis and nephrocalcinosis with progressive renal failure in early adulthood. Female carriers in the family were not hypophosphatemic and lacked any biochemical abnormalities other than hypercalciuria. Three related syndromes have been reported independently: X-linked recessive nephrolithiasis with renal failure, Dent's disease, and low-molecular-weight proteinuria with hypercalciuria and nephrocalcinosis. These syndromes differ in degree from each other, but common themes include proximal tubular reabsorptive failure, nephrolithiasis, nephrocalcinosis, progressive renal insufficiency, and, in some cases, rickets or osteomalacia. Identification of mutations in the voltage-gated chloride-channel gene CLCN5 in all four syndromes has established that they are phenotypic variants of a single disease and are not separate entities [125, 126]. However, the varied manifestations that may be associated with mutations in this gene, particularly the presence of hypophosphatemia and rickets/osteomalacia, underscore that environmental differences, diet, and/or modifying genetic backgrounds may influence phenotypic expression of the disease.

Fanconi's Syndrome

A vitamin D-resistant rachitic/osteomalacic disorder is a part of the Fanconi's syndrome, which results from a generalized dysfunction of the proximal renal tubule, leading to impaired proximal reabsorption of amino acids, glucose, phosphate, urate and bicarbonate, and increased urinary excretion of these solutes [127–130]. The syndrome is associated with various inborn errors of metabolism or acquired through exposure to various toxic agents [131]. The inherited form may occur in isolation (in the absence of any other metabolic disease) or secondary to various primary Mendelian diseases. Regardless, damage to the proximal tubule represents the common underlying disease mechanism. The bone disease in this disorder is likely secondary to hypophosphatemia and/or acidosis, defects which occur in association with abnormally (Fanconi's syndrome, type I) or normally regulated (Fanconi's syndrome, type II) vitamin D metabolism.

Type I

Renal phosphate wasting and hypophosphatemia are the hallmark abnormalities of this disease. Indeed, occurrence of abnormal bone mineralization appears dependent upon the phosphate loss. Thus, disease subtypes in which isolated amino acid, glucose or potassium wasting occurs are not associated with rickets and/or osteomalacia. In many respects this disorder resembles the more common genetic disease, X-linked hypophosphatemic rickets. Thus, in the majority of patients studied, affected subjects similarly exhibit abnormal vitamin D metabolism. Consequently, serum $1{,}25(OH)_2D$ levels are overtly decreased or abnormally low relative to the prevailing serum phosphorus concentration [132–134]. Although cause of the aberrantly regulated calcitriol biosynthesis remains unknown, renal proximal tubule damage and acidosis undoubtedly play important roles. In fact, the acidosis may contribute to the bone disease as well.

In this regard, several studies indicate that acidosis may exert multiple deleterious effects on bone. In some cases the negative sequelae may be related to the loss of bone calcium, which occurs secondary to calcium release for use in buffering [127, 135]. Alternatively, several investigators [136, 137] have reported that acidosis may impair bone mineralization secondary to a direct inhibition of renal 25(OH)D-1α-hydroxylase activity. However, acidosis does not cause rickets or osteomalacia alone but only in association with phosphate wasting. Thus, acidosis cannot be viewed as an independent variable underlying the bone disease in Fanconi's syndrome, type I. Indeed, Brenner et al. [138] reported that the rachitic/osteomalacic component of this disorder occurs only in patients with type 2 renal tubular acidosis and phosphate wasting. In contrast, those with types 1 and 4 renal tubular acidosis displayed no evidence of abnormal bone mineralization. Thus, the interplay of acidosis and phosphate depletion on bone mineralization in this disorder remains poorly understood. Most likely, however, hypophosphatemia and abnormally regulated vitamin D metabolism are the primary factors underlying rickets and osteomalacia in this form of Fanconi's syndrome.

Type II

Tieder et al. [139] have described two siblings (from a consanguineous mating) who presented with classic characteristics of Fanconi's syndrome, including renal phosphate wasting, renal glucosuria, generalized aminoaciduria and increased urinary excretion of uric acid. However, in these patients the serum calcitriol levels were appropriately elevated (relative to the decreased serum phosphorus concentration) and urine calcium was increased despite normal serum parathyroid hormone levels and cyclic AMP excretion. Furthermore, treatment with phosphate alone reduced the serum $1,25(OH)_2D$ concentration in these patients into the normal range and eliminated the associated hypercalciuria. In many regards, this syndrome resembles the genetic disease HHRH, and as such represents a variant of Fanconi's syndrome. The bone disease in affected subjects appears due to the exclusive effects of hypophosphatemia. In any case, the existence of this variant form of disease is likely the result of renal damage in a different segment of the proximal tubule or involvement of a different mechanism at the same site [139]. Further studies will be necessary to distinguish these possibilities.

Treatment

Ideally treatment of the bone disease in Fanconi's syndrome should be directed at correcting the cause of the pathophysiological defect influencing proximal renal tubular function. Unfortunately, in many cases the primary abnormality has not been defined. Moreover, efforts to decrease the tissue levels of toxic metabolites by dietary (such as in fructose intolerance) or pharmacological means (such as in cystonosis and Wilson's syndrome) have met with variable success. Indeed, it remains unknown if the proximal tubule damage is reversible upon relief of the acute toxicity. Regardless, in instances when specific therapies are not available or do not lead to normalization of the primary defect, therapy must be directed at raising the serum phosphorus concentration, replacing calcitriol (in type I disease) and reversing an associated acidosis. Experience with this therapeutic regiment in the management of Fanconi's syndrome, however, is limited. In general such replacement therapy leads to substantial improvement or resolution of the bone disease [140]. However, growth and development, abnormalities more likely associated with the underlying genetic disease, remain substantially impaired [140]. Thus, more efficacious treatment would entail managing the specific pathophysiological disruption causing the various diseases rather than the secondary manifestations. Therefore, only further research into the causes of these disorders will permit improvements in therapy.

Hereditary Hypophosphatemic Rickets with Hypercalciuria

Rarely, patients with genetically transmitted hypophosphatemic rickets have HHRH. Cardinal biochemical features of this disorder include hypophosphatemia due to increased renal phosphate clearance and normocalcemia. In contrast to other diseases in which renal phosphate transport is limited, patients with HHRH exhibit an increased $1,25(OH)_2D$ production rate [141–145]. The resultant elevated serum calcitriol levels enhance the gastrointestinal calcium absorption, which in turn increases the filtered renal calcium load and inhibits parathyroid secretion. These events cause the characteristic hypercalciuria observed in affected patients.

Although initial symptoms generally consist of bone pain and/or deformities of the lower extremeties, presentation is variable. Indeed, additional features of the disease include short stature, muscle weakness and radiographic signs of rickets or osteopenia. These symptoms and signs may exist in variable combination and occur in a mild or severe form. Children generally become symptomatic between the ages of 6 months and 7 years.

Some apparently unaffected relatives of patients with HHRH exhibit an alternative mode of disease expression [145]. These subjects, although without evidence of bone disease, manifest idiopathic hypercalciuria (IH), most evident in postprandial periods, as well as a pattern of biochemical abnormalities similar to those of children with rickets and osteomalacia, albeit quantitatively milder. The absence of bone disease in these patients is ascribed to the relatively mild phosphate depletion.

Only four unrelated kindreds with this disease have been described. However, a phenotypically similar disorder, childhood idiopathic hypercalciuria with bone lesions (rickets) and stunted linear growth, has been independently recognized. In addition, several patients with apparently sporadic occurrence of HHRH have been recognized. In any case, autosomal-recessive transmission of the disease seems consistent with the inheritance pattern in the described kindred. However, if HHRH is an autosomal recessive disease and individuals with IH are heterozygous for the mutant allele, IH must be an incompletely penetrant trait because not all obligate heterozygotes manifest hypercalciuria. Alternatively, it has been suggested that HHRH and IH could be the result of mutations in two different genes [145]. The strongest support against this hypothesis is that when individuals with HHRH are treated with oral P_i, both the hypophosphatemia and the hypercalciuria are corrected. Nevertheless, the variability in clinical presentation in the various described kindreds suggests that mutations in different genes may be involved.

Regardless, the search for a specific gene defect underlying this disease has been unrewarding. In this regard, efforts to implicate an abnormality in the NPT2 gene in patients with HHRH have been unsuccessful [146].

The above notwithstanding the primary inborn error underlying this disorder is likely an expressed abnormality in the renal proximal tubule which impairs phosphate reabsorption. This pivotal defect results in enhanced renal

25(OH)D-1α-hydroxylase, thus promoting the production of $1,25(OH)_2D$ and increasing its serum and tissue levels. Consequently intestinal calcium absorption is augmented, resulting in suppression of parathyroid function and an increase of the renal filtered calcium load. The concomitant prolonged hypophosphatemia diminishes osteoid mineralization and accounts for the ensuing rickets and/or osteomalacia.

The suggestion that abnormal phosphate transport results in increased calcitriol production remains untested. Indeed, the elevation of $1,25(OH)_2D$ in patients with HHRH is a unique phenotypic manifestation of the disease that distinguishes it from other disorders in which abnormal phosphate transport is likewise manifest. Such heterogeneity in the phenotype of these disorders suggests that disease at variable anatomical sites along the proximal convoluted tubule uniformly impairs phosphate transport but not 25(OH)D-1α-hydroxylase activity.

Patients with HHRH have been treated successfully with high-dose phosphorus (1–2.5 g/day in 5 divided doses) alone. In response to therapy bone pain disappears and muscular strength improves substantially. Moreover, the majority of treated subjects exhibit accelerate linear growth and radiologic sings of rickets are completely absent within 4–9 months. Despite this favorable response, limited studies indicate that such treatment does not heal the associated osteomalacia. Therefore, further studies will be necessary to determine if phosphorus alone is truly sufficient for this disorder. Not surprisingly, the complications of phosphorus therapy in this disease are less than those in others. In this regard, secondary hyperparathyroidism and nephrocalcinosis are rarely observed.

References

1 Boskey A: Mineralization, structure and function of bone; in Seibel MJ Sr, Bilezikian JP (eds): Dynamics of Bone and Cartilage Metabolism. San Diego, Academic Press, 1999, pp 153–164.

2 Bordier PJ, Tun Chot S: Quantitative histology of metabolic bone disease. Clin Endocrinol Metab 1972;1:197–215.

3 Parfitt BFaA: Osteomalacia: Current concepts. Ann Intern Med 1978;89:966–982.

4 Mankin H: Rickets, osteomalacia and renal osteodystrophy. J Bone Joint Surg Am 1974;56-A: 101–128.

5 Dent CE, Stamp TCB: Vitamin D, rickets and osteomalacia; in Krane LAaS (ed): Metabolic Bone Diseases. New York, Academic Press, 1977, vol 1, pp 237–248.

6 Econs MJ, Drezner MK: Bone disease resulting from inherited disorders of renal tubule transport and vitamin D metabolism; in Coe FL, Favus MJ (eds): Disorders of Bone and Mineral Metabolism. New York, Raven Press, 1992, pp 935–950.

7 Graham JB, McFalls VW: Familial hypophosphatemia with vitamin D resistant rickets. III. Three additional kindreds of sex-linked dominant type with a genetic analysis of four such families. Am J Hum Genet 1959;11:311–332.

8 Winters RW, Graham JB, Williams TF, McFalls VW, Burnett CH: A genetic study of familial hypophosphatemia and vitamin D-resistant rickets with a review of the literature. Medicine (Baltimore) 1958;37:97–142.

9 Burnett CH, Dent CE, Harper C, et al: Vitamin D resistant rickets: Analysis of 24 pedigrees and hereditary and sporadic cases. Am J Med 1964;36:222–232.

10 Harrison HE, Harrison HC, Lifshitz F, et al: Growth disturbance in hereditary hypophosphatemia. Am J Dis Child 1966;112:290–297.

11 Williams TF, Winters RW: Familial (hereditary) vitamin D-resistant rickets with hypophosphatemia; in Stanbury JB, Wyngaarden JB, Fredrickson DS (eds): The Metabolic Basis of Inherited Disease. New York, McGraw Hill, 1983, pp 1465–1485.

12 Tracey WE, Campbell RA: Dentofacial development in children with vitamin D resistant rickets. J Am Dent Assoc 1968;76:1026–1031.

13 Lyles KW, Burkes EJ Jr, McNamara CR, Harrelson JM, Pickett JP, Drezner MK: The concurrence of hypoparathyroidism provides new insights to the pathophysiology of X-linked hypophosphatemic rickets. J Clin Endocrinol Metab 1985;60:711–717.

14 Polisson RP, Martinez S, Khoury M, Harrell RM, Lyles KW, Friedman N, Harrelson JM, Reisner E, Drezner MK: Calcification of entheses associated with X-linked hypophosphatemic osteomalacia. N Engl J Med 1985;313:1–6.

15 Hardy DC, Murphy WA, Siegel BA, Reid IR, Whyte MP: X-linked hypophosphatemia in adults: Prevalence of skeletal radiographic and scintigraphic features. Radiology 1989;171:403–414.

16 Pierce DS, Wallace WM, Herndon CH: Long term treatment of vitamin D-resistant rickets. J Bone Joint Surg Am 1964;46-A:979–986.

17 Marie PJ, Glorieux FH: Relation between hypomineralized periosteocytic lesions and bone mineralization in vitamin D-resistant rickets. Calcif Tissue Int 1983;35:443–448.

18 Lyles KW, Harrelson JM, Drezner MK: The efficacy of vitamin D_2 and oral phosphorus therapy in X-linked hypophosphatemic rickets and osteomalacia. J Clin Endocrinol Metab 1982;54:307–315.

19 Drezner MK, Lyles KW, Haussler MR, Harrelson JM: Evaluation of a role for 1,25-dihydroxyvitamin D_3 in the pathogenesis and treatment of X-linked hypophosphatemic rickets and osteomalacia. J Clin Invest 1980;66:1020–1032.

20 Steindijk R: On the pathogenesis of vitamin D resistant rickets and primary vitamin D resistant rickets. Helv Paediatr Acta 1962;17:65–85.

21 Stickler GB: External calcium and phosphorus balances in vitamin D-resistant rickets. J Pediatr 1963;63:942–948.

22 Haddad JG, Chyu KJ, Hahn TJ, Stamp TCB: Serum concentrations of 25-hydroxyvitamin D in sex linked hypophosphatemic vitamin D-resistant rickets. J Lab Clin Med 1973;81:22–27.

23 Drezner MK, Haussler MR: Serum 1,25-dihydroxyvitamin D in bone disease. N Engl J Med 1979;300:435.

24 Delvin EE, Glorieux FH: Serum 1,25-dihydroxyvitamin D concentration in hypophosphatemic vitamin D resistant rickets. Calcif Tissue Int 1981:33.

25 Lyles KW, Clark AG, Drezner MK: Serum 1,25-dihydroxyvitamin D levels in subjects with X-linked hypophosphatemic rickets and osteomalacia. Calcif Tissue Int 1982;34:125–130.

26 Hughes MR, Brumbaugh PF, Haussler MR, Wergedal JE, Baylink DJ: Regulation of serum 1,25-dihydroxyvitamin D by calcium and phosphate in the rat. Science 1975;180:578–580.

27 Galante L, Colston KW, Evans IM, Byfield PGH, Matthews EW, MacIntyre I: The regulation of vitamin D metabolism. Nature 1973;244:438–440.

28 Haussler MR, Hughes M, Baylink D, Littledike ET, Cork D, Pitt M: Influence of phosphate depletion on the biosynthesis and circulating level of 1,25-dihydroxyvitamin D. Adv Exp Med Biol 1977;81:233–250.

29 Domininguez JH, Gray RW, Lemann J: Dietary phosphate deprivation in women and men: effects on mineral and acid balances, parathyroid hormone and the metabolism of 25(OH)D. J Clin Endocrinol Metab 1977;43:1056–1068.

30 Gray RW, Wilz DR, Caldas AE, Lemann J: The importance of phosphate in regulating plasma $1,25(OH)_2D$ levels in humans: Studies in healthy subjects, in calcium stone formers and in patients with primary hyperparathyroidism. J Clin Endocrinol Metab 1977;45:299–306.

31 Lyles KW, Drezner MK: Parathyroid hormone effects on serum 1,25-dihydroxyvitamin D levels in patients with X-linked hypophosphatemic rickets: Evidence for abnormal 25-hydroxyvitamin D-1-hydroxylase activity. J Clin Endocrinol Metab 1982;54:638–644.

32 Econs MJ, Lobaugh B, Drezner MK: Normal calcitonin stimulation of serum calcitriol in patients with X- linked hypophosphatemic rickets. J Clin Endocrinol Metab 1992;75:408–411.

33 Nesbitt T, Coffman TM, Griffiths R, Drezner MK: Crosstransplantation of kidneys in normal and Hyp mice: Evidence that the Hyp mouse phenotype is unrelated to an intrinsic renal defect. J Clin Invest 1992;89:1453–1459.

34 McPherson JD, Krane MC, Wagner-McPherson CB, Kos CH, Tenenhouse HS: High resolution mapping of the renal sodium-phosphate cotransporter gene (NPT2) confirms its localization to human chromosome 5q35. Pediatr Res 1977;41:632–634.

35 Francis F, Rowe PS, Econs MJ, See CG, Benham F, O'Riordan JL, Drezner MK, Hamvas RM, Lehrach H: A YAC contig spanning the hypophosphatemic rickets disease gene (HYP) candidate region. Genomics 1994;21:229–237.

36 Econs MJ, Francis F, Rowe PSN, Speer MC, Pericak-Vance MA, Becker PA, O'Riordan J, Lehrach H, Drezner MK: Dinucleotide repeat polymorphism of the microsatellite repeat probe, A0563. Hum Mol Genet 1994;3:680.

37 Econs MJ, Rowe PS, Francis F, Barker DF, Speer MC, Norman M, Fain PR, Weissenbach J, Read A, Davis KE, et al: Fine structure mapping of the human X-linked hypophosphatemic rickets gene locus. J Clin Endocrinol Metab 1994;79:1351–1354.

38 Rowe PS, Goulding JN, Francis F, Oudet C, Econs MJ, Hanauer A, Lehrach H, Read AP, Mountford RC, Summerfield T, Weissenbach J, Fraser W, Drezner MK, Davies KE, O'Riordan JL: The gene for X-linked hypophosphataemic rickets maps to a 200–300 kb region in Xp22.1, and is located on a single YAC containing a putative vitamin D response element (VDRE). Hum Genet 1996;97:345–352.

39 The HYP Consortium: A gene (PEX) with homologies to endopeptidases is mutated in patients with X-linked hypophosphatemic rickets. Nat Genet 1995;11:130–136.

40 Read AP, Thakker RV, Davies KE, Mountford RC, Brenton DP, Davies M, Glorieux F, Harris R, Hendy GN, King A, et al: Mapping of human X-linked hypophosphatemic rickets by multilocus linkage analysis. Hum Genet 1986;73:267–270.

41 Turner AJ, Tanzawa K: Mammalian membrane metallopeptidases: NEP, ECE, KELL, and PEX. FASEB J 1997;11:355–364.

42 Emoto N, Yanagisawa M: Endothelian-converting enzyme-2 is a membrane-bound phosphramidon-sesitive metalloprotease with acidic pH optimum. J Biol Chem 1995;270:15262–15268.

43 Lee S, Zambas ED, Marsh WL, Redman CM: Molecular cloning and primary structure of Kell blood group protein. Proc Natl Acad Sci USA 1991;88:6353–6357.

44 Kiryu-Seo S, Sasaki M, Yokohama H, Nakagomi S, Hirayama T, Aoki S, Wada K, Kiyama H: Damage-induced neuronal endopeptidase (DINE) is a unique metallopeptidase expressed in response to neuronal damage and activates superoxide scavenge. Proc Natl Acad Sci USA 2000; 97:4345–4350.

45 Shimada K, Takahashi M, Turner AJ, Tanzawa K: Rat endothelin-converting enzyme-1 forms a dimer through Cys412 with a similar catalytic mechanism and a distinct substrate binding mechanism compared with neutral endopeptidase-24.11. J Biochem 1996;315:863–867.

46 D'Adamio L, Shipp MA, Masteller EL, Reinherz EL: Organization of the gene encoding common acute lymphoblastic leukemia antigen (neutral endopeptidase 24.11): multiple miniexons and separate 5' untranslated regions. Proc Natl Acad Sci USA 1989;86:7103–7107.

47 Russell F, Davenport A: Evidence for intracellular endothelin-converting enzyme-2 expression in cultured human vascular endothelial cells. Circ Res 1999;84:891–896.

48 Valdenaire O, Richards JG, et al: XCE, a new member of the endothelin-converting enzyme and neutral endopeptidase family, is preferentailly expressed in the CNS. Brain Res Mol Brain Res 1999;64:211–221.

49 Valdenaire O, Rohrbacher E, Langeveld A, Schweizer A, Meijers C: Organization and chromosomal localization of human ECEL1 (XCE) gene encoding a zinc metallopeptidase involved in the nervous control of respiration. Biochem J 2000;346:611–616.

50 Lipman ML, Panda D, Bennett HP, Henderson JE, Shane E, Shen Y, Goltzman D, Karaplis AC: Cloning of human PEX cDNA: Expression, subcellular localization, and endopeptidase activity. J Biol Chem 1998;273:13729–13737.

51 Strom TM, Francis F, Lorenz B, Boddrich A, Econs MJ, Lehrach H, Meitinger T: Pex gene deletions in Gy and Hyp mice provide mouse models for X-linked hypophosphatemia. Hum Mol Genet 1997;6:165–171.
52 Beck L, Soumounou Y, Martel J, Krishnamurthy G, Gauthier C, Goodyer CG, Tenenhouse HS: Pex/PEX tissue distribution and evidence for a deletion in the 3' region of the Pex gene in X-linked hypophosphatemic mice. J Clin Invest 1997;99:1200–1209.
53 Du L, Desbarats M, Viel J, Glorieux FH, Cawthorn C, Ecarot B: cDNA cloning of the murine Pex gene implicated in X-linked hypophosphatemia and evidence for expression in bone. Genomics 1996;36:22–28.
54 Francis F, Strom TM, Hennig S, Boddrich A, Lorenz B, Brandau O, Mohnike KL, Cagnoli M, Steffens C, Klages S, Borzym K, Pohl T, Oudet C, Econs MJ, Rowe PS, Reinhardt R, Meitinger T, Lehrach H: Genomic organization of the human PEX gene mutated in X-linked dominant hypophosphatemic rickets. Genome Res 1997;7:573–585.
55 Rowe PS, Oudet CL, Francis F, Sinding C, Pannetier S, Econs MJ, Strom TM, Meitinger T, Garabedian M, David A, Macher MA, Questiaux E, Popowska E, Pronicka E, Read AP, Mokrzycki A, Glorieux FH, Drezner MK, Hanauer A, Lehrach H, Goulding JN, O'Riordan JL: Distribution of mutations in the PEX gene in families with X-linked hypophosphataemic rickets (HYP). Hum Mol Genet 1997;6:539–549.
56 Holm IA, Nelson AE, Robinson BG, Mason RS, Marsh DJ, Cowell CT, Carpenter TO: Mutational analysis and genotype-phenotype correlation of the PHEX gene in X-linked hypophosphatemic rickets. J Clin Endocrinol Metab 2001;86:3889–3899.
57 Dixon PH, Christie PT, Wooding C, Trump D, Grieff M, Holm I, Gertner JM, Schmidtke J, Shah B, Shaw N, Smith C, Tau C, Schlessinger D, Whyte MP, Thakker RV: Mutational analysis of PHEX gene in X-linked hypophosphatemia. J Clin Endocrinol Metab 1998;83:3615–3623.
58 Filisetti D, Ostermann G, von Bredow M, Strom T, Filler G, Ehrich J, Pannetier S, Garnier JM, Rowe P, Francis F, Julienne A, Hanauer A, Econs MJ, Oudet C: Non-random distribution of mutations in the PHEX gene, and under-detected missense mutations at non-conserved residues. Eur J Hum Genet 1999;7:615–619.
59 Tyynismaa H, Kaitila I, Nanto-Salonen K, Ala-Houhala M, Alitalo T: Identification of fifteen novel PHEX gene mutations in Finnish patients with hypophosphatemic rickets. Hum Mutat 2000;15:383–384.
60 Sabbagh Y, Boileau G, DesGroseillers B, Tenenhouse HS: Turnover and rescue of mutant PHEX proteins sequestered in the endoplasmic reticulum. J Bone Miner Res 2001;16:S227.
61 Christie PT, Harding B, Nesbit MA, Whyte MP, Thakker RV: X-linked hypophosphatemia attributable to pseudoexons of the PHEX gene. J Clin Endocrinol Metab 2001;86:3840–3844.
62 Thompson DL, Sabbagh Y, Tenenhouse HS, Roche PC, Drezner MK, Salisbury JL, Grande JP, Poeschla EM, Kumar R: Ontogeny of Phex/PHEX protein expression in mouse embryo and subcellular localization in osteoblasts. J Bone Miner Res 2002;17:311–320.
63 Meyer MH, Meyer RA Jr: MRNA expression of Phex in mice and rats: The effect of low phosphate diet. Endocrine 2000;13:81–87.
64 Zoidis E, Zapf J, Schmid C: Phex cDNA cloning from rat bone and studies on phex mRNA expression: Tissue-specificity, age-dependency, and regulation by insulin-like growth factor (IGF) I in vivo. Mol Cell Endocrinol 2000;168:41–51.
65 Ruchon AF, Tenenhouse HS, Marcinkiewicz M, Siegfried G, Aubin JE, DesGroseillers L, Crine P, Boileau G: Developmental expression and tissue distribution of Phex protein: Effect of the Hyp mutation and relationship to bone markers. J Bone Miner Res 2000;15:1440–1450.
66 Grieff M, Mumm S, Waeltz P, Mazzarella R, Whyte MP, Thakker RV, Schlessinger D: Expression and cloning of the human X-linked hypophosphatemia gene cDNA. Biochem Biophys Res Commun 1997;231:635–639.
67 Drezner MK: PHEX gene and hypophosphatemia. Kidney Int 2000;57:9–18.
68 Sabbagh Y, Londowski, JM, Mathieson D, Gauthier C, Boileau G, Tenenhouse HS, Poeschia EM, Kumar R: Stable expression of PHEX in hypophosphatemic (Hyp) mouse osteoblasts using a viral vector partially corrects the mutant cell phenotype: Implications for gene therapy. J Am Soc Nephrol 2000;11:413A.

69 Liu S, Guo R, Tu Q, Quarles LD: Overexpression of Phex in osteoblasts fails to rescue the Hyp mouse phenotype. J Biol Chem 2002;277:3686–3697.
70 Ruchon AF, Marcinkiewicz M, Siegfried G, Tenenhouse HS, DesGroseillers L, Crine P, Boileau G: Pex mRNA is localized in developing mouse osteoblasts and odontoblasts. J Histochem Cytochem 1998;46:459–468.
71 Jiang WQ, Chang AC, Satoh M, Furuichi Y, Tam PP, Reddel RR: The distribution of stanniocalcin I protein in fetal mouse tissues suggests a role in bone and muscle development. J Endocrinol 2000;165:457–466.
72 Varghese R, Wong CK, Deol H, Wagner GR, DiMattia GE: Comparative analysis of mammalian stanniocalcin genes. Endocrinology 1998;139:4714–4725.
73 Nesbitt T, Fujiwara I, Thomas R, Xiao ZS, Quarles LD, Drezner MK: Coordinated maturational regulation of PHEX and renal phosphate transport inhibitory activity: Evidence for the pathophysiological role of PHEX in X-linked hypophosphatemia. J Bone Miner Res 1999;14: 2027–2035.
74 Lajeunesse D, Meyer RA Jr, Hamel L: Direct demonstration of a humorally-mediated inhibition of renal phosphate transport in the Hyp mouse. Kidney Int 1996;50:1531–1538.
75 Ecarot B, Glorieux FH, Desbarats M, Travers R, Labelle L: Defective bone formation by Hyp mouse bone cells transplanted into normal mice: Evidence in favor of an intrinsic osteoblast defect. J Bone Miner Res 1992;7:215–220.
76 Xiao ZS, Crenshaw M, Guo R, Nesbitt T, Drezner MK, Quarles LD: Intrinsic mineralization defect in Hyp mouse osteoblasts. Am J Physiol 1998;275:E700–E708.
77 Miyamura T, Tanaka H, Inoue M, Ichinose Y, Seino Y: The effects of bone marrow transplantation on X-linked hypophosphatemic mice. J Bone Miner Res 2000;15:1451–1458.
78 Miao D, Bai X, Panda D, McKee M, Karaplis A, Goltzman D: Osteomalacia in hyp mice is associated with abnormal phex expression and with altered bone matrix protein expression and deposition. Endocrinology 2001;142:926–939.
79 Guo R, Liu S, Spurney RF, Quarles LD: Analysis of recombinant Phex: An endopeptidase in search of a substrate. Am J Physiol Endocrinol Metab 2001;281:E837–E847.
80 Boileau G, Tenenhouse HS, Desgroseillers L, Crine P: Characterization of PHEX endopeptidase catalytic activity: Identification of parathyroid-hormone-related peptide107–139 as a substrate and osteocalcin, PPi and phosphate as inhibitors. Biochem J 2001;355:707–713.
81 The ADHR Consortium: Autosomal dominant hypophosphatemic rickets is associated with mutations in FGF23. Nat Genet 2000;26:345–348.
82 Jonsson KB, Zahradnik R, Larsson T, White KE, Hampson G, Miyauchi A, Econs M, Lavigne J, et al: FGF-23 is a circulating factor that is elevated in oncogenic osteomalacia and X-linked hypophosphatemic rickets. J Bone Miner Res 2002;17:S158.
83 White KE, Jonsson KB, Carn G, Hampson G, Spector TD, Mannstadt M, Lorenz-Depiereux B, Miyauchi A, Yang IM, Ljunggren O, Meitinger T, Strom TM, Juppner H, Econs MJ: The autosomal dominant hypophosphatemic rickets (ADHR) gene is a secreted polypeptide overexpressed by tumors that cause phosphate wasting. J Clin Endocrinol Metab 2001;86:497–500.
84 Shimada T, Mizutani S, Muto T, Yoneya T, Hino R, Takeda S, Takeuchi Y, Fujita T, Fukumoto S, Yamashita T: Cloning and characterization of FGF23 as a causative factor of tumor-induced osteomalacia. Proc Natl Acad Sci USA 2001;98:6500–6505.
85 Bowe AE, Finnegan R, Jan de Beur SM, Cho J, Levine MA, Kumar R, Schiavi SC: FGF-23 inhibits renal tubular phosphate transport and is a PHEX substrate. Biochem Biophys Res Commun 2001;284:977–981.
86 Yamazaki Y, Okazaki R, Shibata M, Hasegawa Y, Satoh K, Tajima T, Takeuchi Y, Fujita T, Nakahara K, Yamashita T, Fukumoto S: Increased circulatory level of biologically active full-length FGF-23 in rickets/osteomalacia. J Clin Endocrinol Metab 2002;87:4957–4960.
87 Rowe PS, de Zoysa PA, Dong R, Wang HR, White KE, Econs MJ, et al: MEPE, a new gene expressed in bone marrow and tumors causing osteomalacia. Genomics 2000;67:54–68.
88 Jan de Beur SM, Finnegan RB, Vassiliadis J, Cook B, Barberio D, Estes S, Manavalan P, Petroziello J, Madden S, Cho JY, Kumar R, Levine MA, Schiavi SC: Tumors associated with oncogenic osteomalacia express markers of bone and mineral metabolism. J Bone Miner Res 2002;17: 1102–1110.

89 Yanagawa N, Shin RN, et al: Identification of an osteoblast-derived phosphaturic factor (ODPF). J Am Soc Nephrol 2001;12:760A.
90 Rasmussen H, Pechet M, Anast C, Mazur A, Gertner J, et al: Long-term treatment of familial hypophosphatemic rickets with oral phosphate and 1a-hydroxyvitamin D_3. J Pediatr 1981;99: 16–25.
91 Rasmussen H, Anast C: Familial hypophosphatemic rickets and vitamin D-dependent rickets; in Stanbury J, Wyngaarden JB, Fredrickson DS, Goldstein JL, Brown M (eds): The Metabolic Basis of Inherited Disease. New York, McGraw Hill, 1983, pp 1743–1773.
92 Glorieux FH, Marie PJ, Pettifor JM, Delvin EE: Bone response to phosphate salts, ergocalciferol, and calcitrol in hypophosphatemic vitamin D resistant rickets. N Engl J Med 1980;303:1023–1031.
93 Costa T, Marie PJ, Scriver CR, Cole DE, Reade TM, Nogrady B, Glorieux FH, Delvin EE: X-linked hypophosphatemia: Effect of calcitriol on renal handling of phosphate, serum phosphate, and bone mineralization. J Clin Endocrinol Metab 1981;52:463–472.
94 Harrell RM, Lyles KW, Harrelson JM, Friedman NE, Drezner MK: Healing of bone disease in X-linked hypophosphatemic rickets/osteomalacia: Induction and maintenance with phosphorus and calcitriol. J Clin Invest 1985;75:1858–1868.
95 Friedman NE, Lobaugh B, Drezner MK: Effects of calcitriol and phosphorus therapy on the growth of patients with X-linked hypophosphatemia. J Clin Endocrinol Metab 1993;76:839–844.
96 Saggerve G, Baronelli G, Butelloni S, Perri G: Long-term growth hormone treatment in children with renal hypophosphatemic rickets: Effects on growth, mineral metabolism and bone density. J Pediatr 1995;127:395–402.
97 Seikaly MG, Brown R, Baum M: The effect of recombinant human growth hormone in children with X- linked hypophosphatemia. Pediatrics 1997;100:879–884.
98 Prader AV, Illig R, Uehilinger E, Stalder G: Rachitis infolge knochentumors. Helv Paediatr Acta 1959;14:554–565.
99 Drezner MK: Tumor-induced osteomalacia; in Favus MJ (ed): Primer on the Metabolic Bone Diseases and Disorders of Mineral Metabolism. Philadelphia, Williams & Wilkins, 1999, pp 331–336.
100 Drezner MK, Feinglos MN: Osteomalacia due to 1,25-dihydroxycholecalciferol deficiency: Association with a giant cell tumor of bone. J Clin Invest 1977;60:1046–1053.
101 Lyles KW, Berry WR, Haussler MR, Harrelson JM, Drezner MK: Hypophosphatemic osteomalacia: Association with prostatic carcinoma. Ann Intern Med 1980;93:275–278.
102 Marie PJ, Glorieux FH: Bone histomorphometry in asymptomatic adults with hereditary hypophosphatemic vitamin D-resistant osteomalacia. Metab Bone Dis Relat Res 1982;4:249–253.
103 Drezner MK, Lyles KW, Harrelson JM: Vitamin D resistant osteomalacia: Evaluation of vitamin D metabolism and response to therapy; in Choh DV, Talmage RV, Matthews JL (eds): Hormonal Control of Calcium Metabolism. Amsterdam, Excerpta Medica, 1980, pp 243–251.
104 Leicht E, Biro G, Langer H-J: Tumor-induced osteomalacia: Pre- and postoperative biochemical findings. Horm Metab Res 1990;22:640–643.
105 Shane E, Parisien M, Henderson JE, Dempster DW, Hardy MA, Tohme JF, Karaplis AC, Clemens TL: Tumor-induced osteomalacia: Clinical and basic studies. J Bone Miner Res 1997;12:1502–1511.
106 Miller MJ, Marel G, Frame B: Adult acquired vitamin D and PTH-resistant hypophosphatemic osteomalacia with multiple skeletal lesions; in Norman AW, Schaefer K, Herrah DV, Grigoleit HG (eds): Vitamin D-Chemical, Biochemical and Clinical Endocrinology of Calcium Metabolism. New York, de Gruyter, 1982, pp 993–995.
107 Dent CE, Gertner JM: Hypophosphatemic osteomalacia in fibrous dysplasia. Q J Med 1976;45: 411–420.
108 Murphy P, Wright G, Rai GS: Hypophosphatemic osteomalacia induced with prostatic carcinoma. Br Med J 1985;290:1945.
109 Hosking DJ, Chamberlain MJ, Whortland-Webb WR: Osteomalacia and carcinoma of prostate with major redistribution of skeletal calcium. Br J Radiol 1975;48:451–456.
110 Taylor AC, Fallon MD, Velasco ME: Oncogenic osteomalacia and inappropriate antidiuretic hormone secretion due to oat-cell carcinoma. Ann Intern Med 1984;101:786–788.
111 Shaker JL, Brickner RC, Divgi AB, Raff H, Findling JW: Case report: Renal phosphate wasting, syndrome of inappropriate antidiuretic hormone and ectopic corticotropin production in small cell carcinoma. Am J Med Sci 1995;310:38–41.

112 Saville PD, Nassim JR, Stevenson FH: Osteomalacia in von Recklinghausen's neurofibromatosis: Metabolic study of a case. Br Med J 1955;1:1311–1313.
113 Carey DE, Drezner MK, Hamdan JA, Mange M, Ashmad MS, Mubarak S, Nyhan WL: Hypophosphatemic rickets/osteomalacia in linear sebaceous nevus syndrome: A variant of tumor-induced osteomalacia. J Pediatr 1986;109:994–1000.
114 Ivker R, Resnick SD, Skidmore RA: Hypophosphatemic vitamin D-resistant rickets, precocious puberty and the epidermal nevus syndrome. Arch Derm 1997;133:1557–1561.
115 Weidner N, Cruz DS: Phosphaturic mesenchymal tumors: A polymorphous group causing osteomalacia or rickets. Cancer 1987;59:1442–1454.
116 Cai Q, Hodgson SF, Kao PC, Lennon VA, Klee GG, Zinsmiester AR, Kumar R: Brief report: Inhibition of renal phosphate transport by a tumor product in a patient with oncogenic osteomalacia. N Engl J Med 1994;330:1645–1649.
117 Tenenhouse HS, Werner A, Biber J, Ma S, Martel J, Roy S, Murer H: Renal Na^{+}-phosphate cotransport in murine X-linked hypophosphatemic rickets: molecular characterization. J Clin Invest 1994;93:671–676.
118 Tenenhouse HS, Martel J, Biber J, Murer H: Effect of P(i) restriction on renal Na(+)-P(i) cotransporter mRNA and immunoreactive protein in X-linked Hyp mice. Am J Physiol 1995;268: F1062–F1069.
119 Lobaugh B, Burch WM Jr, Drezner MK: Abnormalities of vitamin D metabolism and action in the vitamin D resistant rachitic and osteomalacic diseases; in Kumar R (ed): Vitamin D. Boston, Martinus Nijhoff, 1984, pp 665–720.
120 Bianchine JW, Stambler AA, Harrison HE: Familial hypophosphatemic rickets showing autosomal dominant inheritance. Birth Defects Orig Article Ser 1971;7:287–295.
121 Econs MJ, McEnery PT: Autosomal dominant hypophosphatemic rickets/osteomalacia: Clinical characterization of a novel renal phosphate-wasting disorder. J Clin Endocrinol Metab 1997;82:674–681.
122 Econs MJ, McEnery PT, Lennon F, Speer MC: Autosomal dominant hypophosphatemic rickets is linked to chromosome 12p13. J Clin Invest 1997;100:2653–2657.
123 White KE, Carn G, Lorenz-Depiereux B, Benet-Pages A, Strom TM, Econs MJ: Autosomal-dominant hypophosphatemic rickets (ADHR) mutations stabilize FGF-23. Kidney Int 2001;60:2079–2086.
124 Scriver CR, MacDonald W, Reade T, Glorieux RH, Nogrady B: Hypophosphatemic nonrachitic bone disease: an entity distinct from X-linked hypophosphatemia in the renal defect, bone involvement, and inheritance. Am J Med Genet 1977;1:101–117.
125 Scheinman SJ, Pook MA, Wooding C, Pang JT, Frymoyer PA, Thakker RV: Mapping the gene causing X-linked recessive nephrolithiasis to Xp11.22 by linkage studies. J Clin Invest 1997;91: 2351–2357.
126 Scheinman SJ: X-linked hypercalciuric nephrolithiasis: Clinical syndromes and chloride channel mutations. Kidney Int 1998;53:3–17.
127 Chan JCM, Alon U: Tubular disorders of acid-base and phosphate metabolism. Nephron 1985;40: 257–279.
128 Chesney RW: Fanconi syndrome and renal tubular acidosis; in Favus MJ (ed): Primer on Metabolic Bone Diseases and Disorders of Mineral Metabolism. Kelseyville, American Society of Bone and Mineral Research, 1990.
129 De Toni G: Remarks on the relations between renal rickets (renal dwarfism) and renal diabetes. Acta Paediatr Scand 1933;16:479–484.
130 McCune DJ, Mason HH, Clarke HT: Intractable hypophosphatemic rickets with renal glycosuria and acidosis (the Fanconi syndrome). Am J Dis Child 1943;65:81–146.
131 Bergeron M, Gougoux A, Vinay P: The renal Fanconi syndrome; in Scriver CR, Beaudet AL, Sly WS, Valle D (eds): The Metabolic and Molecular Bases of Inherited Disease. New York, McGraw-Hill, 1995, pp 3691–3704.
132 Chesney RW, Rosen JF, Hamstra AJ, DeLuca HF: Serum 1,25-dihydroxyvitamin D levels in normal children and in vitamin D disorders. Am J Dis Child 1980;134:135–139.
133 Steinherz R, Chesney RW, Schulman JD, DeLuca HF, Phelps M: Circulating vitamin D metabolites in nephropathic cystinosis. J Pediatr 1983;102:592–594.
134 Chesney RW, Kaplan BS, Phelps M, DeLuca HF: Renal tubular acidosis does not alter circulating values of calcitriol. J Pediatr 1984;104:51–55.

135 Chevalier RL: Hypercalciuria in a child with primary Fanconi syndrome and hearing loss. Int J Pediatr Nephrol 1983;4:53–57.
136 Lee SW, Russell J, Avioli LV: 25-Hydroxycholecalciferol to 1,25-dihydroxycholecalciferol: conversion impaired by systemic metabolic acidosis. Science 1977;195:994–996.
137 Brewer ED, Tsai HC, Szeto KS, Morris RC: Maleic acid induced impaired conversion of 25(OH)D_3 to 1,25(OH)2D_3: Implications for Fanconi's syndrome. Kidney Int 1977;12:244–252.
138 Brenner RJ, Spring DB, Sebastian A, McSherry EM, Genant HK, Palubinskas AJ, Morris RC: Incidence of radiographically evident bone disease, nephrocalcinosis and nephrolithiasis in various types of renal tubular acidosis. N Engl J Med 1982;307:217–221.
139 Tieder M, Arie R, Modai D, Samuel R, Weissgarten J, Liberman UA: Elevated serum 1,25-dihydroxyvitamin D concentrations in siblings with primary Fanconi's syndrome. N Engl J Med 1988;319:845–849.
140 Schneider JA, Schulman JD: Cystinosis; in Stanbury JB, Wyngaarden JB, Fredrickson DS, Goldstein JL, Brown MS (eds): The Metabolic Basis of Inherited Disease. New York, McGraw-Hill, 1983, pp 1844–1866.
141 Tieder M, Modai D, Samuel R, Arie R, Halabi A, Bab I, Gabizon D, Liberman UA: Hereditary hypophosphatemic rickets with hypercalciuria. N Engl J Med 1985;312:611–617.
142 Sermet-Gaudelus I, Garabedian M, Dechaux M, Lenoir G, Rey J, et al: Hereditary hypophosphatemic rickets with hypercalciuria: Report of a new kindred. Nephron 2001;88:83–86.
143 Tieder M, Arie R, Bab I, Maor J, et al: A new kindred with hereditary hypophosphatemic rickets with hypercalciuria: Implications for correct diagnosis and treatment. Nephron 1992;62:176–181.
144 Gazit D, Tieder M, Liberman UA, Passi-Even L, et al: Osteomalacia in hereditary hypophosphatemic rickets with hypercalciuria: A correlative clinical-histomorphometric study. J Clin Endocrinol Metab 1991;72:229–235.
145 Tieder M, Modai D, Shaked U, Samuel R, Arie R, Halabe A, Maor J, Weissgarten J, Averbukh Z, Cohen N: 'Idiopathic' hypercalciuria and hereditary hypophosphatemic rickets: Two phenotypical expressions of a common genetic defect. N Engl J Med 1987;316:125–129.
146 Jones A, Tzenova J, Frappier D, Crumley M, Roslin N, Kos C, Tieder M, Langman C, Proesmans W, Carpenter T, Rice A, Anderson D, Morgan K, Fujiwara T, et al: Hereditary hypophosphatemic rickets with hypercalciuria is not caused by mutations in the Na/P_i cotransporter NPT2 gene. J Am Soc Nephrol 2001;12:507–514.

Mark K. Drezner, MD
H4/554, Clinical Science Center, University of Wisconsin Medical School
600 Highland Avenue, Madison, WI 53792–5148 (USA)
Tel. +1 608 262 9288, Fax +1 608 263 9983, E-Mail mkd@medicine.wisc.edu

Hochberg Z (ed): Vitamin D and Rickets.
Endocr Dev. Basel, Karger, 2003, vol 6, pp 156–174

Vitamin D Biosynthesis and Vitamin D 1α-Hydroxylase Deficiency

Walter L. Miller, Anthony A. Portale

Department of Pediatrics, University of California San Francisco, San Francisco, Calif., USA

Contents

Vitamin D

The diagnosis and treatment of rickets and the understanding of its pathophysiology requires a thorough understanding of the biosynthesis of vitamin D. Recent work has elucidated this pathway at a molecular level. Vitamin D exists in two chemical forms: ergocalciferol (vitamin D_2) produced by plants, and cholecalciferol (vitamin D_3) produced in animal tissues and by the action of near-ultraviolet (290–310 nm) light on 7-dehydrocholesterol in human skin. Both are biologically inactive pro-hormones which differ only in the arrangement of the cholesterol side chain, and that must undergo 25-hydroxylation and 1α-hydroxylation before they can bind to and activate the vitamin D receptor (fig. 1). The 25-hydroxylation of vitamin D in the liver is probably catalyzed by more than one enzyme, including the mitochondrial cytochrome P450c27 enzyme that also hydroxylates carbons 26 and 27 to initiate bile acid synthesis.

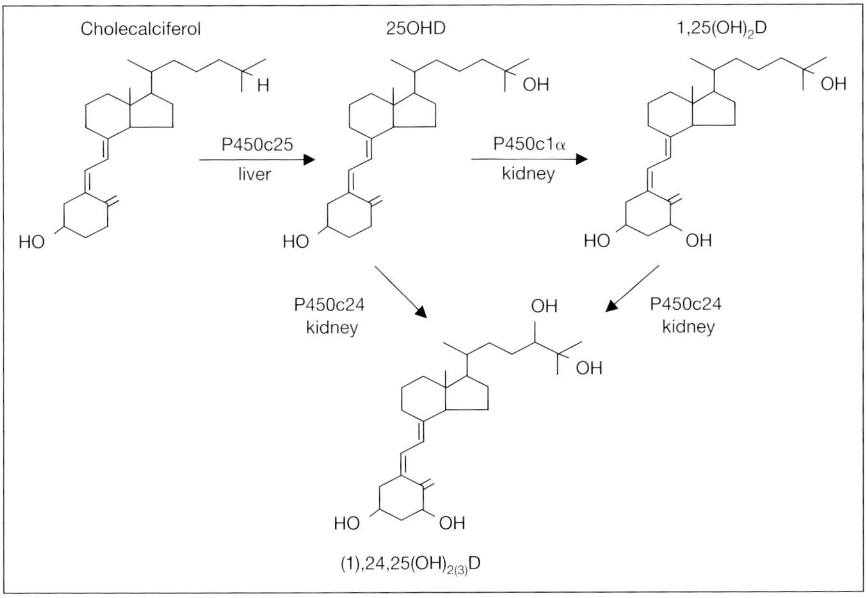

Fig. 1. Biosynthesis of vitamin D_3. Ultraviolet light (290 to 320 nm) cleaves the B ring of 7-dehydrocholesterol in the skin to yield cholecalciferol (vitamin D_3). Vitamin D, which circulates in blood bound to 56 kD vitamin D-binding protein, undergoes 25-hydroxylation in the liver. The resulting 25(OH)D, which is the most abundant form of vitamin D in the human circulation, can undergo 1α-hydroxylation in the kidney by P450c1α to yield the active hormonal compound $1,25(OH)_2D$. Both 25(OH)D and $1,25(OH)_2D$ also can undergo 24-hydroxylation in the kidney by P450c24 to yield either $24,25(OH)_2D$ or $1,24,25(OH)_3D$, respectively.

The circulating concentration of 25-hydroxyvitamin D (25(OH)D) is about 10^{-7} M, and is determined mainly by dietary intake and exposure to sunlight. About 75% of circulating vitamin D is 25-hydroxylated on a single pass through the liver, but this catalytic activity is not under tight hormonal regulation. Like vitamin D itself, 25(OH)D has minimal capacity to bind to the vitamin D receptor and elicit a biologic response.

The hormonally active form of vitamin D is 1,25-dihydroxyvitamin D ($1,25(OH)_2D$), formed by the 1α-hydroxylation of 25-OHD (fig. 1). Although circulating concentrations of $1,25(OH)_2D$ primarily reflect its synthesis in the kidney, 1α-hydroxylase activity is also found in placenta, brain, keratinocytes, macrophages and osteoblasts. Renal 1α-hydroxylase activity is tightly regulated by parathyroid hormone (PTH), calcium, phosphorus, and $1,25(OH)_2D$ itself [1, 2]. This is the hormonally regulated, rate-limiting, obligatorily bio-activating step. Because of its importance in calcium physiology and because it can be disordered in chronic renal failure, X-linked hypophosphatemic rickets, Fanconi syndrome in autosomal recessive 1α-hydroxylase deficiency (vitamin D-dependent rickets, type 1) and in other diseases, 1α-hydroxylase has been the subject of intense study for about 30 years.

Cytochrome P450

The known vitamin D metabolizing enzymes are all type I (mitochondrial) forms of cytochrome P450, which function as oxidases using electrons from NADPH and molecular oxygen [3, 4]. For catalysis by a type I P450, electrons from NADPH are first taken up by a flavoprotein termed ferredoxin reductase, which is bound to the inner mitochondrial membrane; ferredoxin reductase then passes the electrons to ferredoxin, an iron-sulfur protein that may be loosely associated with the inner membrane or may be in solution in the mitochondrial matrix. Ferredoxin can donate electrons to any mitochondrial form of cytochrome P450. The P450 moiety binds the substrate, receives electrons and molecular oxygen, and catalyzes the reaction using the iron of the heme group to coordinate the oxygen. Type II cytochrome P450 enzymes, such as the steroidogenic 17α-hydroxylase, 21-hydroxylase, and aromatase enzymes, and the hepatic enzymes involved in drug metabolism, are found in the endoplasmic reticulum, where they receive electrons from P450 oxidoreductase which is a different flavoprotein, occasionally facilitated by cytochrome b_5 [5], and without the need for an iron-sulfur protein. Most P450 enzymes can catalyze multiple reactions, and many reactions can be catalyzed by more than one distinct P450 enzyme.

Vitamin D 25-Hydroxylase

Uncertainty remains about the enzyme(s) catalyzing vitamin D 25-hydroxylation. The hepatic 25-hydroxylase was initially thought to be a microsomal enzyme. Studies of bile acid 26-hydroxylation led to the cloning of a rat liver mitochondrial P450 that had bile acid 26-hydroxylase activity, and vitamin D 25-hydroxylase activity [6–12]. When expressed in transfected cells this single P450 can catalyze both vitamin D 25-hydroxylation or cholesterol 26-hydroxylation. The corresponding human cDNA was cloned in 1991 [13] and is now termed P450c27, as it can hydroxylate both carbons 26 and 27 of cholesterol. However, genetic evidence indicates that other enzymes besides P450c27 probably catalyze vitamin D 25-hydroxylase activity. Mutations of P450c27 cause cerebrotendinous xanthomatosis [14], but a disorder of vitamin D biosynthesis has not been described in these patients. Furthermore, a single patient has been described with apparent vitamin D 25-hydroxylase deficiency but who lacked cerebrotendinous xanthomatosis [15]. A microsomal P450 with vitamin D 25-hydroxylase activity has been cloned from pig liver [16]; this enzyme shares 76% amino acid sequence identity with human P4502B6, but P4502B6 is not expressed in 5–10% of normal people. Thus, if P4502B6 is a human 25-hydroxylase, its activity is not indispensable. Thus, much remains to be determined about the biochemistry and genetics of vitamin D 25-hydroxylation. There may be more than one hepatic vitamin D 25-hydroxylase, so that the lack of a single enzyme may not cause a syndrome of 25-hydroxylase deficiency, accounting for the apparent absence of this hypothetical disease.

Vitamin D 24-Hydroxylase

The vitamin D 24-hydroxylase, P450c24, was cloned by purifying P450c24 from renal mitochondria, raising a polyclonal antiserum, and screening a rat kidney cDNA expression library [17]. This facilitated cloning the rat gene [18] and the human cDNA and gene [19, 20]. Studies with the purified rat renal enzyme [17] and with cells expressing the transfected human cDNA [19] show that P450c24 can catalyze the 24 hydroxylation of either 25(OH)D or 1,25$(OH)_2$D. The conversion 1,25$(OH)_2$D to 1,24,25$(OH)_3$D is inducible to 1,25$(OH)_2$D itself providing an important mechanism by which 1,25$(OH)_2$D regulates its own abundance by regulating its catabolism [21]. Thus P450c24 is the first step in the degradation of 1,25$(OH)_2$D via the C-24 side chain oxidation pathway, a major catabolic pathway for 1,25$(OH)_2$D in target tissues [22, 23]. 24-Hydroxylase activity is found in kidney, intestine, lymphocytes, fibroblasts, bone, skin, macrophages, and possible other tissues [24]. The gene for P450c24 is structurally related to the genes for the mitochondrial steroidogenic P450 enzymes, P450scc (the cholesterol side chain cleavage enzyme), and the two isozymes of P450c11: P450c11β (11β-hydroxylase) and P450c11AS (aldosterone synthetase) [18], suggesting that all of the mitochondrial P450s are closely related. This was confirmed by cloning the 1α-hydroxylase.

Vitamin D 1α-Hydroxylase

Although the 25 and 24-hydroxylases were cloned in 1990 and 1991, the 1α-hydroxylase was not cloned until the second half of 1997, when four independent groups using different approaches reported cloning the mouse, rat, and human vitamin D 1α-hydroxylase, P450c1α [25–30; for review, see 31]. The cloning of P450c1α was difficult because there is very little P450c1α protein in the kidney. Although physiologic maneuvers such as raising animals on a D-deficient, low-phosphorus diet in the absence of UV light will indeed increase 1α-hydroxylase activity, efforts to purify the enzyme as had been done for the 24- and 25-hydroxylases were consistently unsuccessful.

Kato's group increased P450c1α expression by using mice lacking the vitamin D receptor (VDR) [30]. Because these animals cannot respond to $1,25(OH)_2D$, they behave as though they are deficient in $1,25(OH)_2D$, and hence over-produce $1,25(OH)_2D$ by increasing P450c1α synthesis 10-fold. Cloning of the corresponding renal cDNA into cells that express a fusion of the ligand-binding domain of VDR and the yeast GAL4 DNA-binding domain, provided a vitamin-D based selection system. When these cells were also transfected with vectors for the ferredoxin and ferredoxin reductase needed by P450c1α, those expressing P450c1α could produce $1,25(OH)_2D$, thus activating the VDR/GAL4 fusion [30].

Two other groups [28, 29] prepared cDNA from the kidneys of rats raised on low calcium, low phosphorus, vitamin D-depleted diets. This physiologic manipulation stimulates 1α-hydroxylase activity while suppressing 24-hydroxylase activity. One group screened the corresponding cDNA library with a fragment of P450c24 cDNA corresponding to the relatively well-conserved heme-binding site, yielding a P450c1α clone [29]. The other group used oligonucleotides based on the conserved ferredoxin-binding and heme-binding sites of P450c24 and P450c25 for PCR amplification of the rat renal cDNA. This PCR product was cloned and used to screen a rat renal cDNA library identifying a P450c1α cDNA [28].

To circumvent the problem of the low renal abundance of P450c1α, we used cultured human keratinocytes [25], which have substantial vitamin D 1α-hydroxylase activity when grown in serum-free medium with very low concentrations of calcium [32–34]. These cells gave us a 100-fold enriched source of human P450c1α mRNA. Based on the relatively-well conserved sequences of the ferredoxin-binding site and heme-binding site of other mitochondrial P450 enzymes, we designed several sets of degenerate-sequence primers to amplify a 300-bp human keratinocyte cDNA fragment whose sequence resembled that of other mitochondrial P450s. We then prepared a human keratinocyte cDNA library, screened it with the 300-bp fragment and identified a 1.9-kb clone whose 5′ end was obtained by primer extension to yield the full-length 2.4-kb cDNA [25].

To establish that the keratinocyte P450 enzyme we had cloned was identical to the renal 1α-hydroxylase, rather than being an unrelated keratinocyte P450 that had gratuitous 1α-hydroxylase activity, we did four separate experiments [25].

First, we expressed our keratinocyte cDNA in mouse Leydig MA-10 cells, and found that the encoded enzyme catalyzed the conversion of 25(OH)D to 1,25$(OH)_2$D. The 1,25$(OH)_2$D product of this reaction was measured by a radioreceptor assay and its chemical identity was inferred by co-migration with authentic 1,25$(OH)_2$D standards on HPLC using two different solvent systems; furthermore, this reaction had a K_m of 2.7×10^{-7}, which is similar to the circulating concentrations of 25(OH)D. Second, we proved that the product of this reaction was authentic 1,25$(OH)_2$D, and not some other metabolite of vitamin D. Because the mouse Leydig MA-10 cells we used contain abundant ferredoxin and ferredoxin reductase, which are needed by all mitochondrial forms of cytochrome P450 [35]; expression of mitochondrial P450s in these cells yields 100- to 1,000-fold more activity than is achieved in non-steroidogenic cells [36]. This permitted us to prepare and purify enough of the 1,25$(OH)_2$D product to prove its complete chemical identity by gas chromatography/mass spectrometry. Third, we used reverse transcription/polymerase chain reaction (RT-PCR) to show that the same sequences we had cloned from keratinocytes were expressed in the human kidney, as well as in other tissues. Fourth, we obtained keratinocytes from a patient with vitamin D-dependent rickets, type I (VDDR-I), used RT-PCR to clone the patient's P450c1α cDNA and showed that the patient was a compound heterozygote for two different frameshift mutations. This provided definitive genetic proof that the same P450c1α is expressed in keratinocytes and in renal tubules, and provided the first proof that VDDR I is caused by mutations in P450c1α [25].

We then cloned and sequenced the human gene (now officially termed CYP27B1), localized it to chromosome 12 by somatic cell hybrid analysis, identified its transcriptional start site, and compared the structures of the genes for the four mitochondrial P450s now available (P450c1α, P450c24, P450scc, P450c11) [26]. The gene location on chromosome 12 was expected, as Labuda and coworkers had previously mapped VDDR-I to chromosome 12q13–14 by genetic linkage analysis [37] and then to a single YAC clone in chromosome 12q13.13 microsatellite haplotyping [38]. At about the same time, two other group also mapped the gene to 12q13.3 by fluorescence in situ hybridization (FISH) analysis [29, 39]. There is only one copy of the human P450c1α gene; it consists of 9 exons and 8 introns and, although it is substantially smaller than the genes for the other mitochondrial P450 enzymes, its intron/exon organization is very similar, especially to that of P450scc [26]. This strongly suggests that all the mitochondrial P450 enzymes belong to a single evolutionary lineage even though they have only 30–40% amino acid sequence identity with each other. At about the same time, Saruta's group also cloned the human P450c1α cDNA and gene [27] and soon thereafter, Kato's group reported the structure of the human P450c1α gene and four additional mutations causing VDDR-1 [39].

1α-Hydroxylase Deficiency

The first reported case of 1α-hydroxylase deficiency appears to be that of Prader et al. [40] who described a new form of rickets characterized by its appearance in the first year of life, presence of severe hypocalcemia but only moderate hypophosphatemia, and reversal of the clinical and laboratory findings of rickets by daily administration of high doses of vitamin D. Initially termed 'hereditary pseudo-vitamin D deficiency rickets' (PDDR), 'vitamin D dependency' because of its responsiveness to vitamin D, or vitamin D-dependent rickets type I, this disease is now known to be caused by loss-of-function mutations in P450c1α. And hence is now better termed vitamin D 1α-hydroxylase deficiency [25].

Patients with 1α-hydroxylase deficiency usually come to medical attention in the first 24 months of life with growth retardation, poor gross motor development, or generalized muscle weakness. Some infants are irritable when held, presumably due to bone pain, or develop pneumonia or seizures. Physical findings are similar to those observed in rickets due to simple vitamin D deficiency, and include enlargement of the costochondral junction of the ribs ('rachitic rosary'), enlargement of the wrists or ankles, genu varus, and in some cases, hypotonia, frontal bossing, enlarged sutures and fontanelles, or craniotabes (softening of the parieto-occipital area). Muscle traction on the softened rib cage can give rise to thoracic deformity, including pectus carinatum. Dental development is often affected, with delayed eruption, enamel hypoplasia, and early caries.

Radiographic examination of the long bones reveals the typical abnormalities of rickets, with widening of the metaphysis, fraying, cupping and widening of the zone of provisional calcification, and diffuse demineralization. Radiographs of the chest may reveal enlargement of the costochondral junctions, and older children may have bowing of the tibia and femur.

Most patients will have hypocalcemia, hypophosphatemia, and increased serum alkaline phosphatase activity and parathyroid hormone (PTH) concentrations are observed [40–47], as is typical of patients with vitamin D deficiency. When severe, hypocalcemia can cause tetany and seizures. Metabolic balance studies show that patients with 1α-hydroxylase deficiency have malabsorption of calcium and phosphorus and reduced urinary calcium excretion [42, 43, 46, 48]. Some patients also have the renal tubular abnormalities of hyperchloremic metabolic acidosis and generalized hyperaminoaciduria [40, 41, 43–46], findings that are also seen in patients with vitamin D deficiency [49].

The hallmarks of 1α-hydroxylase deficiency include reduced serum concentrations of $1,25(OH)_2D$ despite normal concentrations of 25(OH)D, and

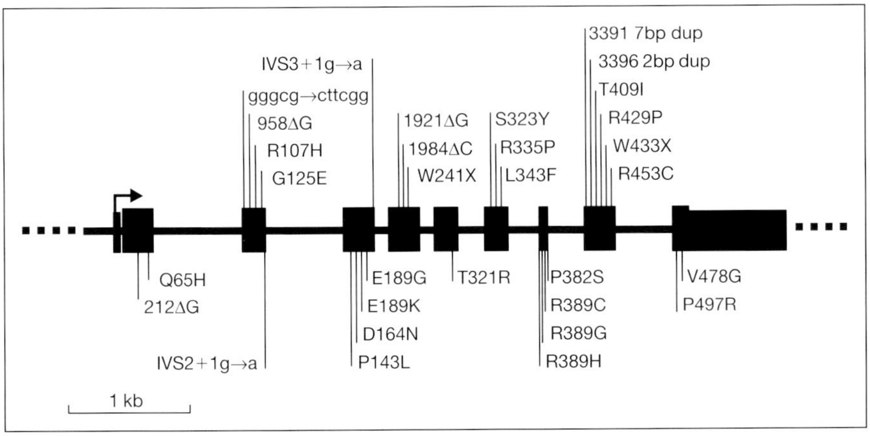

Fig. 2. Scale diagram of the intron/exon organization of the human P450c1α gene, as reported by Fu et al. [26]. All mutations causing 1α-hydroxylase deficiency reported through late 2002 are shown.

the reversal of clinical and laboratory abnormalities by administration of physiologic replacement doses of 1,25(OH)$_2$D [47, 50, 51]. These findings distinguish patients with 1α-hydroxylase deficiency from those with nutritional vitamin D deficiency in whom serum concentrations of 25(OH)D are reduced, or hereditary 1,25(OH)$_2$D-resistant rickets (vitamin D dependent rickets type II) in whom serum 1,25(OH)$_2$D is greatly increased. In some patients with 1α-hydroxylase deficiency, serum concentrations of 1,25(OH)$_2$D are nominally within the normal range [48, 52], although such values are inappropriately low given the reduced serum concentrations of calcium and phosphorus and increased concentrations of PTH, all of which should increase renal production of 1,25(OH)$_2$D. Indeed, administration of parathyroid extract failed to increase the serum concentration of 1,25(OH)$_2$D in a child with 1α-hydroxylase deficiency, in contrast to the increase induced in control subjects [53].

Molecular Genetics of 1α-Hydroxylase Deficiency

With the cloning of the 1α-hydroxylase gene, the molecular genetics of 1α-hydroxylase deficiency has now been studied thoroughly by several groups (fig. 2) [25, 39, 52, 55–57]. We identified the first P450c1α in a Caucasian-American girl with 1α-hydroxylase deficiency who was a compound heterozygote for two deletion/frameshift mutations in exon 2 of the gene, predicting

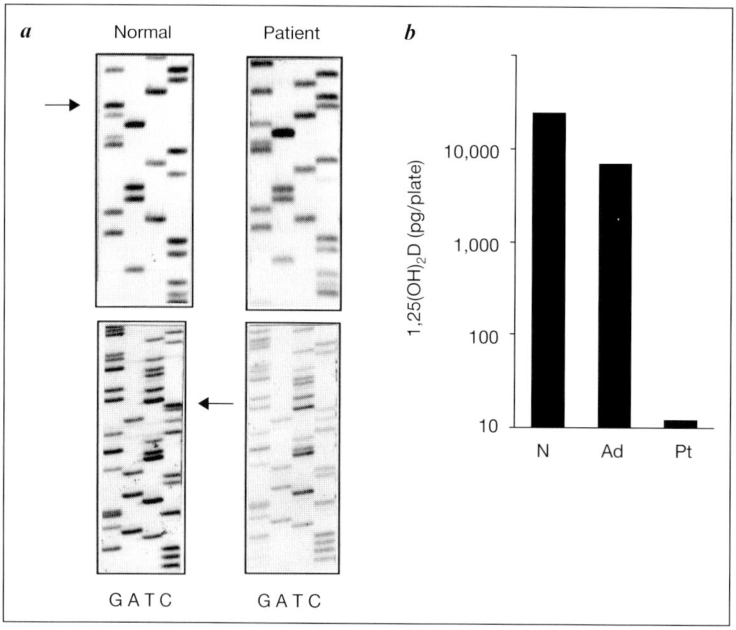

Fig. 3. Mutation of P450c1α causes 1α-hydroxylase deficiency. ***a*** Keratinocytes from a healthy person and from a patient with 1α-hydroxylase deficiency were used to prepare mRNA, which was reverse-transcribed, and the P450c1α cDNA was PCR-amplified using specific primers. The upper panel displays normal (left) and patient (right) cDNA sequence in the region of codon 211, showing that the G (arrow) in the normal sequence is deleted in the patient. The lower panel displays cDNA sequence in the region of codon 211, showing that the normal C (arrow) is deleted in the patient. Thus the patient was a compound heterozygote for two deletion/frameshift mutations. ***b*** 1α-Hydroxylase activity in keratinocytes from human neonatal foreskin (N), adult skin (Ad), and skin from a patient with 1α-hydroxylase deficiency (Pt). No activity was detected in the patient. The scale is logarithmic and begins at the level of detection of the assay.

premature truncation of the protein (fig. 3a) [25]. Cultured skin keratinocytes from the patient were devoid of 1α-hydroxylase activity (fig. 3b) [25]. Study of four unrelated Japanese patients studied confirmed that mutations in the 1α-hydroxylase gene could cause the clinical syndrome of 1α-hydroxylase deficiency [39]. However, several questions remained. It was not yet known whether all patients with the typical clinical syndrome of 1α-hydroxylase deficiency had the same disease. Furthermore, although it was known that 1α-hydroxylase deficiency was common in French Canada [54], it was not known whether such patients had two distinct mutations, as had been suggested by linkage analysis [38]. Finally, there was no information relating enzyme structure to its function.

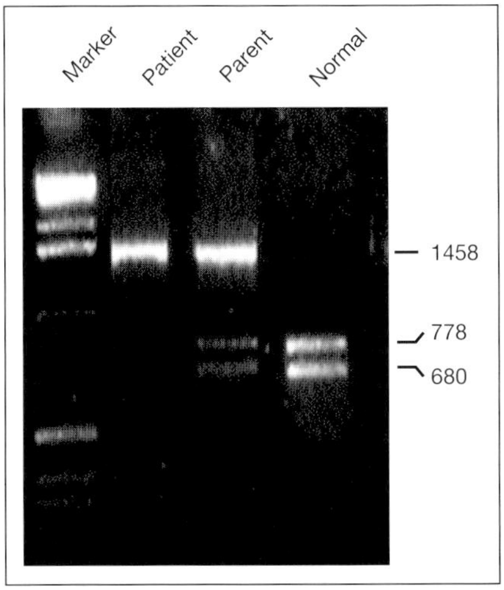

Fig. 4. Genetic diagnosis of the ΔG958 mutation commonly found among the Charlevoix French Canadian population. Mutation ΔG958 deletes a *Tai*I site. A 1,458-bp fragment was amplified from genomic DNA from a homozygously affected patient, an obligately heterozygous parent, and a homozygously unaffected normal control, and digested with *Tai*I. The patient's DNA, carrying ΔG958 on both alleles, is not cut; half of the parent's DNA is cut, and the normal DNA is cut to completion.

We first studied the P450c1α genes of nineteen patients with 1α-hydroxylase deficiency from seventeen families representing multiple ethnic groups, [52]. All of the patients were healthy at birth but came to medical attention within the first 24 months of life, most commonly because of growth retardation or poor gross motor development. All patients had typical laboratory findings of 1α-hydroxylase deficiency: hypocalcemia, hypophosphatemia, increased serum concentrations of alkaline phosphatase and parathyroid hormone, normal serum concentrations of 25(OH)D, and low or undetectable concentrations of $1,25(OH)_2$ D. All patients had radiographic evidence of rickets and all responded to physiologic replacement doses of $1,25(OH)_2D$. We identified the parental origin of each P450c1α mutation and correlated the mutations with microsatellite haplotyping of chromosome 12q13, using the markers D12S90, D12S305, and D12S104. Among the five French-Canadian families in our population, nine of ten unique alleles carried the 4-7-1 microsatellite haplotype identified by Labuda's group as found in the Charlevoix region of Quebec, and all nine of these carried a deletion of guanosine at position 958 (ΔG958), in codon 88. This changes the reading frame and leads to premature termination of translation. This mutation deletes the G in the sequence 5′ACGT3′, destroying the sequence normally recognized by the endonucleases *Tai*I and *Mae*II, permitting a rapid, accurate PCR-based diagnostic test that can detect this mutation in genomic DNA from any source (fig. 4) [52].

Another group had characterized the P450c1α genes of four French-Canadian patients [21], finding the homozygous ΔG958 mutation in three and

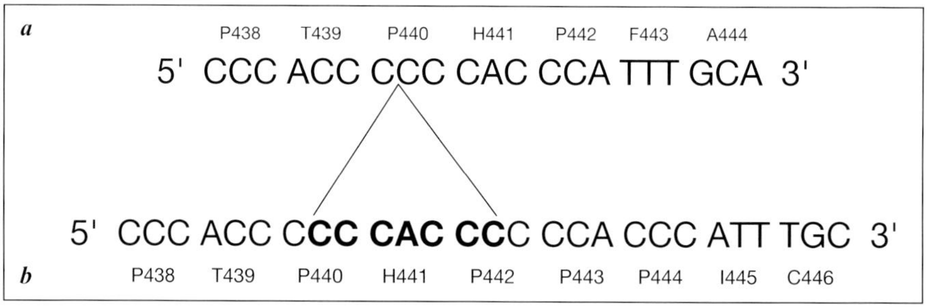

Fig. 5. The 7-bp duplication. ***a*** The sequence CCCACCC is normally duplicated in exon 8, encoding residues 438 to 442 (Pro-Thr-Pro-His-Pro). ***b*** The mutation involves the insertion of a third copy of the CCCACCC sequence, which changes the reading frame, beginning with residue 443. The *triplication* is arbitrarily shown as an insert at codon 440 between the two normal copies of the CCCACCC sequence. It is not possible to specify which of the three copies in the mutant sequence is new.

the homozygous duplication of a 7-bp sequence in exon 8 in the fourth, and suggested that mutation ΔG958 is the Charlevoix mutation and that the 7-bp duplication is the Acadian mutation, but they did not perform microsatellite haplotyping to confirm this [58]. However, we found this 7-bp duplication on seven separate alleles in six families (fig. 5) [38]. Four of these alleles carried the haplotype 9-7-2 but were found in Polish, Chinese, and Hispanic patients. The other three alleles bearing the 7-bp duplication carried the haplotypes 9-6-2, 9-3-3, and 6-6-1, and were found among Filipino, Caucasian-American, and African-American patients. Only one patient (from Poland) carried the 'Acadian' 6-7-2 haplotype, but that allele carried the missense mutation P497R, rather than the 7-bp duplication. Smith et al. [55] also identified two unrelated patients from the United Kingdom who were homozygous for this same 7-bp duplication. Thus, the 7-bp duplication arose de novo among many different ethnic groups, and the identity of the 'Acadian' mutation remains to be established.

There is considerable clinical phenotypic variation among patients with 1α-hydroxylase deficiency; hence, there has been considerable interest in correlating P450c1α mutations with varying degrees of enzymatic activity and with varying degrees of clinical severity. Among the 14 mutations we found in our initial cohort of 19 patients, 7 were missense mutations [52]. East of these was recreated in a P450c1α expression vector, expressed in MA-10 cells, and analyzed for 1α-hydroxylase activity. However, we were surprised to find that none of these conferred activity significantly greater than the low level of activity normally found in MA-10 cells [52]. Similarly, two other groups examined two British patients [55] and 8 Japanese patients [56], including one who had mild clinical findings, yet none of the missense mutations identified in these

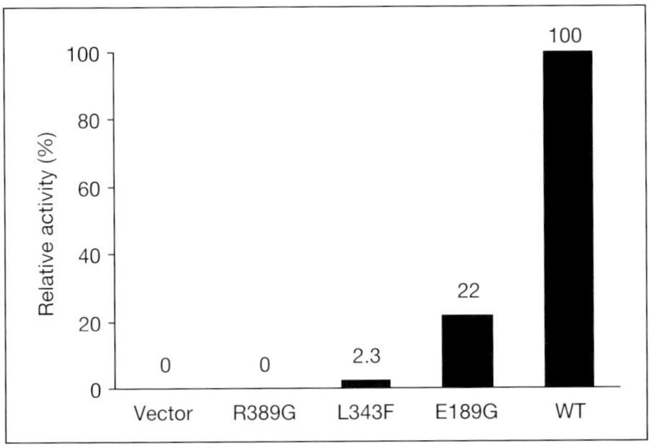

Fig. 6. 1α-Hydroxylase activity of the P450c1α mutants. The 3 novel missense mutations, R389G, L343F and E189G, were recreated in a P450c1α cDNA expression vector and transfected into mouse Leydig MA-10 cells. The mutation R389G had no 1α-hydroxylase activity, as did the vector control (vector), mutation L343F retained 2.3% of wild-type activity (WT), and mutation E189G retained 22% of wild-type activity [57]. Data are expressed as a percentage of the activity of the wild-type cDNA.

10 patients could be shown to retain any activity, although the assays employed differed from ours, and their sensitivities cannot be compared. However, we recently analyzed six additional patients, four of whom had classic findings, but two of whom had mild hypocalcemia and normal serum $1,25(OH)_2D$ concentrations [57]. We found the mutations in each, including three new missense mutations. One of these, R389G, was totally inactive, but mutant L343F retained 2.3% of wild-type activity, and mutant E189G retained 22% of wild-type activity (fig. 6). The two mutations that confer partial enzyme activity in vitro were found in the 2 patients with mild laboratory abnormalities, indicating that such mutations contribute to the variable phenotype observed in patients with 1α-hydroxylase deficiency [57].

The patient who was homozygous for the E189G mutation came to medical attention because of hypotonia and a leg deformity and had secondary hyperparathyroidism, but serum concentrations of calcium, phosphorus, and $1,25(OH)_2D$ were not reduced. The diagnosis of 1α-hydroxylase deficiency was considered when the patient failed to respond to large doses of vitamin D but showed rapid improvement with administration of 0.25 μg per day of $1,25(OH)_2D$. In the patient whose mutation retained 2.3% of wild type activity, serum concentrations of 25(OH)D and $1,25(OH)_2D$ were not reduced, but the diagnosis was more apparent because of hypophosphatemia and increased concentrations of alkaline phosphatase and PTH. Such patients demonstrate that the classical laboratory criteria for the diagnosis of 1α-hydroxylase deficiency may fail to identify patients with partial but significant defects in this enzyme, and hence 1α-hydroxylase deficiency syndromes may be more common than previously appreciated.

Structure and Function of 1α-Hydroxylase

Although the tertiary structures of mitochondrial cytochrome P450 have not yet been determined, most bacterial P450s are also class I, and the structures of several bacterial P450 enzymes have been determined by X-ray crystallography [59–61]. Comparisons of the structures of these enzymes reveals remarkable conservation of their topology and tertiary structure, despite low amino acid sequence identity [62]. Using a computer algorithm that aligns sequences on the basis of regions of predicted secondary structure rather than amino acid sequence identity, we aligned P450c1α with three bacterial class I P450 enzymes, permitting preliminary assignment of the locations of the amino acid replacement mutations and a prediction of the likely mechanisms by which such mutations disrupt enzyme activity (fig. 7).

Mutation Q65H is in α-helix A', T409I is in strand 3 of β-sheet 1, and R389H is in strand 4 of β-sheet 1. Although distant from one another in the linear amino acid sequence, these residues are clustered in the β-sheet domain that probably interacts with the inner mitochondrial membrane and defines the substrate entry channel. Their locations suggest that these mutations probably disrupt substrate binding rather than disrupting the catalytic site. E189L lies in the E-helix and would disrupt the four-helix bundle consisting of the D, E, I, and L helices, and thus would significantly disrupt the structure of 1α-hydroxylase. R429P inserts a proline at the junction of the K' helix and the meander, changing the direction of the carbon backbone causing a major conformational change. R453C, which is two residues away from the thiolate cysteine at position 455, probably disrupts a salt bridge that interacts with one of the heme propionate groups, much like the corresponding P440C mutation in P450c17, which causes complete 17α-hydroxylase deficiency [63], and like the R435C mutation in P450arom, which causes complete aromatase deficiency [64]. Mutant P497R lies near strand 3 of β-sheet 3, which participates in defining the top of the substrate-binding pocket; again, any mutation inserting or deleting a proline will change the direction of the carbon backbone, causing a conformational mutant.

Three different missense mutations have been described in codon 389, R389G [57], R389H [52] and R389C [56], all three of which are inactive. R389 aligns with the highly conserved arginine in the β1–4 helix of type 1 P450 proteins [52]; this arginine coordinates one of the heme propionate side chains [62, 65] and hence is probably essential for catalytic activity. It is not known

```
cα     MTQTLKYASRVFHRVRWAPELGASLGYREYHSA----------RRSLADIPGPSTPSFLAELFCKGGLS   59
cam    -------------------------------MTTETIQSNANLAPLPPHVPEHLVFDFDMYNPSNLSA-   37
terp   -------------------------------------------MDARATIPEHIARTVILPQGYA----   22
eryF   ---------------------------------------------------MTTVPDLESDSFHV----   14
                                                                  αA'
          ▽Q65H                                         ▽R107H
c1α    RLHELQVQGAAHFG---PVWLASFG-TVRTVYVAAPALVEELLRQEGPRPER--CS-----------FSPWTEHRRCRQRAC  124
cam    GVQEAWAVLQESNV--PDLVWTRCNG--GHWIATRGQLIREAYEDYRHFSSE--CP-----------FIPREAGEAY-----  97
terp   -DDEVIYPAFKWLRDEQPLAMAHIEGYDPMWIATKHADVMQIGKQPGLFSNAEGSE-----------ILYDQNNEAFMRSIS  92
eryF   ----DWYRTYAELRETAPVTPVRFLGQD-AWLVTGYDEAKAALSDLRLSSDPKKKYPGVEVEFPAYLGFPEDVRNYFA----  87
           αA          β1-1           β1-2     αB        β1-5                        αB'
           ▽G125E                ▽P125L                ▽D164N                      ▽E189G/K
c1α    -------GLLTAEG-EEWQRLRSLLAPLLLRPQAAARYAGTLNNVVCDLVRRLRRQRGRGTGPPALVRDVAGEFYKFGLEGIAAVLLG  204
cam    ------DFIPTSMDPPEQRQFRALANQVVGMPVVDK----LENRIQELACSLIESLRP----Q-GQCNFTEDYAEPFPIRIFMLLAGL  170
terp   GGCPHVIDSLTSMDPPTHTAYRGLTLNWFQPASIRK----LEENIRRIAQASVQRLLDF---D-GECDFMTDCALYYPLHVVMTALGV  172
eryF   -------TNMGTSDPPTHTRLRKLVSQEFTVRRVEAM----RPRVEQITAELLDEVGD----S-GVVDIVDRFAHPLPIKVICELLGV  159
                         αC          αC'              αD                β3-1  αE'          αE

c1α    SRLGCLEAQVPPDTETFIRAVGSVFVSTLLTM------AMPHWLRHLVPGPWGRLCRDWDQMFAFAQRHVERR  271
cam    -----PEEDIPHLKYLTDQMTR----------PD--GSM-----------TFAEAKEALYDYLIPIIEQRRQK  215
terp   -----PEDDEPLMLKLTQDFFGVHEPDEQAVA------APRQSADEAAR-RFHETIATFYDYFNGFTVDRRSC  233
eryF   -----DEKYRGEFGRWSSEILV----------MDPERAE-----------QRGQAAREVVNFILDLVERRRTE  206

              αF                                        T321R▽ ▽S323YS αG   ▽R335P   ▽L343F
c1α    EAEAAMRNGGQPEKDLESGAHLT-HFLFR--E-ELPAQSILGNVTELLLAGVDTVSNTLSWALYELSRHPEVQTALHSEITAALSPGSS 356
cam    PGTDAISIVAN-------------GQV--NGR-PITSDEAKRMCGLLLVGGLDTVVNFLSFSMEFLAKSPEHRQELIERP--------- 279
terp   PKDDVMSLLAN-------------SKL--DGN-YIDDKYINAYYVAIATAGHDTTSSSSGGAIIGLSRNPEQLALAKSDP--------- 297
eryF   PGDDLLSALIRVQ-------------D--DDDGRLSADELTSIALVLLLAGFEASVSLIGIGTYLLLTHPDQLALVRRDP--------- 271
          αH                     β5-1   β5-2               αI                        αJ
                                 ▽P382S  ▽R389C/G/H          ▽T409I                   ▽R429P
c1α    AYPSATVLSQLPLLKAVVKEVLRLYPVVPGNSR-VPDKDIHVGDYIIPKNTLVTLCHYATSRDPAQFPEPNSFRPARWLGEG-P----T 439
cam    -----------ERIPAACEELLRRFSLV-ADGRILTSDYEFHG-VQLKKGDQILLPQMLSGLDERENACPMHVDFSRQKVS-------- 347
terp   -----------ALIPRLVDEAVRWTAPVKSFMRTALADTEVRG-QNIKRGDRIMLSYPSANRDEEVFSNPDEFDITRFPNR-------- 366
eryF   -----------SALPNAVEEILRYIAPPETTTRFAAEEVEIRG-VAIPQYSTVLVANGAANRDPKQFPDPHRFDVTRDTRG-------- 340
                  αK               β1-4       β2-1  β2-2     β1-3      αK'       Meander
              ▽R453C                         ▽V478G                       ▽P497R
c1α    PHPFASLPFGFGKRSCMGRRLAELELQMALAQILTHFEV--QPEPG-AAPVR-PKTRTVLVPERSINLQFLDR---   508
cam    -----HTTFGHGSHLCLGQHLARREIIVTLKEWLTRIPDFSIAPGA-QIQHK-S-GIVSGVQALPLVWDPATTKAV   414
terp   -----HLGFGWGAHMCLGQHLAKLEMKIFFEELLPKLK--SVELSG-PPRLV-ATNFVGGPKNVPIRFTKA-----   428
eryF   -----HLSFGQGIHFCMGRPLAKLEGEVALRALFGRFPALSLGIDADDVVWRRS-LLLRGIDHLPVRLDG------   404
          Cys-pocket             αL                β3-3      β4-1       β4-2  β3-2
```

Fig. 7. Alignment of the sequence of human P450c1α (top) with the sequences of the crystallographically solved bacterial class I P450 proteins P450cam, P450trp, and P450eryF [52]. The names of the various α-helices and β-sheets are given below, with the α-helices highlighted in boldface and the β-sheets underlined. The location of the 'meander' and Cys pocket also are shown. The location of the known amino acid replacement mutations in P450c1α are shown above its sequence with downward pointing arrows.

whether these mutants can even bind heme. The mutation L343F [57] changes leucine, a small uncharged residue to phenylalanine, into a bulky one. L343 lies in the J helix, which is a structurally conserved region that is important structurally, but not catalytically. The mutation L343F could disrupt activity by creating a conformational mutant. The mutation E189G, which retained 22% of wild type activity [57] lies in the E-helix. A change from glutamic acid to glycine removes a 3-carbon side chain and replaces an acidic residue with a neutral one;

such a change could cause a conformational disturbance that still permits substrate binding and interaction with ferredoxin, albeit at decreased efficiency.

Another group recently analyzed P450c1α using essentially the same sequence alignments that we had used [66]. They suggested that mutations of residues R107, G125, and P497, which are located in the substrate-recognition region, would abolish enzyme activity by disrupting the tertiary structure of the substrate-heme pocket. They also suggested that R389 and R453 are involved in heme-propionate binding, and that D164, which is negatively charged and located in the D-helix, would stabilize the four-helix bundle, possibly by forming a salt bridge. Residue T321 was thought to be required for the activation of molecular oxygen [66].

Treatment

In the earliest reports, 1α-hydroxylase deficiency was treated with large doses of vitamin D_2, 50,000–200,000 units per day, which reversed the clinical, chemical, and radiographic abnormalities, and improved growth [40, 41–43]. However, the availability of activated forms of vitamin D has now rendered such therapy obsolete. Hypocalcemia and hyperparathyroidism are reversed and rickets are healed by administration of 1–3 μg/day (80–100 ng/kg) of $1\alpha(OH)D_3$ [67], a 1α-hydroxylated analogue of vitamin D that requires 25-hydroxylation in the liver. The synthetic analogue dihydrotachysterol (DHT) is not 1α-hydroxylated, but carries a hydroxyl group in the 3α-position; rotation of the A-ring about the 6–7 carbon bond brings this group into a 'pseudo-1α-hydroxyl' configuration, so that DHT is active in the absence of 1α-hydroxylation. Typical doses are 50 mg/kg/day in infancy or 0.5–1.0 mg/day in adults.

Most authorities currently use physiologic replacement doses of $1,25(OH)_2D_3$ (calcitriol), the most potent and most rapidly acting form of vitamin D. Oral administration of 0.25–2.0 μg/day (10–400 ng/kg/day) of $1,25(OH)_2D$ induced rapid correction of hypocalcemia, secondary hyperparathyroidism and rickets, restoration of bone mineral content, and repair of bone architecture [47]. The maintenance dose of $1,25(OH)_2D$ typically is lower than that needed to initiate healing of rickets; therapy must be life-long and is predictably successful [52]. Regardless of the form of vitamin D therapy, it is essential to monitor serum calcium, phosphorus and parathyroid hormone concentrations. A substantial calcium intake must be ensured, especially during the bone healing that accompanies the initial phase of therapy. One generally aims to increase the total serum calcium concentration into the low-normal range (8.5–9 mg/dl), sufficient to suppress the parathyroid hormone concentration to values just below the upper limit of normal; higher calcium values increase the risk of hypercalciuria and nephrocalcinosis. It is important to monitor the excretion of urinary calcium. The ratio of urinary calcium to urinary creatinine in a single urine specimen should remain less than 0.25; the 24-hour urinary excretion of calcium should remain below 4 mg/kg.

References

1 Kumar R: Metabolism of 1,25-dihydroxy vitamin D_3. Physiol Rev 1984;64:478–504.

2 Breslau NA: Normal and abnormal regulation of 1,25$(OH)_2$D synthesis. Am J Med Sci 1988;296: 417–425.

3 Nebert DW, Gonzalez FJ: P450 genes: Structure, evolution and regulation. Ann Rev Biochem 1987;56:945–993.

4 Black SD, Coon MJ: P-450 cytochromes: Structure and function. Adv Enzymol Relat Areas Mol Biol 1987;60:35–87.

5 Auchus RJ, Lee TC, Miller WL: Cytochrome b_5 augments the 17,20 lyase activity of human P450c17 without direct electron transfer. J Biol Chem 1998;73:3158–3165.

6 Andersson S, Davis D, Dahlback H, Jornvall H, Russel D: Cloning structure, and expression of the mitochondrial cytochrome P-450 sterol 26-hydroxylase, a bile acid biosynthetic enzyme. J Biol Chem 1989;264:8222–8229.

7 Dahlback H, Wikvall K: 25-Hydroxylation of vitamin D by a cytochrome P-450 from rabbit liver mitochondria. J Biochem 1988;252:207–213.

8 Masumoto O, Ohyama Y, Okuda K: Purification and characterization of vitamin D 25-hydroxylase from rat liver mitochondria. J Biol Chem 1988;263:14256–14260.

9 Shayiq R, Avadhani N: Purification and characterization of a hepatic mitochondrial cytochrome P450 active in aflatoxin B1 metabolism. Biochemistry 1989;28:7546–7554.

10 Wikvall K: Hydroxylations in biosynthesis of bile acids: Isolation of a cytochrome P-450 from rabbit liver mitochondria catalyzing 26-hydroxylation of C-27 steroids. J Biol Chem 1984;259: 3800–3804.

11 Usui E, Noshiro M, Okuda K: Molecular cloning of cDNA for vitamin D_3 25-hydroxylase from rat liver mitochondria. FEBS Lett 1990;262:135–138.

12 Su P, Rennert H, Shayiq RM, Yamamoto R, Zheng Y, Addya S, Strauss JF III, Avadhani NG: A cDNA encoding a rat mitochondrial cytochrome P450 catalyzing both the 26-hydroxylations of cholesterol and 25-hydroxylation of vitamin D_3: Gonadotropic regulation of the cognate mRNA in ovaries. DNA Cell Biol 1990;9:657–665.

13 Cali JJ, Russell DW: Characterization of human sterol 27-hydroxylase: A mitochondrial cytochrome P-450 that catalyzes multiple oxidation reaction in bile acid biosynthesis. J Biol Chem 1991;266: 7774–7778.

14 Garuti R, Lelli N, Barozzini M, Dotti MT, Frederico A, Bertolini S, Calandra S: Partial deletion of the gene encoding sterol 27-hydroxylase in a subject with cerebrotendinous xanthomatosis. J Lipid Res 1996;37:662–672.

15 Casella SJ, Reiner BJ, Chen TC, Holick MF, Harrison HE: A possible genetic defect in 25-hydroxylation as a cause of rickets. J Pediatr 1994;124:929–932.

16 Postlind H, Axen E, Bergman T, Wikvall K: Cloning, structure and expression of a cDNA encoding vitamin D_3 25-hydroxylase. Biochem Biophys Res Commun 1997;241:491–497.

17 Ohyama Y, Noshiro M, Okuda K: Cloning and expression of cDNA encoding 25-hydroxyvitamin D_3 24-hydroxylase. FEBS Lett 1991;278:195–198.

18 Ohyama Y, Noshior M, Eggertsen G, Gotoh O, Kato Y, Bjorkhem I, Okuda K: Structural characterization of the gene encoding rat 25-hydroxyvitamin D_3 24-hydroxylase. Biochemistry 1993;32: 76–82.

19 Chen KS, Prahl JM, DeLuca HF: Isolation and expression of human 1,25-dihydroxyvitamin D_3 24-hydroxylase cDNA. Proc Natl Acad Sci USA 1993;90:4543–4547.

20 Chen KS, DeLuca HF: Cloning of the human 1α-25-dihydroxyvitamin D_3–24-hydroxylase gene promoter and identification of two vitamin D-responsive elements. Biochim Biophys Acta 1995;1263:1–9.

21 Xie Z, Munson SJ, Huang N, Portale AA, Miller WL, Bikle DD: The mechanism of 1,25-dihydroxyvitamin D_3 autoregulation in keratinocytes. J Biol Chem 2002;277:36987–36990.

22 Makin G, Lohnes D, Byford V, Ray R, Jones G: Target cell metabolism of 1,25 dihydroxyvitamin D_3 to calcitroic acid. Biochem J 1989;262:173–180.

23 Tomon M, Tenenhouse H, Jones G: 1,25-Dihydroxyvitamin D_3-induced catabolism of vitamin D metabolites in mouse intestine. Am J Physiol 1990;258:G557–G563.

24 Ambrecht H, Okuda K, Wongsurawat N, Nemani R, Chen M, Boltz M: Characterization and regulation of vitamin D hydroxylases. J Steroid Biochem Mol Biol 1992;43:1073–1081.

25 Fu GK, Lin D, Zhang MYH, Bikle DD, Shackleton CHL, Miller WL, Portale AA: Cloning of human 25-hydroxy vitamin D-1α-hydroxylase and mutations causing vitamin D-dependant rickets type I. Mol Endocrinol 1997;11:1961–1970.

26 Fu GK, Portale AA, Miller WL: Complete structure of the human gene for the vitamin D 1α-hydroxylase, P450c1a. DNA Cell Biol 1997;16:1499–1507.

27 Monkawa T, Yoshida T, Wakino S, Shinki T, Anazawa H, DeLuca HF, Suda T, Hayashi M, Saruta T: Molecular cloning of cDNA and genomic DNA for human 25-hydroxyvitamin D_3 1α-hydroxylase. Biochem Biophys Res Commun 1997;239:527–533.

28 Shinki T, Shimada H, Wakino S, Anazawa H, Hayashi M, Saruta T, DeLuca H: Cloning and expression of rat 25-hydroxyvitamin D_3–1α-hydroxylase cDNA. Proc Natl Acad Sci USA 1997;94: 12920–12925.

29 St-Arnaud R, Messerlian S, Moir JM, Omdahl JL, Glorieux FH: The 25-hydroxyvitamin D 1α-hydroxylase gene maps to the pseudovitamin D-deficiency rickets (PDDR) disease locus. J Bone Miner Res 1997;12:1552–1559.

30 Takayama K, Kitanaka S, Sato T, Kobori M, Yanagisawa J, Kato S: 25-Hydroxyvitamin D_3 1α-hydroxylase and vitamin D synthesis. Science 1997;277:1827–1830.

31 Miller WL, Portale AA: Genetic disorders of vitamin D biosynthesis. Endocrinol Metab Clin North Am 1999;28:825–840.

32 Bikle DD, Nemanic MK, Gee E, Elias P: 1,25-Dihydroxyvitamin D_3 production by human keratinocytes. J Clin Invest 1986;78:557–566.

33 Bikle D, Nemanic M, Whitney J, Elias P: Neonatal human foreskin keratinocytes produce 1,25-dihydroxyvitamin D_3. Biochemistry 1986;25:1545–1548.

34 Bikle D, Pillai S: Vitamin D, calcium and epidermal differentiation. Endocr Rev 1993;14:3–19.

35 Miller WL: Molecular biology of steroid hormone synthesis. Endocr Rev 1988;9:295–318.

36 Fardella CE, Hum DW, Rodriguez H, Zhang G, Barry F, Bloch CA, Miller WL: Gene conversion in the CYP11B2 gene encoding aldosterone synthase (P450c11AS) is associated with, but does not cause, the syndrome of corticosterone methyl oxidase II deficiency. J Clin Endocrinol Metab 1996;81:321–326.

37 Labuda M, Morgan K, Glorieux FH: Mapping autosomal recessive vitamin D dependency type 1 to chromosonal 12q14 by linkage analysis. Am J Hum Genet 1990;47:28–36.

38 Labuda M, Labuda D, Korab-Laskowska M, Cole DEC, Zietkiewicz E, Weissenbach J, Popowska E, Pronicka E, Root AW, Glorieux FH: Linkage disequilibrium analysis in young populations: Pseudo-vitamin D-deficiency rickets and the founder effect in French Canadians Am J Hum Genet 1996;59:633–643.

39 Kitanaka S, Takeyama K, Murayama A, Sato T, Okumura K, Nogami M, Hasegawa Y, Niimi H, Yanagisawa J, Tanaka T, Kato S: Inactivating mutations in the 25-hydroxyvitamin D_3 1α-hydroxylase gene in patients with pseudovitamin D-deficiency rickets. N Engl J Med 1998;338:653–661.

40 Prader A, Illig R, Heierli E: Eine besondere form des primare vitamin-D-resistenten rachitis mit hypocalcamie und autosomal-dominanten erbgang: Die hereditare pseudomangelrachitis. Helv Paediatr Acta 1961;16:452–468.

41 Stoop JW, Schraagen MJ, Tiddens HA: Pseudo vitamin D deficiency rickets Report of four new cases. Acta Paediatr Scand 1967;56:607–616.

42 Dent CE, Friedman M, Watson L: Hereditary pseudo-vitamin D deficiency rickets ('Hereditare pseudo-mangelrachitis'). J Bone Joint Surg Br 1968;50:708–719.

43 Matsuda I, Sugai M, Ohsawa T: Laboratory findings in a child with pseudo-vitamin D deficiency rickets. Helv Paediatr Acta 1969;24:329–336.

44 Fanconi A, Prader A: Hereditary pseudo-vitamin D deficiency rickets. Helv Paediatr Acta 1969;24: 423–447.

45 Arnaud C, Maijer R, Reade T, Scriver CR, Whelan DT: Vitamin D dependency: an inherited postnatal syndrome with secondary hyperparathyroidism. Pediatrics 1970;46:871–880.

46 Hamilton R, Harrison J, Fraser D, Radde I, Morecki R, Paunier L: The small intestine in vitamin D dependent rickets. Pediatrics 1970;45:364–373.

47 Delvin EE, Glorieux FH, Marie PJ, Pettifor JM: Vitamin D dependency: Replacement therapy with calcitriol. J Pediatr 1981;99:26–34.

48 Balsan S: Hereditary pseudo-deficiency rickets or vitamin D-dependency type I; in Glorieux FH (ed): Rickets. New York, Vevey/Raven Press, 1991, pp 155–165.

49 Fraser D, Kooh SW, Scriver CR: Hyperparathyroidism as the cause of hyperaminoaciduria and phosphaturia in human vitamin D deficiency. Pediatr Res 1967;1:425–435.

50 Fraser D, Kooh SW, Kind HP, Holick MF, Tanaka Y, DeLuca HF: Pathogenesis of hereditary vitamin-D-dependent rickets: An inborn error of vitamin D metabolism involving defective conversion of 25-hydroxyvitamin D to 1α,25-dihydroxyvitamin D. N Engl J Med 1973;289: 817–822.

51 Scriver CR, Reade TM, DeLuca HF, Hamstra AJ: Serum 1,25-dihydroxyvitamin D levels in normal subjects and in patients with hereditary rickets or bone disease. N Engl J Med 1978;299:976–979.

52 Wang JT, Lin CJ, Burridge SM, Fu GK, Labuda M, Portale AA, Miller WL: Genetics of vitamin D 1α-hydroxylase deficiency in 17 families. Am J Hum Genet 1998;63:1694–1702.

53 Aarskog D, Aksnes L, Markestad T: Effect of parathyroid hormone on cAMP and 1,25-dihydroxyvitamin D formation and renal handling of phosphate in vitamin D-dependent rickets. Pediatrics 1983;1:59–63.

54 De Braekeleer M, Larochelle J: Population genetics of vitamin D-dependent rickets in northeastern Quebec. Ann Hum Genet 1991;55:283–290.

55 Smith SJ, Rucka AK, Berry JL, Davies M, Mylchreest S, Paterson CR, Heath DA, Tassabehji M, Read AP, Mee AP, Mawer EB: Novel mutations in the 1α-hydroxylase (P450c1) gene in three families with pseudovitamin D-deficiency rickets resulting in loss of functional enzyme activity in blood-derived macrophages. J Bone Miner Res 1999;14:730–739.

56 Kitanaka S, Murayama A, Sakaki T, Inouye K, Seino Y, Fukumoto S, Shima M, Yukizane S, Takayanagi M, Niimi H, Takeyama K, Kato S: No enzyme activity of 25-hydroxyvitamin D_3 1α-hydroxylase gene product in pseudovitamin D deficiency rickets including that with mild clinical manifestation. J Clin Endocrinol Metab 1999;84:4111–4117.

57 Wang X, Zhang MYH, Miller WL, Portale AA: Novel gene mutations in patients with 1α-hydroxylase deficiency that confer partial enzyme activity in vitro. J Clin Endocrinol Metab 2002;87:2424–2430.

58 Yoshida T, Monkawa T, Tenenhouse H, Goodyear P, Shinki T, Suda T, Wakino S, Hayashi M, Saruta T: Two novel 1α-hydroxylase mutations in French-Canadians with vitamin D dependency rickets type I. Kidney Int 1998;54:1437–1443.

59 Poulos TL, Finzel BC, Howard AJ: High-resolution crystal structure of cytochrome P450cam. J Mol Biol 1987;195:687–700.

60 Hasemann CA, Ravichandran KG, Peterson JA, Deisenhofer J: Crystal structure and refinement of cytochrome P450terp at 2.3 A resolution. J Mol Biol 1994;236:1169–1185.

61 Cupp-Vickery JR, Poulos TL: Structure of cytochrome P450eryF involved in erythromycin biosynthesis. Nat Struct Biol 1995;2:144–153.

62 Hasemann CA, Kurumbail RG, Boddupalli SS, Peterson JA, Deisenhofer J: Structure and function of cytochromes P450: A comparative analysis of three crystal structures. Structure 1995;3: 41–62.

63 Fardella CE, Hum DW, Homoki J, Miller WL: Point mutation of Arg440 to His in cytochrome P450c17 causes severe 17α-hydroxylase deficiency. J Clin Endocrinol Metab 1994;79:160–164.

64 Conte FA, Grumbach MM, Ito Y, Fisher CR, Simpson ER: A syndrome of female pseudohermaphrodism, hypergonadotropic hypogonadism, and multicystic ovaries associated with missense mutations in the gene encoding aromatase (P450arom). J Clin Endocrinol Metab 1994;78:1287–1292.

65 Auchus RJ, Miller WL: Molecular modeling of human P450c17 (17α-hydroxylase/17,20-lyase): Insights into reaction mechanisms and effects of mutations. Mol Endocrinol 1999;13:1169–1182.
66 Sawada N, Sakaki T, Kitanaka S, Kato S, Inouye K: Structure-function analysis of CYP27B1 and CYP27A1 Studies on mutants from patients with vitamin D-dependent rickets type I (VDDR-I) and cerebrotendinous xanthomatosis (CTX). Eur J Biochem 2001;268:6607–6615.
67 Reade TM, Scriver CR, Glorieux FH, Nogrady B, Delvin E, Poirier R, Holick F, DeLuca HF: Response to crystalline 1α-hydroxyvitamin D_3 in vitamin D dependency. Pediatr Res 1975;9: 593–599.

Prof. Walter L. Miller
Bldg. MR-IV, Room 209, University of California San Francisco
San Francisco, CA 94143–0978 (USA)
Tel. +1 415 476 2598, Fax +1 415 476 6286, E-Mail wlmlab@itsa.ucsf.edu

Hochberg Z (ed): Vitamin D and Rickets.
Endocr Dev. Basel, Karger, 2003, vol 6, pp 175–199

Hereditary 1,25-Dihydroxyvitamin D-Resistant Rickets

Peter J. Malloy, David Feldman

Department of Medicine, Stanford University School of Medicine, Stanford, Calif., USA

Contents

Supported by NIH grant DK 42482.

This review will focus on the clinical syndrome of hereditary vitamin D-resistant rickets (HVDRR), also known as vitamin D-dependent rickets, type II (VDDR-II). HVDRR is a rare genetic disease caused by a generalized resistance to 1α,25-dihydroxyvitamin D [$1,25(OH)_2D_3$], the hormonally active form of vitamin D. $1,25(OH)_2D_3$ actions are mediated by the vitamin D receptor (VDR), a member of the steroid-thyroid-retinoid family of nuclear hormone receptors [1]. In target cells the $1,25(OH)_2D_3$-VDR complex regulates the expression of specific genes that give rise to the biological responses elicited by the hormone [2]. In HVDRR, target organ resistance to vitamin D is caused by a heterogeneous group of defects in the VDR. A variety of mutations in the VDR gene cause the receptor to be nonfunctional or decrease the activity of the receptor. In this chapter, we will describe the clinical syndrome and the molecular defects in the VDR that give rise to HVDRR. An extensive review of HVDRR was published earlier [3].

In 1978, Brooks et al. [4] and Marx et al. [5] described patients having osteomalacia, rickets and high serum levels of $1,25(OH)_2D_3$. The clinical findings were similar to patients with vitamin D-dependent rickets, type I (VDDR-I) except for the high serum levels of $1,25(OH)_2D_3$. They postulated that the rickets was due to an end-organ resistance to $1,25(OH)_2D_3$ and they named the syndrome vitamin D-dependent rickets, type II (VDDR-II). The cause of VDDR-I is now known to be due to mutations in the gene encoding 1α-hydroxylase [6], the renal enzyme that converts $25(OH)D_3$ to $1,25(OH)_2D_3$ [7,8] and so we choose to refer to this entity as 1α-hydroxylase deficiency. Similarly, we prefer to use the term hereditary 1,25-dihydroxyvitamin D-resistant rickets (HVDRR) instead of VDDR-II since it is now known that the disease is caused by genetic defects in the VDR that ultimately cause resistance to the action of $1,25(OH)_2D_3$ [3]. It should be noted that in the Online Mendelian Inheritance in Man web site (http://www.ncbi.nlm.nih.gov/omim/) this disease is also referred to as vitamin D-resistant rickets with end-organ unresponsiveness to 1,25-dihydroxycholecalciferol, rickets-alopecia syndrome, VDDR-II with alopecia, and hypocalcemic vitamin D-resistant rickets.

The Clinical Syndrome of HVDRR

HVDRR is caused by a generalized resistance to $1,25(OH)_2D_3$. The major clinical findings are hypocalcemia and rickets, which are due to defective mineralization of newly formed bone and preosseous cartilage. The rickets ranges from mild to severe and is exhibited usually within months of birth. Patients suffer from bone pain, muscle weakness, hypotonia and occasionally convulsions from the hypocalcemia. Children are often growth retarded and in some cases they develop severe dental caries or exhibit hypoplasia of the teeth [9]. Some infants have died from pneumonia caused by poor respiratory movement due to severe rickets of the chest wall. Many children with HVDRR have sparse body hair and some have total scalp and body alopecia including eyebrows and in some cases eyelashes. Hair loss usually occurs during the first year of life. Consanguinity is highly associated with the disease and multiple family members are often affected [3].

The clinical findings include low serum levels of calcium and phosphate and elevated serum alkaline phosphatase activity. The patients develop secondary hyperparathyroidism and exhibit substantial increases in serum PTH. Importantly, the serum $1,25(OH)_2D_3$ levels are elevated. This clinical feature distinguishes HVDRR from 1α-hydroxylase deficiency since the serum $1,25(OH)_2D_3$ values in 1α-hydroxylase deficiency are depressed. HVDRR follows an autosomal-recessive pattern of inheritance with males and females equally affected. The recessive nature of the disease is evident from the parents of affected children who are heterozygous for the genetic trait. The heterozygotes show no symptoms of the disease and have normal bone development.

HVDRR is almost always caused by mutations in the VDR that result in end-organ resistance to $1,25(OH)_2D_3$ action. The major effect of the defective VDR on the vitamin D endocrine system is to decrease intestinal calcium and phosphate absorption that results in decreased bone mineralization and rickets. Secondary hyperparathyroidism contributes to the hypophosphatemia. Since 1978, over 100 cases of HVDRR have been reported [3]. In all cases, the diagnosis of HVDRR has been based on resistance to the action of vitamin D in combination with high circulating levels of $1,25(OH)_2D_3$. Of these, a number of cases have been analyzed at the molecular level. The findings were that the disease was caused by defects in VDR function that result from heterogeneous mutations in the VDR gene.

Analysis of the syndrome of HVDRR provides many interesting insights into vitamin D physiology and the role of the VDR in mediating $1,25(OH)_2D_3$ action. VDR have been found in many tissues in the body widening the scope of potential vitamin D target cells. In addition to maintaining calcium homeostasis, $1,25(OH)_2D_3$ regulates a number of other cellular processes [2]. Important biological actions for vitamin D have been postulated in many of these sites particularly in the immune and endocrine systems. VDRs have been found in endocrine glands such as pituitary, pancreas, parathyroid, gonads and placenta, and $1,25(OH)_2D_3$ has been shown to regulate hormone synthesis and secretion from these glands [10]. VDRs have also been found in hematolymphopoietic cells and $1,25(OH)_2D_3$ has been shown to regulate cell differentiation and the production of interleukins and cytokines [11]. However, despite the many processes shown to be regulated by $1,25(OH)_2D_3$, children with HVDRR only exhibit symptoms that relate to their calcium deficiency and alopecia [12]. Hochberg et al. [10] examined hormone secretion in patients with HVDRR and found no abnormalities in insulin, TSH, PRL, GH and testosterone levels in serum. Even et al. [13] showed that urinary cAMP and renal excretion of potassium, phosphorous and bicarbonate were normal in HVDRR patients treated with PTH. However, PTH failed to decrease urinary calcium and sodium excretion in these patients to the extent found in the control patients. This suggests that 1,25$(OH)_2D_3$ may selectively modulate the renal response to PTH and facilitate the PTH-induced reabsorption of calcium and sodium. Although minor aberrations have been noted in the fungicidal activity of neutrophils from HVDRR patients, the patients do not exhibit any clinically apparent immunologic defects [14].

Regulation of Gene Expression by 1,25-Dihydroxyvitamin D

How does 1,25$(OH)_2D$ regulate gene transcription? A simplified model of 1,25$(OH)_2D$ activated gene transcription is shown in figure 1. After being synthesized to the active form in the kidney, 1,25$(OH)_2D$ circulates in the blood mostly bound to DBP with a small fraction of hormone in the free state. The free, fat-soluble hormone readily enters target cells through the lipid bilayer of the cell membrane. Once inside the cell 1,25$(OH)_2D_3$ binds to the VDR and translocates to the nucleus whereupon a series of changes occur that enables the VDR to activate gene transcription [15]. One event that occurs upon 1,25$(OH)_2D$ binding is that the VDR becomes phosphorylated at serine 208 in the LBD [16]. Although phosphorylation is thought to participate in the transactivation process, its precise role in the activation of the VDR is not clear. The unoccupied VDR may also be loosely associated with DNA and its partner protein, the retinoid X receptor (RXR). Ligand binding on the other hand, causes the association with RXR to become stronger and tightly bound to DNA. The VDR-RXR heterodimer complex binds with high affinity to specific DNA sequences termed vitamin D response elements (VDREs) that are located in the promoter regions of target genes [1]. The typical VDRE is two imperfect hexanucleotides arranged as direct repeats separated by 3 nucleotide bases, a so-called DR3 motif. 1,25$(OH)_2D_3$ also contacts specific amino acid residues in the VDR ligand-binding pocket [17]. In doing so, the ligand's signal is transmitted via these amino acids allowing the VDR LBD to recruit coactivators [18]. A coactivator-binding cleft is formed when helix H12 folds back upon the LBD. Following the recruitment of other transcription factors and coactivators, the VDR-RXR heterodimer drives the transcription of 1,25$(OH)_2D$-responsive genes. The target genes encode proteins that determine the nature of the cellular response to the hormone. One target gene in particular encodes 24-hydroxylase. This enzyme is responsible for the initial step leading to the inactivation of 1,25$(OH)_2D_3$. 1,25$(OH)_2D$ can also down-regulate the expression of specific genes. This

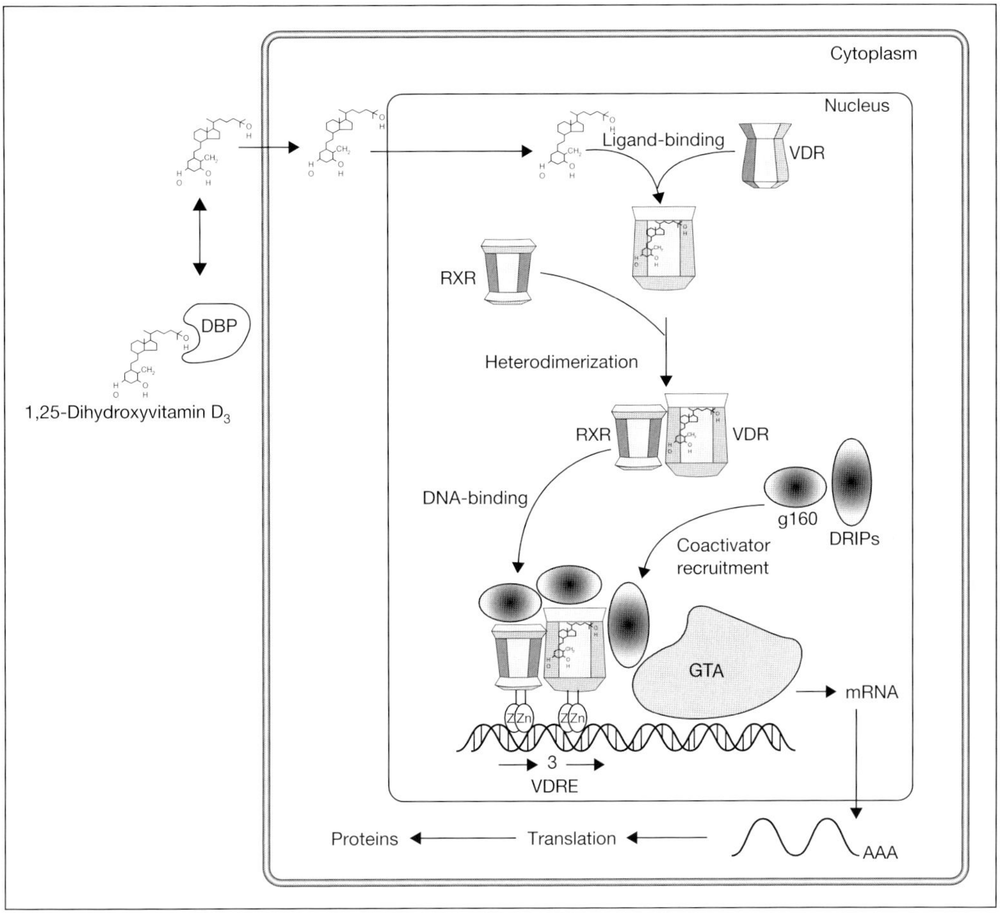

Fig. 1. Mechanism of 1,25$(OH)_2D_3$ action. 1,25-Dihydroxyvitamin D_3 circulates in the blood mainly bound to the DBP with a small amount in equilibrium with the free or unbound state. The free ligand enters the cell and binds with high affinity to the VDR. Ligand binding allows the VDR to heterodimerize with RXR and bind to VDRE in promoter sequences of target genes. Once bound to DNA the VDR-RXR heterodimer recruit coactivator proteins. These factors are involved in the modification of chromatin through acetylation or deacetylation of histones. Proteins that may play a role include the g160 family of coactivators such as SRC-1 and the vitamin D receptor interacting proteins or DRIPs as well as unknown proteins. The VDR-RXR-coactivator complex then interacts with the GTA and initiates gene transcription. The newly synthesized proteins then elicit the physiologic response to the hormone. Reproduced in part from Endocr Rev 1999;20:156–188.

negative regulatory activity is perhaps best illustrated by the ability of $1,25(OH)_2D$ to inhibit parathyroid hormone (PTH) gene expression.

The Vitamin D Receptor

The VDR is a ligand-activated nuclear transcription factor and a member of the steroid-thyroid-retinoid receptor gene superfamily [19]. The VDR is similar in overall structure to the other members of the steroid-thyroid-retinoid superfamily having a highly conserved DNA-binding domain (DBD) and a more variable ligand-binding domain (LBD).

The VDR DNA-Binding Domain

The VDR DBD is located between amino acids 24–90 and contains 9 highly conserved cysteine residues, which enable this region to fold into two loops or modules of 12–13 amino acids each (fig. 2). Each module contains four cysteine residues that coordinate the binding of one zinc atom and thus yields a two 'zinc-finger' structure. In the N-terminal zinc finger module the P-box an α-helix composed of amino acids 40–46 makes contact with specific nucleotide bases in promoters of target genes. In the C-terminal zinc finger module two additional α-helices form the D and T boxes. The D-box (residues 61–65) appears to be involved in DNA-binding and the T-box (residues 91–114) is important in heterodimerization with RXR and transactivation [20].

The VDR Ligand-Binding Domain

The structure of the VDR LBD that stretches over two-thirds of the protein from amino acids 123–427 has been determined by x-ray crystallography [17]. The VDR LBD is formed by 12 α-helices (H1–H12) and three β-sheets (S1–S3) (fig. 2). The LBD also has a variable length region between helix H1 and helix H3 (loop 1–3). Conserved residues located in a 34 amino acid cluster from the C-terminus of helix H3 to the middle of helix H5 form the hydrophobic core. These residues hold together H3, H4, H5, H8, and H9, and the interhelical loops 3–4 and 8–9. Residues in H1, H3, H5, β-turn, loop 6–7, H11, loop 11–12 and H12 form the framework for a 3-dimensional pocket that the ligand occupies. Helix H12 is thought to form a retractable lid that traps and holds the ligand in position. Once inside the ligand-binding pocket, the ligand makes contact with specific amino acid residues of the various α-helices that line the face of the pocket to transmit its signal. Ligand binding causes a conformational change in the VDR that allows the receptor to form protein heterodimers with RXR. Ligand binding also activates DNA-binding. In addition to forming the ligand-binding pocket, the LBD contains several structural elements that are

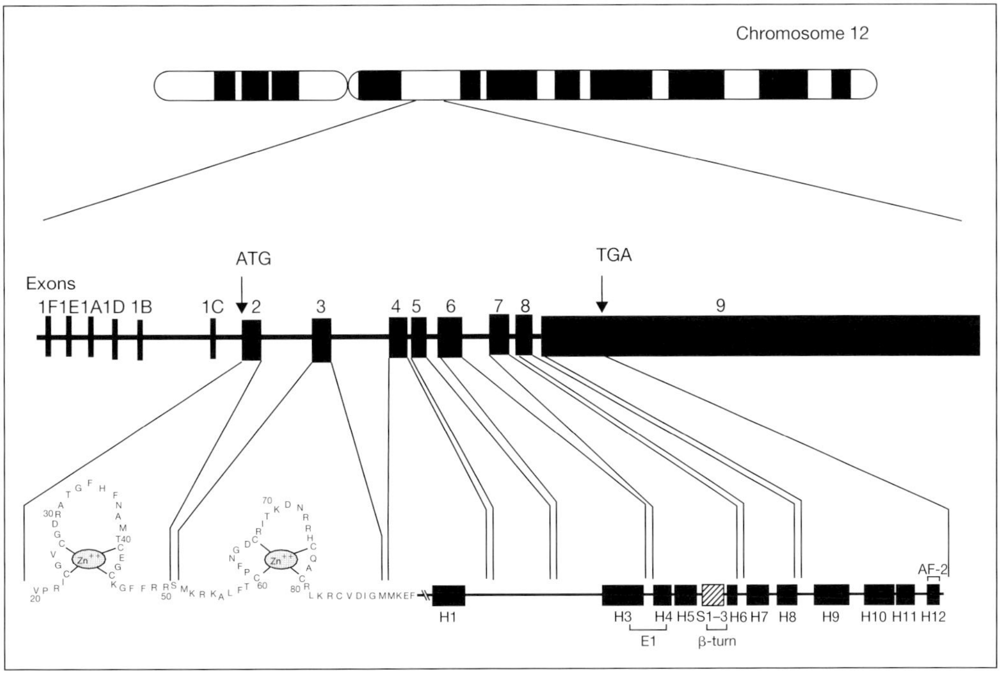

Fig. 2. The human VDR chromosomal gene and protein. The structural organization of the human VDR gene located on chromosome 12 is shown. The gene spans approximately 80 kb of DNA and is comprised of at least 14 exons. The locations of the start (ATG) and termination (TGA) codons are indicated. The boundaries of these exons and their corresponding locations within the VDR protein are indicated. Reproduced in part from Endocr Rev 1999;20:156–188.

involved in heterodimerization and transactivation (fig. 2). Mutational analysis of the VDR LBD has shown that H9, H10 and an E1 domain that overlaps H4 and H5 are required for RXR heterodimerization. Two regions of the VDR LBD are essential for transactivation function. These regions include the AF-2 domain that encompasses H12 (residues 416–424) and the region between amino acids 232–272 encompassing H3 and H4 [17]. Repositioning of helix H12 after ligand binding is critical to forming a hydrophobic cleft that can accommodate the LxxLL motif of coactivators and allow them to bind to the receptor.

The Cellular Basis of HVDRR

Studies to elucidate the mechanism of vitamin D resistance in children with HVDRR began after it was shown that the VDR was expressed in human skin and that regulation of 24-hydroxylase activity by $1,25(OH)_2D_3$ could be studied in dermal fibroblasts cultured from skin biopsies [21]. In the first study by Feldman et al. [22], using cultured fibroblasts from a patient with the HVDRR, the authors showed that specific $[^3H]1,25(OH)_2D_3$-binding was absent in cell extracts. They also demonstrated that the fibroblasts were resistant to $1,25(OH)_2D_3$ action since the cells failed to induce 24-hydroxylase enzyme activity when treated with high doses of the hormone. The parent's of the children with HVDRR had no sign of the disease or bone abnormalities. When the fibroblasts from the patient's parents were examined they showed a normal level of $[^3H]1,25(OH)_2D_3$-binding and a normal 24-hydroxylase induction by $1,25(OH)_2D_3$. These findings help account for the normal phenotype presented by the parents.

A number of HVDRR cases were subsequently examined using cultured skin fibroblasts [3]. In some cases no specific $[^3H]1,25(OH)_2D_3$-binding was found while others had normal $[^3H]1,25(OH)_2D_3$-binding but their cells were still resistant to $1,25(OH)_2D_3$ treatment as measured by 24-hydroxylase induction. The conclusion reached was that the HVDRR syndrome was caused by cellular resistance to $1,25(OH)_2D_3$ action and was due to at least two types of defects in the VDR. One class of defects impairs ligand binding and one class of defects retains ligand binding but causes resistance to $1,25(OH)_2D_3$ because of defective VDR binding to DNA or impairment of other steps in the hormone action pathway.

Although cultured skin fibroblasts have been the main source for studying HVDRR, a number of other cells have been used to study this disease including peripheral mononuclear cells, phytohemagglutinin-stimulated lymphocytes, myeloid progenitor cells, Epstein-Barr virus immortalized B lymphoblasts, and HTLV-1 virus immortalized T lymphoblasts [3].

Based on the concept that VDR binding to DNA is essential for activity, Hirst et al. [23] showed that defective DNA-binding could be the cause of resistance in cases that had normal ligand-binding. In a study of a family from Haiti with two sisters with HVDRR and an unaffected sister they showed that the fibroblasts from the affected individuals had normal $[^3H]1,25(OH)_2D_3$-binding but were resistant to $1,25(OH)_2D_3$ treatment. Using DNA-cellulose chromatography they demonstrated that the VDR from the HVDRR fibroblasts bound weakly to DNA while VDR from an unaffected sister as well as control subjects bound strongly to DNA. The authors concluded that the VDR defect was probably located in the DBD that caused the VDR to have a decreased affinity for DNA. A similar DNA-binding defect in the VDR was demonstrated in other cases of HVDRR that exhibited normal $[^3H]1,25(OH)_2D_3$-binding [3]. In addition, the parents from one family exhibited two forms of the VDR, one that had a normal affinity for DNA (wild-type) and one that had a low affinity

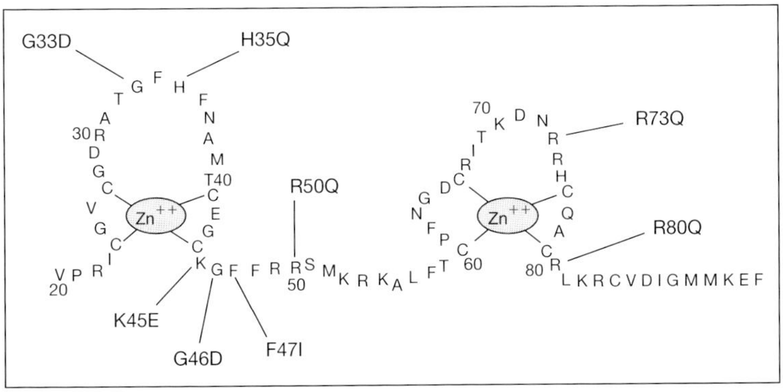

Fig. 3. Mutations in the VDR DNA-binding domain. The two zinc finger modules and the amino acid composition of the DBD are shown. The locations of the missense mutations are indicated.

for DNA (mutant VDR similar to the affected children) [24]. Both forms of the receptor had the same size as the normal VDR suggesting the defect was probably caused by a point mutation in the DBD. Since the parents were heterozygous for the defective VDR, but showed a normal response to hormone, this demonstrated that the genetic defect was recessive in nature.

Molecular Basis for HVDRR

First Genetic Defect to Be Identified in the Steroid-Thyroid-Retinoid Receptor Superfamily

Based upon the biochemical and cellular data obtained from the earlier studies of the HVDRR cases, investigation was begun into the molecular causes of this disease. The HVDRR cases that exhibited normal $[^3H]1,25(OH)_2D_3$ binding but abnormal binding to DNA were suspected to result from point mutations in the DBD. In 1988, Hughes et al. [25] used the polymerase chain reaction (PCR) to amplify the VDR gene from two families with the disease. In one family a unique single base change G to A was identified in exon 3. This missense mutation replaced arginine with glutamine at amino acid residue 73 in the second zinc finger module (R73Q) (fig. 3). In the second family, a G to A transition was identified in exon 2. This missense mutation changed glycine to aspartic acid at amino acid residue 33 in the first zinc finger module (G33D) (fig. 3). The unique base changes were found in the children with HVDRR while their parents had both a normal and a mutant sequence. The mutations found by Hughes et al. [25] were the first genetic defects identified in any member of the steroid-thyroid-retinoid receptor superfamily.

To demonstrate that the unique base changes found in these families were the cause of the HVDRR phenotype, the defects were recreated in the wild type VDR cDNA [26]. The recreated mutant VDRs expressed in COS-1 cells exhibited normal [^{3}H]1,25(OH)$_2$D$_3$-binding and abnormal DNA-binding properties. The recreated mutant receptors had also lost their ability to activate gene transcription. These data proved that the missense mutations caused the VDR to be transcriptionally inactive and therefore led to the 1,25(OH)$_2$D$_3$ resistance seen in the patients.

Since the original report by Hughes et al. [25] a number of mutations have been identified in the VDR in patients with HVDRR. Over 100 cases of HVDRR have been recorded and a number of these have been analyzed at the biochemical and molecular level [3]. Several genetic abnormalities have been found in the VDR gene, usually missense and nonsense mutations, but also a partial gene deletion, and splice site mutations. A description of these mutations and the consequences of the abnormality in the VDR will be discussed below. Because of space limitations, many original references describing the individual mutations cannot be cited but they can be found in our previous review [3]. More current references will be included as space allows.

Mutations in the VDR DNA-Binding Domain

A number of missense mutations have been identified in the VDR DBD [3]. The mutations and the location in the zinc-finger modules of the VDR are summarized in fig. 3. Like the cases described by Hughes et al. [25], all of the missense mutations in the DBD exhibit intact [^{3}H]1,25(OH)$_2$D$_3$-binding but are defective in binding to DNA. Although two of these mutations (K45E and G46D) fall within the P box [3], a region of the DBD thought to be critical for DNA binding, other mutations are dispersed throughout the two zinc-finger structure. The DBD mutations appear to alter the DNA-binding ability of the VDR preventing normal VDR-DNA interactions. In each case, the mutation caused complete resistance to 1,25(OH)$_2$D$_3$ as well as alopecia.

Mutations Causing Premature Termination of the VDR

The first molecular analysis of an HVDRR case in which the patient's fibroblasts exhibited no [^{3}H]1,25(OH)$_2$D$_3$-binding was reported by Ritchie et al. [27]. A single unique base change C to A was identified in exon 8. This single

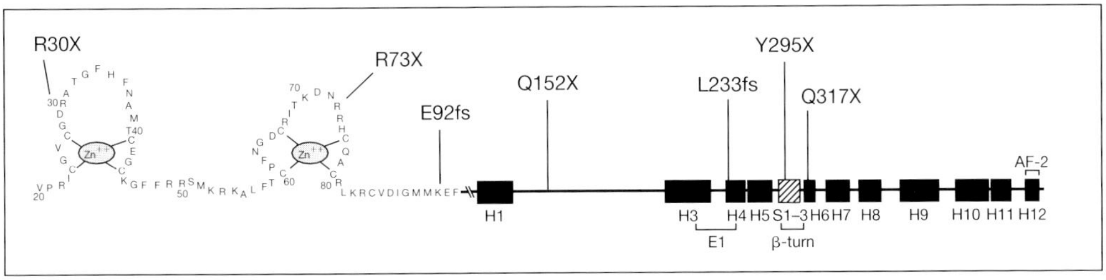

Fig. 4. Mutations causing premature termination of the VDR. The locations of the premature stop mutations and frameshift (Fs) mutations are shown.

base substitution changed the codon for tyrosine (TAC) to an ochre termination codon (TAA) (Y295X) (fig. 4). The location of the premature stop at amino acid 295 truncates the VDR to a molecular size of 32,000 Daltons, approximately 18,000 Daltons shorter than the native protein and results in the loss of $[^3H]1,25(OH)_2D_3$-binding. The recreated mutant VDR containing the ochre mutation exhibited a molecular size of 32,000 Daltons and was unable to bind $[^3H]1,25(OH)_2D_3$. The truncated VDR also failed to activate gene transcription demonstrating that this mutation was the cause of the hormone resistant state in the patients.

The three families studied by Ritchie et al. [27] and four additional related families comprise a large kindred in which as many as 8 offspring had HVDRR and where consanguineous marriages were common. An analysis of an *Rsa*I restriction fragment length polymorphism created by the mutation showed that all of the patients with HVDRR were homozygous for the Y295X mutation and that their parents were heterozygous for the mutant allele [28]. This study also showed that the mutant VDR mRNA was absent in all but one family in which it was greatly diminished. The absence of RNA transcripts has been reported in a number of other genetic diseases where premature stop mutations were found. In those cases in which it has been studied, the decreased or absent transcript has been attributed to instability of the abnormal mRNA harboring a nonsense mutation. Interestingly, the Y295X mutation was also found in two children that lived in the same town as the extended kindred described above but apparently are unrelated to the large kindred [3]. The same mutation was also found in two related patients from Saudi Arabia who were unrelated to the other cases [3]. It is not clear whether Y295X mutation represents a mutational 'hot spot' in the VDR gene or whether these cases all descended from a common founder mutation.

Since the report by Ritchie et al. [27] a number of premature stop mutations have been identified in the VDR from patients with HVDRR [3]. The locations of these mutations are shown in figure 4. A Moroccan patient was shown to have a mutation in exon 3 that replaced arginine (CGA) with an opal termination codon (TGA) (R73X). Interestingly, the R73X mutation occurs in the same codon that gives rise to the R73Q mutation but at a different nucleotide base. In two related patients of Turkish origin a mutation was found in exon 4 that changed glutamine (CAG) to an amber termination codon (TAG) (Q152X). In two unrelated cases, a patient of French-Canadian origin and in a patient from Brazil, a unique C to T base substitution was found in exon 2 which changed arginine (CGA) to an opal stop codon (TGA) at amino acid 30 (R30X). Also, an Iranian girl was shown to have a mutation in exon 8 that changed the codon for glutamine to a termination codon (Q317X) [29]. All of the nonsense mutations in the VDR eliminate $[^3H]1,25(OH)_2D_3$-binding and cause complete hormone resistance.

Other Mutations Causing Premature Termination of the VDR

Splice Site Mutations

A single base change in the intron between exons 3 and 4 in the VDR gene was found to cause HVDRR due to exon skipping [3]. The patient's RNA sequence diverged from the normal sequence at nucleotide 147 where the sequence for exon 4 was deleted and exon 5 continued in its place. The mutation occurred in the 5′-donor splice site consensus sequence (normal sequence: GTA/GAGT; mutant sequence: GTA/GACT) and caused a reading frameshift that resulted in the introduction of a premature stop codon in exon 5. The mutant protein which contained 92 amino acids of the wild-type sequence and an additional 6 amino acids due to the frameshift (Glu92fs) was functionally inactive (fig. 4).

A splice site mutation was also identified in a patient whose fibroblasts showed no specific $[^3H]1,25(OH)_2D_3$-binding or induction of 24-hydroxylase activity [3]. The mutation occurred in exon 6 that changed the sequence GT<u>C</u>AGT to GT<u>G</u>AGT and created a cryptic 5′ donor splice site. The mutation caused a 56 bp deletion that led to a frameshift 15 bases into exon 7. The mutant protein contains 233 amino acids of the wild-type sequence and an additional 4 amino acids due to the frameshift (Leu233fs) (fig. 4). The mutation caused the truncation of 194 amino acids of the VDR leading to a loss of $1,25(OH)_2D_3$ binding and hormone responsiveness.

Gene Deletion

There has been one case reported in which a major structural defect in the VDR gene was found to cause HVDRR [3]. The defect found by PCR and

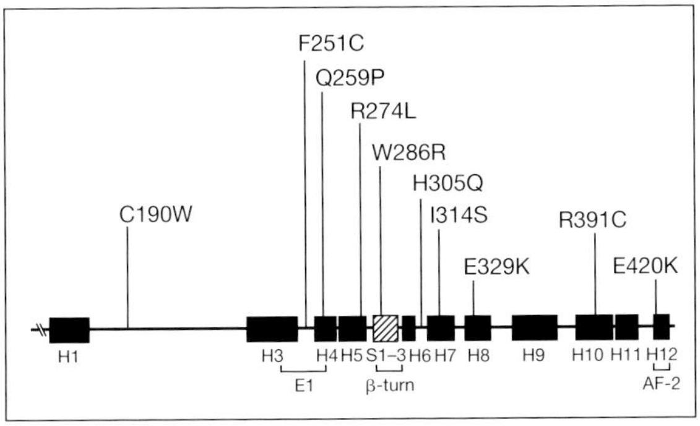

Fig. 5. Mutations in the VDR ligand-binding domain. The α-helices (H1–H12) of the VDR LBD are represented as rectangles and the β-turns (S1–3) are drawn as a hatched rectangle. The E1 and AF-2 regions are shown below the α-helices. The locations of the missense mutations are indicated. Reproduced in part from Endocr Rev 1999;20:156–188.

Southern blotting was a deletion in the VDR gene that eliminated exons 7, 8, and 9. This is the only case reported thus far in which a partial deletion in the VDR gene has been shown to cause HVDRR.

Mutations in the VDR Ligand-Binding Domain

Mutations that Affect 1,25(OH)$_2$D$_3$ Binding

A number of missense mutations causing single amino acid substitutions in the LBD have been described (fig. 5). The first description of a missense mutation in the VDR LBD was in a patient from Kuwait who exhibited no [^{3}H]1,25(OH)$_2$D$_3$-binding or 24-hydroxylase activity [3]. A unique G to T single base change was found in exon 7 that replaced a positively charged arginine with a neutral leucine at amino acid 274 (R274L) (fig. 5). The R274L mutation occurs in H5. Based on the crystal structure of the holo-VDR, R274 makes contact with the 1-hydroxyl group of 1,25(OH)$_2$D$_3$ [17]. Thus the R274L mutation would be expected to affect ligand binding. In transactivation experiments, the recreated R274L mutant VDR required 1,000-fold more 1,25(OH)$_2$D$_3$ to achieve the same activity attained by the wild type receptor. Although the resistance caused by the defective VDR could be overcome treating with high concentrations of 1,25(OH)$_2$D$_3$ in vitro, the patient failed to respond to massive does of the hormone and eventually died of pneumonia.

A second missense mutation in the VDR LBD was found in a patient who, in addition to having HVDRR, also had two other rare genetic disorders, congenital total lipodystrophy and persistent Müllerian duct syndrome [30].

Analysis of [^{3}H]1,25(OH)$_2$D$_3$-binding experiments showed that the patient's VDR had a slightly lower affinity for 1,25(OH)$_2$D$_3$ than the wild-type receptor. In addition, induction of 24-hydroxylase mRNA by the patient's fibroblasts required approximately 5-fold more hormone to achieve maximal activity as compared to control cells. A unique single C to G base change was found in exon 8 [3]. This mutation resulted in the replacement of histidine with glutamine at amino acid 305 (H305Q). In transactivation assays, the recreated H305Q mutant VDR exhibited the same hyporesponsiveness to 1,25(OH)$_2$D$_3$ as seen in the patient's fibroblasts. The H305Q mutation occurs in the inter-helical loop between H6–H7. From the crystallographic studies of the holo-VDR, H305 makes contact with the 25-hydroxyl group in 1,25(OH)$_2$D$_3$. It is apparent that the disruption of the ligand contact point by the H305Q mutation is the basis for HVDRR in this patient. No explanation was forthcoming for the presence of three genetic defects in a single individual. The congenital total lipodystrophy has been shown to be caused by a mutation in the seipin gene [31]. No cause has been found for the persistent Müllerian duct syndrome.

An Algerian boy and his younger sister both with HVDRR were shown to have a mutation in exon 7 that changed a tryptophan to an arginine at amino acid 286 (W286R) [32]. The fibroblasts from the patient expressed a normal size VDR but no specific [^{3}H]1,25(OH)$_2$D$_3$-binding was observed and the cells were totally unresponsive to 1,25(OH)$_2$D$_3$ treatment. The W286R mutation occurs in the β1 sheet of the three-stranded β sheet between helices H5–H6. From the crystallographic studies of the VDR, W286 makes contact with the α face of the C ring in 1,25(OH)$_2$D$_3$ and is involved in forming the hydrophobic channel where the conjugated triene connecting the A and the C rings fits [17]. The W286R mutation, therefore, directly alters VDR contact with the ligand and causes the loss of 1,25(OH)$_2$D$_3$-binding [32].

Mutations that Affect RXR Heterodimerization

As mentioned above, the VDR requires heterodimerization with RXR for activity. Several mutations have been described that affect heterodimerization. In one patient with HVDRR and alopecia a C to T base change in exon 9 was found that changed an arginine to a cysteine at amino acid 391 (R391C) [3]. The R391C mutation occurs in H10. Helix H10 provides a surface interface for RXR binding (fig. 5). In transactivation experiments, the R391C mutant receptor not only required high concentrations of 1,25(OH)$_2$D$_3$ for activity but required increased levels of RXR in order to achieve a normal response. These studies showed the importance of both 1,25(OH)$_2$D$_3$-binding and RXR heterodimerization in VDR mediated gene transactivation. This was the first reported case of HVDRR in which a mutation in the VDR interferes with RXR binding.

A second patient with HVDRR who exhibited normal $[^3H]1,25(OH)_2D_3$-binding but was hormone insensitive revealed a single base change that substituted a proline for glutamine at amino acid 259 (Q259P) [3]. The Q259P mutation occurs in helix H4 (fig. 5). Although Q259P had no apparent affect on ligand binding there was evidence of impaired VDR-RXR-VDRE formation. Transactivation experiments demonstrated that the recreated Q259P mutant VDR was functionally inactive.

In a third case, studies of a patient with HVDRR showed that the patient's fibroblasts were approximately 1,000-fold less responsive to calcitriol than control fibroblasts confirming target organ resistance. Analyses of the VDR demonstrated a normal size receptor but with decreased abundance and affinity for $1,25(OH)_2D_3$. The mutant VDR also exhibited reduced binding to RXR. A missense mutation was identified in exon 6 that changed a phenylalanine to cysteine at amino acid 251 (F251C) [33].

The F251C mutation occurs in the E1 region (aa 244–263) of the VDR LBD (fig. 5). The E1 region overlaps the C-terminal portion of helix H3, loop 3–4 and the N-terminal portion of helix H4. This structural motif is highly conserved throughout the nuclear receptor superfamily. A cluster of hydrophobic amino acids within the E1 region is critical to the 3-dimensional folding and formation of the ligand-binding pocket [34]. At the center of this region is an invariant aromatic phenylalanine residue which corresponds to F251 in the VDR. Since F251 is in such a critical site in the LBD, replacing the aromatic amino acid phenylalanine with a small hydrophilic cysteine residue likely disrupts the ligand-binding pocket of the VDR and interferes with the fundamental conformation required for optimal function. From the crystallographic studies, F251 does not form a direct contact point with the bound ligand. Indeed, at 4°C normal ligand binding was observed. However, at elevated temperatures, the binding affinity was severely decreased suggesting that the F251C mutation disrupted the folding of the ligand-binding pocket [33].

From crystallographic studies of RXRα, RAR-RXRα, and PPARγ-RXRα, the dimer interface is formed from helix H9 and helix H10 and the interhelical loops between H7–H8 and H8–H9 [17]. Although the interhelical loop between H3–H4, where the F251C mutation is located, is not part of the dimer interface, the loop does appear to be positioned beneath the H8–H9 loop and helix H9. In this critical location the mutation therefore appears to disrupt the heterodimer interface in addition to disrupting the folding of the ligand-binding pocket. The F251C mutation results in a decreased ability of the receptor to heterodimerize with RXRα at physiologic hormone concentrations. The single amino acid defect provides evidence for the interdependency of ligand-binding and heterodimer-binding to achieve transactivation.

Mutations that Affect Coactivator Binding

A novel E420K mutation in helix H12 in the VDR LBD (fig. 5) was the molecular basis for another patient with HVDRR [35]. The E420K mutant VDR exhibited normal ligand binding, heterodimerization with RXR, and DNA binding. However, the mutation prevented the coactivators SRC-1 and DRIP205 from binding to the VDR and caused complete resistance to $1,25(OH)_2D_3$ [35].

It is now clear from crystallographic studies of the VDR and other members of the steroid receptor superfamily that repositioning of helix H12 is a critical event that occurs as a consequence of ligand binding and is essential for transactivation [17]. The repositioning of helix 12 upon ligand binding is critical for the formation of the hydrophobic cleft for coactivator binding. The polar interactions that stabilize the positioning of helix H12 involve a conserved salt-bridge between K264 in helix H4 and E420 in helix H12 and a hydrogen bond between S235 in helix H3 and T415 in helix H12. The E420K mutation prevents the correct repositioning of helix H12 after binding the ligand. The substitution of the negatively charged glutamic acid (E420) with a positively charged lysine residue (K420) would prevent the polar interaction with the positively charged lysine (K264) salt bridge partner. A charge clamp formed by K246, K264 and E420 enables the VDR to recruit and bind coactivators through their LxxLL motifs. The K246 in helix 3 and E420 in helix 12 are thought to be indispensable for binding the LxxLL peptide on the coactivator. The E420K mutation disrupts coactivator binding and causes the hormone resistance seen in the patient. This case represents the first description of a naturally occurring mutation in the VDR that disrupts coactivator interaction and causes HVDRR [35].

Other Mutations in the VDR LBD

A mutation in exon 5 has been described in the VDR LBD that changed a cysteine to tryptophan at amino acid 190 (C190W) [3]. The Cys190Trp mutation occurs in the loop between H1 and H3 (fig. 5). The effect of this mutation on the VDR and further details about this case were not reported.

Fibroblasts from one patient that had normal $[^3H]1,25(OH)_2D_3$-binding showed a reduced response to hormone induction of 24-hydroxylase activity. A single T to G substitution was found in exon 8 that replaced isoleucine with serine at amino acid 314 (I314S) [3]. In transactivation experiments, the I314S mutant receptor required higher concentrations of $1,25(OH)_2D_3$ to achieve a normal response. The I314S mutation occurs in H7 (fig. 5). The mutation causes a subtle defect in heterodimerization with RXR and decreased response to $1,25(OH)_2D_3$ in transactivation assays. Interestingly, this patient who did not have alopecia showed a nearly complete cure when treated with pharmacological doses of 25-hydroxyvitamin D.

There has been one report of a patient with HVDRR that was a compound heterozygote having two mutations in the VDR gene [36]. One mutation in exon 8 changed a glutamic acid to lysine at amino acid 329 (E329K) (fig. 5). The second mutation, a single base deletion of a cytosine at nucleotide 366 (366delC) causes a frameshift and introduces a premature termination codon in exon 4. The premature termination codon would be expected to delete most of the LBD. The affects of the E329K mutation on VDR functions were not reported.

Description of HVDRR without Mutations in the VDR

Resistance to 1,25(OH)$_2$D$_3$ exhibited by HVDRR patients is caused by mutations in the VDR. However, although the VDR is the principle factor in the 1,25(OH)$_2$D$_3$ action pathway, there exists the possibility that target organ resistance to 1,25(OH)$_2$D$_3$ may be caused by mutations in other proteins that participate in the transactivation process such as RXR or coactivators. Hewison et al. [37] have described a case of HVDRR which may be caused by a defect in a protein other than the VDR. The patient, a young girl, exhibited all the hallmarks of HVDRR including alopecia. Examination of the patient's fibroblasts showed that they expressed a normal size VDR transcript and VDR that had a normal binding affinity for [^{3}H]1,25(OH)$_2$D$_3$. However, no 24-hydroxylase activity could be detected after treating the fibroblasts with up to 1 μM 1,25(OH)$_2$D$_3$. Although the cells were clearly resistant to 1,25(OH)$_2$D$_3$, the authors could not find a mutation in the coding region of the VDR gene. Their data suggest that hormone resistance and HVDRR may be caused by mutations in an essential protein that participates in the 1,25(OH)$_2$D$_3$ hormone action pathway.

Therapy for Patients with HVDRR

As opposed to 1α-hydroxylase deficiency, most patients with HVDRR do not respond to treatment with calcitriol or vitamin D analogs, even at supraphysiological and pharmacological doses. Many therapies using combinations of calcium and active vitamin D metabolites have been tried to ameliorate symptoms of this disease. In a few of the early reports, HVDRR patients responded clinically and X-rays showed improvement in rickets following administration of pharmacological doses of vitamin D ranging from 5,000 to 40,000 IU/day, 20 to 200 μg of 25(OH)D/day, and 17–20 μg of 1,25(OH)$_2$D$_3$/day. It is possible that these patients had minor aberrations in the VDR that resulted in a decreased binding affinity for 1,25(OH)$_2$D$_3$. Treatment with high doses of the vitamin D metabolite could well have been successful in overcoming the binding defect. However, the molecular basis of some of these earlier cases of HVDRR has not been determined and the diagnosis of cellular resistance was therefore not confirmed.

The patients with the R274L and H305Q mutations, contact points for 1-hydroxyl and 25-hydroxyl groups of $1,25(OH)_2D_3$, respectively, were treated with massive doses $1,25(OH)_2D_3$. The patient with the R274L mutation did not respond to the treatment and eventually died of pneumonia. Interestingly, the recreated R274L mutant VDR did exhibit transcriptional activity when high doses of hormone were given. The patient with the H305Q mutation, on the other hand, showed some improvement in the rickets when treated with high doses of $1,25(OH)_2D_3$ (30 μg/day). However, the patient died from complications resulting from his other conditions.

High dose calcium administration has also been used to treat HVDRR patients. A patient who failed to respond to calciferols, was treated with 3–4 grams of elemental calcium orally per day. The patient showed clinical improvement within the 4 months of therapy [38].

The most successful therapy for HVDRR is long term intravenous calcium infusions. Balsan et al. [39] showed the beneficial effects of intravenous calcium infusions in a child with HVDRR who did not respond to prior treatment with large doses of vitamin D derivatives or oral calcium supplements. The child received high doses of calcium intravenously during the nocturnal hours over a 9-month period. Relief from bone pain was observed within the first 2 weeks of intravenous therapy and within 7 months the child gained weight and height. Similar clinical improvement was seen following calcium infusion therapy by al-Aqueel et al. [40] and Hochberg et al. [41]. Intravenous calcium infusions by-passed the calcium absorption defect in the intestine caused by the disease. To maintain normal serum calcium concentrations after radiological healing of the rickets by i.v. calcium infusion, high dose oral calcium has been shown to be an effective therapy. Children with HVDRR are now routinely started on this two-step protocol at 2 years of age [41].

In a few cases of HVDRR, a 'spontaneous cure' has been observed. The improvement occurred after long-term ineffective treatment with vitamin D metabolites and mineral replacement or after the treatment was stopped. It is interesting to note that fibroblasts taken from HVDRR patients after spontaneous healing remained resistant to $1,25(OH)_2D_3$. Spontaneous improvement occurred in patients with the Y295X mutation as well as with the R73Q mutation [3]. The patients who showed spontaneous improvement, however, nevertheless had no improvement in their alopecia.

The use of potent vitamin D analogs to induce responses in mutant VDR from HVDRR patients is currently being investigated. Gardezi et al. [42] examined several VDRs with LBD mutations and showed that 20-epi analogs of $1,25(OH)_2D_3$ could greatly enhance the transactivation of the defective

VDRs compared to 1,25(OH)$_2$D$_3$. This was especially true for mutations in the VDR that disrupt contact points for 1- and 25-hydroxyl groups. This potential therapy has not yet been attempted in patients.

HVDRR and Alopecia

Alopecia is found in many of the cases of HVDRR reported to date [3]. In those cases examined at the molecular level, alopecia has been associated with all patients with DBD mutations and premature stop mutations. These mutations result in complete hormone resistance. On the other hand, the presence of alopecia is variable in patients that have missense mutations in the VDR LBD.

Alopecia was not associated with the disease when the molecular cause of HVDRR was the result of mutations that affect ligand binding (R274L, H305Q, I314S, and W286R). Three of these residues R274, H305, W286, and are contact points for 1,25(OH)$_2$D$_3$ (the 1-hydroxyl and 25-hydroxyl groups and the C ring, respectively). Since the patients with the H305Q and I314S mutations were somewhat responsive to vitamin D therapy, it is reasonable to speculate that the limited VDR function may have prevented the development of alopecia after birth. These patients responded to treatment with high doses of vitamin D or 25(OH)D. On the other hand, the patients with the R274L and W286R mutations did not exhibit any [^{3}H]1,25(OH)$_2$D$_3$-binding and were totally resistant to 1,25(OH)$_2$D$_3$.

In the patients with mutations in the VDR LBD that affects heterodimerization with RXRα (F251C, Q259P and R391C) alopecia was present. Both the F251C and R391C mutations caused 1,25(OH)$_2$D$_3$ resistance although the function of the VDR could be restored by supra-physiological doses of the hormone in vitro.

Interestingly, the patient with the E420K mutation does not have alopecia. The E420K mutation affects coactivator binding but not ligand binding, RXR heterodimerization nor DNA-binding. The patient's cells were totally resistant to high doses of hormone.

In the 1α-hydroxylase knockout mouse model, abnormalities develop in skeletal, reproductive and immune function [43]. However, the 1α-hydroxylase knockout mice do not develop alopecia nor do patients with 1α-hydroxylase deficiency. These findings suggest that 1,25(OH)$_2$D$_3$ itself is not required for hair development. On the other hand, VDR knockout mice develop alopecia indicating that the VDR is essential for hair growth [44, 45]. Furthermore, targeting of the WT VDR to keratinocytes of the VDR knockout mouse prevents alopecia [46]. These finding raise the question of how vitamin D and the VDR are involved in regulating hair growth. Our analysis of HVDRR cases and the types of mutations associated with alopecia suggest that patient's who have a VDR that can bind to RXR and to DNA will not develop alopecia. We speculate that patients with HVDRR will develop alopecia when the molecular cause of the disease compromises the ability of the VDR to heterodimerize with RXR or to bind to DNA. The data on the VDR mutations combined with the findings in the 1-hydroxylase knockout mouse model, suggest the possibility that the VDR represses the expression of some genes in a ligand-independent manner and requires RXR heterodimerization and DNA binding but not interaction with coactivators for this activity. Since the VDR is a negative regulator of a number of genes, loss of a negative regulatory activity by the unliganded VDR could potentially lead to the loss of repression of those genes and this activity could then lead to alopecia.

Clinical Ramifications and Conclusions

HVDRR is a rare recessive disorder caused by mutations in the gene encoding the VDR resulting in end-organ resistance to $1,25(OH)_2D_3$ action. The major effect of the VDR mutations on the vitamin D endocrine system is to decrease intestinal calcium and phosphate absorption that results in hypocalcemia, hypophosphatemia, secondary hyperparathyroidism and decreased bone mineralization and rickets. Since 1978, more than 100 cases of HVDRR have been reported [3]. In all cases, the diagnosis of HVDRR has been based on a clinical picture of rickets and hypocalcemia in the face of elevated circulating levels of $1,25(OH)_2D$ indicating resistance to vitamin D action. Many of the cases have been analyzed for $[^3H]1,25(OH)_2D_3$-binding and bioactivity that revealed that the disease was caused by heterogeneous defects in the VDR that result from mutations in the VDR gene. A number of cases of HVDRR have not yet been examined for mutations. Since some of these cases presented late in life, they may be due to non-hereditary resistance to $1,25(OH)_2D$.

Analysis of the syndrome of HVDRR provides many interesting insights into vitamin D physiology and the role of the VDR in mediating $1,25(OH)_2D$ action. VDRs have been found in many tissues in the body widening the scope of potential vitamin D target cells. In addition to maintaining calcium homeostasis, $1,25(OH)_2D$ regulates a number of other biological processes including the rate of cellular proliferation, the state of differentiation and immunosuppression [2]. VDRs have been found in endocrine glands such as pituitary, pancreas, parathyroid, gonads and placenta, and $1,25(OH)_2D_3$ has been shown to regulate hormone synthesis and secretion from these glands. VDRs have also been found in hematolymphopoietic cells and $1,25(OH)_2D_3$ has been shown to regulate cell differentiation and the production of interleukins and cytokines. VDRs are present in many malignant cells including, breast, prostate and colon cancer cells and $1,25(OH)_2D_3$ action is to inhibit cellular proliferation.

However, despite the many pleiotropic processes shown to be regulated by $1,25(OH)_2D_3$, children with HVDRR only exhibit symptoms that relate to their calcium deficiency, rickets and alopecia [3]. We speculate that the pleiotropic actions of $1,25(OH)_2D_3$ are also regulated by many other factors in vivo. Thus in HVDRR, other redundant regulatory factors must compensate for the absence of $1,25(OH)_2D_3$ action and the defects potentially attributable to $1,25(OH)_2D_3$ resistance, are not manifested clinically. However, the potential application of these pleiotropic actions of vitamin D or its analogs in a therapeutic manner is an exciting area of current research [2].

The improvement of rickets in HVDRR cases in response to treatment with chronic i.v. calcium infusions or high dose oral calcium raises interesting questions about the role of vitamin D in bone homeostasis and PTH regulation [3, 12]. In respect to bone, correction of hypocalcemia and secondary hyperparathyroidism leads to healing of the rickets as assessed by X-ray and bone biopsy. Thus, although there are many well defined actions of vitamin D on osteoblasts, the calcium treatment data suggest that $1,25(OH)_2D_3$ actions on osteoblasts are not essential in order to form normally mineralized bone. The implication from this finding is that the critical $1,25(OH)_2D_3$ action takes place predominantly in the intestinal cells on mineral absorption to provide calcium and phosphate for bone mineralization. The same conclusion was reached by Underwood and DeLuca [47]. They showed that the development of rickets could be prevented in totally vitamin D-deficient rats by calcium infusions in the absence of vitamin D. Similar findings have been documented in two models of HVDRR in VDR null mice [44, 48].

In respect to PTH regulation, although $1,25(OH)_2D_3$ is an inhibitor of PTH production in many in vitro and in vivo settings, in the HVDRR children, normalizing serum calcium by i.v. infusion is sufficient to suppress their secondary hyperparathyroidism. It is possible that inactivation of the VDR causes a loss of repression of the PTH gene and that this, together with hypocalcemia, triggers the secondary hyperparathyroidism. The correction of serum calcium concentration by i.v. infusions could then signal through the calcium-sensing receptor on the parathyroid glands to down-regulate the PTH gene and suppress the secondary hyperparathyroidism, even in the absence of $1,25(OH)_2D_3$ action. In addition, i.v. calcium therapy without concomitant phosphate administration is adequate to correct all of the metabolic abnormalities in children with HVDRR including the hypophosphatemia. This suggests that the hypophosphatemia in these patients is mainly the result of secondary hyperparathyroidism.

A prenatal diagnosis of HVDRR is now possible in pregnant women from high risk families. Cultured cells from chorionic villus samples or amniotic fluid have been used to ascertain whether the fetus has HVDRR using $[^3H]1,25(OH)_2D_3$ binding and induction of 24-hydroxylase activity [49, 50].

In many cases, the mutations were found to cause altered restriction fragment length polymorphisms which could be used to readily identify carriers of the mutant allele. The method of PCR amplification followed by restriction enzyme digestion provides a convenient diagnostic test to genotype family members.

A final point is the interesting dilemma regarding the spontaneous improvement in some HVDRR children as they get older. One hypothesis to explain the normalization of the $1,25(OH)_2D_3$ endocrine system in the face of inactive VDRs, is that some other transcription factor can substitute for the defective system. Possibly RAR, RXR or TR can substitute for a nonfunctional VDR and activate the appropriate target genes to reverse the hypocalcemia and restore the bones to normal. This hypothetical explanation remains to be tested.

The biochemical and genetic analysis of the VDR in the HVDRR syndrome has yielded important insights into the structure and function of the receptor in mediating $1,25(OH)_2D_3$ action. Similarly, studies of the affected children with HVDRR continue to provide further insight into the biological role of $1,25(OH)_2D_3$ in vivo. A concerted investigative approach of HVDRR at the clinical, cellular and molecular level has proven exceedingly valuable in understanding the mechanism of action of $1,25(OH)_2D_3$ and improving the diagnostic and clinical management of this rare genetic disease.

References

1 Haussler MR, Whitfield GK, Haussler CA, Hsieh J, Thompson PD, Selznick SH, Dominguez CE, Jurutka PW: The nuclear vitamin D receptor: Biological and molecular regulatory properties revealed. J Bone Min Res 1998;13:325–349.

2 Feldman D, Malloy PJ, Gross C: Vitamin D: Biology, action, and clinical implications; in Marcus R, Feldman D, Kelsey J (eds): Osteoporosis. San Diego, Academic Press, 2001, vol 1, pp 257–303.

3 Malloy PJ, Pike JW, Feldman D: The vitamin D receptor and the syndrome of hereditary 1,25-dihydroxyvitamin D-resistant rickets. Endocr Rev 1999;20:156–188.

4 Brooks MH, Bell NH, Love L, Stern PH, Orfei E, Queener SF, Hamstra AJ, DeLuca HF: Vitamin-D-dependent rickets type II. Resistance of target organs to 1,25-dihydroxyvitamin D. N Engl J Med 1978;298:996–999.

5 Marx SJ, Spiegel AM, Brown EM, Gardner DG, Downs RW Jr, Attie M, Hamstra AJ, DeLuca HF: A familial syndrome of decrease in sensitivity to 1,25-dihydroxyvitamin D. J Clin Endocrinol Metab 1978;47:1303–1310.

6 Takeyama K, Kitanaka S, Sato T, Kobori M, Yanagisawa J, Kato S: 25-Hydroxyvitamin D_3 1alpha-hydroxylase and vitamin D synthesis. Science 1997;277:1827–1830.

7 Fu GK, Lin D, Zhang MY, Bikle DD, Shackleton CH, Miller WL, Portale AA: Cloning of human 25-hydroxyvitamin D-1 alpha-hydroxylase and mutations causing vitamin D-dependent rickets type 1. Mol Endocrinol 1997;11:1961–1970.

8 Kitanaka S, Takeyama K, Murayama A, Sato T, Okumura K, Nogami M, Hasegawa Y, Niimi H, Yanagisawa J, Tanaka T, Kato S: Inactivating mutations in the 25-hydroxyvitamin D_3 1(alpha)-hydroxylase gene in patients with pseudovitamin D-deficiency rickets. N Engl J Med 1998; 338:653–661.

9 Laufer D, Benderly A, Hochberg Z: Dental pathology in calcitirol resistant rickets. J Oral Med 1987;42:272–275.

10 Hochberg Z, Borochowitz Z, Benderli A, Vardi P, Oren S, Spirer Z, Heyman I, Weisman Y: Does 1,25-dihydroxyvitamin D participate in the regulation of hormone release from endocrine glands? J Clin Endocrinol Metab 1985;60:57–61.
11 Tsoukas CD, Provvedini DM, Manolagas SC: 1,25-dihydroxyvitamin D_3: a novel immunoregulatory hormone. Science 1984;224:1438–1440.
12 Feldman D, Malloy PJ: Hereditary 1,25-dihydroxyvitamin D resistant rickets: Molecular basis and implications for the role of $1,25(OH)_2D_3$ in normal physiology. Mol Cell Endocrinol 1990; 72:C57–C62.
13 Even L, Weisman Y, Goldray D, Hochberg Z: Selective modulation by vitamin D of renal response to parathyroid hormone: A study in calcitriol-resistant rickets. J Clin Endocrinol Metab 1996; 81: 2836–2840.
14 Etzioni A, Hochberg Z, Pollak S, Meshulam T, Zakut V, Tzehoval E, Keisari Y, Aviram I, Spirer Z, Benderly A, Weisman Y: Defective leukocyte fungicidal activity in end-organ resistance to 1,25-dihydroxyvitamin D. Pediatr Res 1989;25:276–279.
15 Racz A, Barsony J: Hormone-dependent translocation of vitamin D receptors is linked to transactivation. J Biol Chem 1999;274:19352–19360.
16 Jurutka PW, Hsieh JC, MacDonald PN, Terpening CM, Haussler CA, Haussler MR, Whitfield GK: Phosphorylation of serine 208 in the human vitamin D receptor: The predominant amino acid phosphorylated by casein kinase II, in vitro, and identification as a significant phosphorylation site in intact cells. J Biol Chem 1993;268:6791–6799.
17 Rochel N, Wurtz JM, Mitschler A, Klaholz B, Moras D: The crystal structure of the nuclear receptor for vitamin D bound to its natural ligand. Mol Cell 2000;5:173–179.
18 Freedman LP: Increasing the complexity of coactivation in nuclear receptor signaling. Cell 1999;97:5–8.
19 Mangelsdorf DJ, Thummel C, Beato M, Herrlich P, Schutz G, Umesono K, Blumberg B, Kastner P, Mark M, Chambon P, et al.: The nuclear receptor superfamily: the second decade. Cell 1995;83: 835–839.
20 Hsieh JC, Jurutka PW, Selznick SH, Reeder MC, Haussler CA, Whitfield GK, Haussler MR: The T-box near the zinc fingers of the human vitamin D receptor is required for heterodimeric DNA binding and transactivation. Biochem Biophys Res Commun 1995;215:1–7.
21 Feldman D, Chen T, Hirst M, Colston K, Karasek M, Cone C: Demonstration of 1,25-dihydroxyvitamin D_3 receptors in human skin biopsies. J Clin Endocrinol Metab 1980;51:1463–1465.
22 Feldman D, Chen T, Cone C, Hirst M, Shani S, Benderli A, Hochberg Z: Vitamin D resistant rickets with alopecia: Cultured skin fibroblasts exhibit defective cytoplasmic receptors and unresponsiveness to $1,25(OH)_2D_3$. J Clin Endocrinol Metab 1982;55:1020–1022.
23 Hirst MA, Hochman HI, Feldman D: Vitamin D resistance and alopecia: a kindred with normal 1,25-dihydroxyvitamin D binding, but decreased receptor affinity for deoxyribonucleic acid. J Clin Endocrinol Metab 1985;60:490–495.
24 Malloy PJ, Hochberg Z, Pike JW, Feldman D: Abnormal binding of vitamin D receptors to deoxyribonucleic acid in a kindred with vitamin D-dependent rickets, type II. J Clin Endocrinol Metab 1989;68:263–269.
25 Hughes MR, Malloy PJ, Kieback DG, Kesterson RA, Pike JW, Feldman D, O'Malley BW: Point mutations in the human vitamin D receptor gene associated with hypocalcemic rickets. Science 1988;242:1702–1705.
26 Sone T, Scott RA, Hughes MR, Malloy PJ, Feldman D, O'Malley BW, Pike JW: Mutant vitamin D receptors which confer hereditary resistance to 1,25-dihydroxyvitamin D_3 in humans are transcriptionally inactive in vitro. J Biol Chem 1989;264:20230–20234.
27 Ritchie HH, Hughes MR, Thompson ET, Malloy PJ, Hochberg Z, Feldman D, Pike JW, O'Malley BW: An ochre mutation in the vitamin D receptor gene causes hereditary 1,25-dihydroxyvitamin D_3-resistant rickets in three families. Proc Natl Acad Sci USA 1989;86:9783–9787.
28 Malloy PJ, Hochberg Z, Tiosano D, Pike JW, Hughes MR, Feldman D: The molecular basis of hereditary 1,25-dihydroxyvitamin D_3 resistant rickets in seven related families. J Clin Invest 1990;86:2071–2079.
29 Malloy PJ, Zhu W, Bouillon R, Feldman D: A novel nonsense mutation in the ligand binding domain of the vitamin D receptor causes hereditary 1,25-dihydroxyvitamin D-resistant rickets. Mol Genet Metab 2002;77:314–318.

30 Van Maldergem L, Bachy A, Feldman D, Bouillon R, Maassen J, Dreyer M, Rey R, Holm C, Gillerot Y: Syndrome of lipoatrophic diabetes, vitamin D resistant rickets, and persistent Müllerian ducts in a Turkish boy born to consanguineous parents. Am J Med Genet 1996;64:506–513.
31 Magre J, Delepine M, Khallouf E, Gedde-Dahl T Jr, Van Maldergem L, Sobel E, Papp J, Meier M, Megarbane A, Bachy A, Verloes A, d'Abronzo FH, Seemanova E, Assan R, Baudic N, Bourut C, Czernichow P, Huet F, Grigorescu F, de Kerdanet M, Lacombe D, Labrune P, Lanza M, Loret H, Matsuda F, Navarro J, Nivelon-Chevalier A, Polak M, Robert JJ, Tric P, Tubiana-Rufi N, Vigouroux C, Weissenbach J, Savasta S, Maassen JA, Trygstad O, Bogalho P, Freitas P, Medina JL, Bonnicci F, Joffe BI, Loyson G, Panz VR, Raal FJ, O'Rahilly S, Stephenson T, Kahn CR, Lathrop M, Capeau J: Identification of the gene altered in Berardinelli-Seip congenital lipodystrophy on chromosome 11q13. Nat Genet 2001;28:365–370.
32 Nguyen TM, Adiceam P, Kottler ML, Guillozo H, Rizk-Rabin M, Brouillard F, Lagier P, Palix C, Garnier JM, Garabedian M: Tryptophan missense mutation in the ligand-binding domain of the vitamin D receptor causes severe resistance to 1,25-dihydroxyvitamin D. J Bone Miner Res 2002;17:1728–1737.
33 Malloy PJ, Zhu W, Zhao XY, Pehling GB, Feldman D: A novel inborn error in the ligand-binding domain of the vitamin D receptor causes hereditary vitamin D-resistant rickets. Mol Genet Metab 2001;73:138–148.
34 Wurtz JM, Bourguet W, Renaud JP, Vivat V, Chambon P, Moras D, Gronemeyer H: A canonical structure for the ligand-binding domain of nuclear receptors. Nat Struct Biol 1996;3: 87–94.
35 Malloy PJ, Xu R, Peng L, Clark PA, Feldman D: A novel mutation in helix 12 of the vitamin D receptor impairs coactivator interaction and causes hereditary 1,25-dihydroxyvitamin D-resistant rickets without alopecia. Mol Endocrinol 2002;16:2538–2546.
36 Miller J, Djabali K, Chen T, Liu Y, Ioffreda M, Lyle S, Christiano AM, Holick M, Cotsarelis G: Atrichia caused by mutations in the vitamin D receptor gene is a phenocopy of generalized atrichia caused by mutations in the hairless gene. J Invest Dermatol 2001;117:612–617.
37 Hewison M, Rut AR, Kristjansson K, Walker RE, Dillon MJ, Hughes MR, O'Riordan JL: Tissue resistance to 1,25-dihydroxyvitamin D without a mutation of the vitamin D receptor gene. Clin Endocrinol 1993;39:663–670.
38 Sakati N, Woodhouse NJY, Niles N, Harfi H, de Grange DA, Marx S: Hereditary resistance to 1,25-dihydroxyvitamin D: Clinical and radiological improvement during high-dose oral calcium therapy. Hormone Res 1986;24:280–287.
39 Balsan S, Garabedian M, Larchet M, Gorski AM, Cournot G, Tau C, Bourdeau A, Silve C, Ricour C: Long-term nocturnal calcium infusions can cure rickets and promote normal mineralization in hereditary resistance to 1,25-dihydroxyvitamin D. J Clin Invest 1986;77:1661–1667.
40 Al-Aqeel A, Ozand P, Sobki S, Sewairi W, Marx S: The combined use of intravenous and oral calcium for the treatment of vitamin D dependent rickets type II (VDDR-II). Clin Endocrinol 1993;39:229–237.
41 Hochberg Z, Tiosano D, Even L: Calcium therapy for calcitriol-resistant rickets. J Pediatr 1992; 121:803–808.
42 Gardezi SA, Nguyen C, Malloy PJ, Posner GH, Feldman D, Peleg S: A rationale for treatment of hereditary vitamin D-resistant rickets with analogs of 1-alpha,25-dihydroxyvitamin D_3. J Biol Chem 2001;276:29148–29156.
43 Panda DK, Miao D, Tremblay ML, Sirois J, Farookhi R, Hendy GN, Goltzman D: Targeted ablation of the 25-hydroxyvitamin D 1alpha-hydroxylase enzyme: evidence for skeletal, reproductive, and immune dysfunction. Proc Natl Acad Sci USA 2001;98:7498–7503.
44 Li YC, Pirro AE, Amling M, Delling G, Baron R, Bronson R, Demay MB: Targeted ablation of the vitamin D receptor: an animal model of vitamin D-dependent rickets type II with alopecia. Proc Natl Acad Sci USA 1997;94:9831–9835.
45 Yoshizawa T, Handa Y, Uematsu Y, Takeda S, Sekine K, Yoshihara Y, Kawakami T, Arioka K, Sato H, Uchiyama Y, Masushige S, Fukamizu A, Matsumoto T, Kato S: Mice lacking the vitamin D receptor exhibit impaired bone formation, uterine hypoplasia and growth retardation after weaning. Nat Genet 1997;16:391–396.

46 Chen CH, Sakai Y, Demay MB: Targeting expression of the human vitamin D receptor to the keratinocytes of vitamin D receptor null mice prevents alopecia. Endocrinology 2001;142: 5386–5389.
47 Underwood JL, DeLuca HF: Vitamin D is not directly necessary for bone growth and mineralization. Am J Physiol 1984;246:E493–E498.
48 Masuyama R, Nakaya Y, Tanaka S, Tsurukami H, Nakamura T, Watanabe S, Yoshizawa T, Kato S, Suzuki K: Dietary phosphorus restriction reverses the impaired bone mineralization in vitamin D receptor knockout mice. Endocrinology 2001;142:494–497.
49 Weisman Y, Jaccard N, Legum C, Spirer Z, Yedwab G, Even L, Edelstein S, Kaye AM, Hochberg Z: Prenatal diagnosis of vitamin D-dependent rickets, type II: response to 1,25-dihydroxyvitamin D in amniotic fluid cells and fetal tissues. J Clin Endocrinol Metab 1990;71:937–943.
50 Weisman Y, Malloy PJ, Krishnan AV, Jaccard N, Feldman D, Hochberg Z. Prenatal diagnosis of calcitriol resistant rickets (CRR) by 1,25(OH)$_2$D$_3$ binding, 24-hydroxylase induction and RFLP analysis. Ninth workshop on Vitamin D, Orlando, 1994, p 106.

David Feldman, MD, Stanford University School of Medicine
Division of Endocrinology, Gerontology and Metabolism
Stanford University Medical Center, Room S005
Stanford, CA 94305–5103 (USA)
Tel. +1 650 725 2910, Fax +1 650 725 7085, E-Mail feldman@cmgm.stanford.edu

Hochberg Z (ed): Vitamin D and Rickets.
Endocr Dev. Basel, Karger, 2003, vol 6, pp 200–219

Rickets in Transgenic Animals

Geert Carmeliet, Sophie Van Cromphaut, Christa Maes, Tim Raemaekers, Roger Bouillon

Laboratory for Experimental Medicine and Endocrinology, Katholieke Universiteit Leuven, Belgium

Contents

Mouse genetic studies have been a major driving force in elucidating bone biology at the molecular level and they often mimic bone pathology found in humans. Both rickets and osteomalacia show in mice histological features resembling those observed in humans. During development, a defective chondrocyte mineralization occurs at the growth plates and contributes to disorganization of chondrocyte arrangement. This leads to epiphyseal widening, a typical hallmark of rickets, retardation of longitudinal bone growth and skeletal deformities. In osteomalacia, the characteristic pathological changes involve bone remodeling. Impaired mineralization of bone matrix or osteoid is manifested by a decrease in the mineralizing surface (the percentage of bone surface undergoing calcification) and mineralization rate. This results in the accumulation of large surfaces of unmineralized osteoid in thick seams with numerous active osteoblasts overlying the osteoid seams.

As in humans, the various types of rickets and osteomalacia in mice can be divided into diseases characterized by calciopenia, phosphopenia or normal mineral availability. This chapter will concentrate only on the types of rickets or osteomalacia caused by genetic defect and not the diseases that are acquired or secondary to renal or gastrointestinal dysfunction. In addition, since most genetic studies are performed in mice only this transgenic animal model will be discussed.

Calciopenic Rickets

The currently recognized forms of calciopenic rickets due to genetic defects include disorders with abnormal vitamin D metabolism or resistance to the effects of the active form of vitamin D. It is generally accepted that vitamin D, either from dietary intake or synthesized in skin by ultraviolet exposure, is one of the main hormones for calcium homeostasis and bone mineralization.

Over the last years it was recognized that vitamin D undergoes sequential hydroxylation to 25(OH)D in the liver and to $1,25(OH)_2D$ [$1,25(OH)_2D_3$] in the kidney. The latter is the biologically active form of vitamin D. The ligand $1,25(OH)_2D_3$ will bind to the nuclear vitamin D receptor (VDR), which heterodimerizes with the retinoid X receptor and interacts with specific DNA sequences on target genes [1].

Genetic defects are found at several steps of this pathway but rickets are part of the clinical picture in only two disorders. The 25-hydroxylation step is guaranteed by a multifunctional hepatic CYP27 enzyme or through alternative pathways. Patients with cerebrotendinous xanthomatosis due to deficiency of CYP27 do not suffer from rickets, neither does the CYP27 KO mouse [2]. A specific hereditary defect in the gene coding for the 25-hydroxyvitamin D-1α-hydroxylase [1α(OH)ase] or CYP27B1 impairs the final, critical step in the biosynthesis of $1,25(OH)_2D_3$ resulting in vitamin D-dependent rickets type I (VDDR-I), also called pseudo-vitamin D-deficiency (PDDR) [3]. Mutations in the VDR are responsible for vitamin D-dependent rickets type II (VDDR-II) also called hereditary hypocalcemic vitamin D resistant rickets (HVDRR) [4]. Both these diseases display an autosomal-recessive trait, but clinical features and response to administrated $1,25(OH)_2D_3$ are distinct. The phenotypes of mice with targeted ablation of 1α(OH)ase or VDR exhibit the clinical abnormalities observed in the VDDR-I and -II patients, respectively, and offered the opportunity to investigate in vivo functions of $1,25(OH)_2D_3$ and the molecular basis of its actions. Gene ablation of 25-hydroxyvitamin D-24-hydroxylase (CYP24), the key effector of $1,25(OH)_2D_3$ catabolic breakdown in mice, results in increased levels of $1,25(OH)_2D$ that lead to deficient mineralization of intramembranous bone, but rickets are not observed [5].

Defect in Vitamin D Receptor-Effector System (Vitamin D-Dependent Rickets Type II)

Generation of VDR Null Mice

VDR null or VDR mutant mice have been created by 4 different groups (Tokyo, Boston, Leuven and München, respectively [6–9]) by either ablation of exon II/first zinc finger [6, 8–9] or exon III/second zinc finger [7] in the DNA-binding site of this nuclear receptor. The Leuven VDR null mice were generated using the Cre-lox system. The VDR mutant mice (München) are a phenocopy of the mice totally lacking the VDR protein and will be discussed together. VDR null mice of the Boston, Leuven and München strains exhibit nearly normal survival rates for up to 6 months, while affected homozygotes of the Tokyo strain die within 15 weeks. The differing survival times are not completely related to diet or environmental variations, but may partly be related to strain differences: the Tokyo VDR null mice housed in the facilities of the Leuven VDR null mice still suffer from a more important failure to thrive compared with the Leuven strain. However, all VDR null mice show a growth retardation starting after weaning.

Mineral Homeostasis and Rickets of VDR Null Mice

VDR null mice are born phenotypically normal, despite expression of VDR in fetal life from embryonic day 10.5 onwards in several tissues of WT mice. After weaning, VDR null mice acquire hypocalcemia and hyperparathyroidism, as evidenced by elevated parathyroid (PTH) levels in serum, an increase in the size of the parathyroid gland as well as an increase in PTH mRNA levels. Concomitant hypophosphatemia develops and $1,25(OH)_2D_3$

serum levels become 10- to 100-fold elevated, coincident with extremely low 24,25$(OH)_2D_3$ serum levels. These latter data are consistent with earlier findings that the activities of 1α(OH)ase and 24-hydroxylase are regulated negatively and positively, respectively, by 1,25$(OH)_2D_3$ [10, 11]. Inspection and X-ray analysis of long bones showed a reduced length and the typical features of rickets including widening of epiphyseal growth plates, thinning of the cortex, cupping and widening of the metaphysis. The time of onset of symptoms at 3 weeks of age fits with the observation that in neonatal rats intestinal calcium absorption occurs by a 1,25$(OH)_2D_3$-independent mechanism and is gradually replaced by a 1,25$(OH)_2D_3$-dependent mechanism [12]. This also suggests that the vitamin D endocrine system is principally required for maintaining bone mineral homeostasis when the organism is deprived of a consistent and plentiful supply of calcium, such as occurs after weaning in mammals.

Amling et al. [13] studied histomorphometric and biomechanical parameters in Boston VDR null mice, fed regular chow. They found by the age of 70 days: (a) 85% of bone surface covered with osteoid (osteoid/bone surface); (b) a marked increase in bone volume, due to increased osteoid; (c) an increase in osteoblast number and increased surface of bone covered by osteoblasts; (d) normal osteoclast number and surface of bone covered by osteoclasts; (e) impaired mineral apposition rate; (f) reduced stiffness and increased ultimate deformation; (g) expansion of length of growth plate (+48%) and disorganization of the chondrocyte columns and increased matrix.

However, normalization of mineral ion homeostasis (calcemia and phosphatemia) by feeding these mice a diet enriched with 2% calcium, 20% lactose and 1.25% phosphorus (the so-called 'rescue diet') prevented hyperparathyroidism and rickets [13, 14]. Normal morphology in the growth cartilage and adjacent metaphysis and normal biomechanical competence of cortical bone were demonstrated. Also, in humans is the bone pathology of VDRR type II cured by frequent intravenous calcium infusions and prevented by high oral doses of calcium.

These data suggest that, in an ideal metabolic environment, the VDR is not essential for the development or maintenance of normal bone, although 1,25$(OH)_2D_3$ has been shown to have significant effects on the expression of genes by osteoblasts and osteoclasts. Thus, the principle action of the VDR in skeletal growth, maturation and remodeling is its role in intestinal calcium absorption and/or renal calcium reabsorption.

Mechanisms Underlying the Disorganization of Growth Plate

Rickets or the expansion and disorganization of the growth plate are a characteristic feature of VDR inactivation (fig. 1). Analysis of growth plate

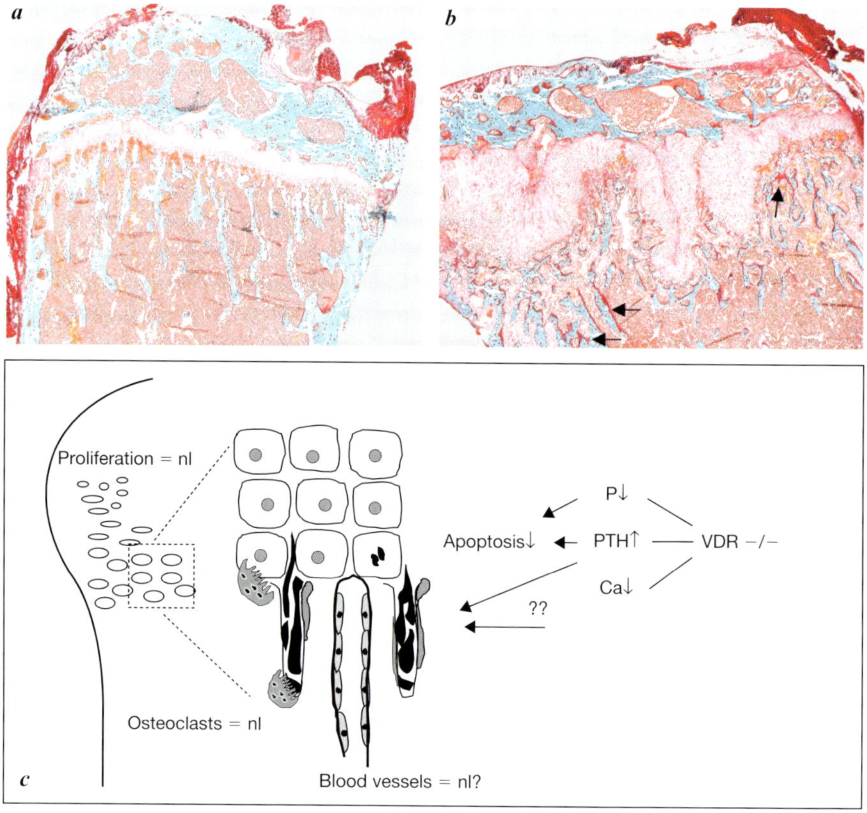

Fig. 1. Bone histomorphometry and molecular mechanisms of bone pathology in VDR null mice. ***a***, ***b*** The growth plate is manifestly disorganized and osteoid (arrow) is increased in the tibia of 8-week-old VDR null mice (***b***) compared to WT mice (***a***). ***c*** Model of molecular mechanisms of rickets in VDR null mice. Inactivation of VDR leads to increased bone volume, mainly due to increased osteoid, which normalizes when a rescue diet is given. The molecular mechanism of increased osteoid is not yet fully understood. The disorganization of the growth plate in VDR null mice is not secondary to osteoclast formation and proliferation of chondrocytes which are both normal in these mice. VEGF gene expression by hypertrophic chondrocytes is normal suggesting normal vascular invasion of the growth plate. Rather apoptosis of hypertrophic chondrocytes is decreased possibly as a consequence of hypophosphatemia although the effect of increased PTH levels can not be excluded.

morphology demonstrated normal resting and proliferating chondrocyte layers, but expansion of the hypertrophic chondrocyte layer. This latter finding could potentially be a consequence of an osteoclast defect, since $1,25(OH)_2D_3$ has been shown to be a potent inducer of the osteoclast differentiating factor, RANKL produced by osteoblasts [15]. This signal facilitates osteoclast differentiation via interaction with RANK present on the osteoclast. However, histomorphometric analyses have demonstrated normal numbers of osteoclasts in the metaphyses of several strains of VDR null mice. In addition, osteoblasts/stromal cells from WT mice did support $1,25(OH)_2D_3$ induced osteoclastogenesis of VDR null spleen cells in vitro, using the co-culture system, whereas the reverse experiment (VDR null osteoblasts/stromal cells and WT mouse spleen cells) did not result in the production of osteoclasts upon exposure of the coculture to $1,25(OH)_2D_3$ [16]. These data demonstrated that other osteoclast activating factors such as PTH and interleukin-1α are capable of inducing the formation of mature, resorbing osteoclasts in vivo in the absence of the VDR showing that the VDR is not essential for osteoclast-mediated bone resorption. This also suggests that the expansion of the hypertrophic chondrocyte layer is not secondary to an osteoclast defect. Osteoclasts are brought to the hypertrophic chondrocytes concomitant with vascular invasion. This process is initiated by secretion of vascular endothelial growth factor (VEGF), a signaling molecule produced by hypertrophic chondrocytes. No impairment of VEGF RNA production by these cells was observed in VDR null mice indicating that hypertrophic chondrocytes were capable of signaling vascular invasion [17].

Alternatively, the expansion of the hypertrophic chondrocyte layer may be due to altered chondrocyte development in VDR null mice, but present data are not conclusive at this moment. A recent study shows that in (Boston) VDR null mice, this feature is not secondary to increased chondrocyte proliferation or impaired differentiation but rather a consequence of decreased apoptosis [17]. The authors also postulate that hypophosphatemia, rather than hypocalcemia, is the major determinant of decreased chondrocyte apoptosis. However, excess PTH secretion in these mice might mimic the PTHrP paracrine effects on chondrocyte survival [18]. In contrast, no manifest alteration in the number of apoptotic cells or in the expression of apoptosis-related genes was detected in another VDR null strain [19].

A Second VDR and/or Nongenomic Actions?

After interaction with its ligand, VDR binds as a heterodimer with one of three retinoid X receptors (RXRα, -β, and -γ) to vitamin D-responsive elements in the promoters of vitamin D target genes [1]. To investigate the possibility of a functionally redundant VDR, mice deficient in both VDR and RXRγ were generated since RXRγ null mice exhibit no discernible abnormalities [19]. The phenotype observed in double null mutant mice was basically similar to those in VDR null mice, except that growth plate development was more severely impaired and was not prevented by dietary supplementation. A selective impairment of hypertrophic chondrocyte development was observed despite normalized mineral homeostasis produced by the high mineral diet. These findings indicate that the combined actions of VDR- and RXRγ-mediated signals are essential for normal development of growth plate cartilage and might be explained by a functional, but redundant, VDR-like receptor in growth plate chondrocytes.

Most of the actions of $1,25(OH)_2D_3$ are considered to result from regulation of gene transcription. However, a number of cellular and tissue responses to vitamin D metabolites have been described that occur within seconds to minutes. The exact mechanism explaining these rapid, nongenomic actions of $1,25(OH)_2D_3$ are not yet clearly defined. Interestingly, the rapid increase in intracellular calcium concentrations after addition of $1,25(OH)_2D_3$ to primary osteoblasts was absent in VDR mutant mice [9]. These data suggest that the classical VDR interacts with as yet unknown proteins to elicit rapid, non-genomic effects in osteoblasts.

Calcium Absorption in VDR Null Mice

The beneficial effect of the rescue diet aroused the question whether intestinal calcium absorption was indeed impaired in VDR null mice.

Calcium is absorbed through two different pathways in the small intestine [20]. On the one hand, the passive, paracellular pathway through tight junctions is more prominent in distal parts of the small intestine when calcium intake is high. On the other hand, the active, transcellular pathway is considered typical of duodenal calcium absorption and would rather intervene when calcium supply is low (fig. 2a). The latter is metabolically driven and positively regulated by $1\alpha,25(OH)_2D_3$ genomic actions [21]. Active calcium absorption was assessed in the Leuven and Tokyo VDR null strains by measuring appearance of ^{45}Ca in serum between 2 and 10 min after oral gavage [8]. The area under the curve was used to quantify the absorption. This area under the curve was, compared to the respective WT mice, reduced to one third of normal, whether measured in the Leuven VDR null mice (on a low calcium diet) or in Tokyo VDR null mice (kept on a normal calcium diet).

Subsequently, attempts were made to unravel the molecular basis of this impaired active calcium absorption. Possible target genes of active duodenal calcium absorption are: (a) calcium influx, which was elusive until the epithelial calcium channel ECaC1 (TRPV5, 22) and the calcium transport protein type 1 CaT1 (TRPV6, 23) were described as possible gatekeepers for calcium entering the cell; (b) intracellular calcium transfer by means of calbindin-D_{9K} [24]; (c) calcium extrusion which is guaranteed by the plasma membrane calcium ATPase ($PMCA_{1b}$) [25].

Former studies learned that $1,25(OH)_2D_3$ repletion of vitamin deficient chickens or rats led to an increase in calbindin-D_{9K} and PMCA expression [26].

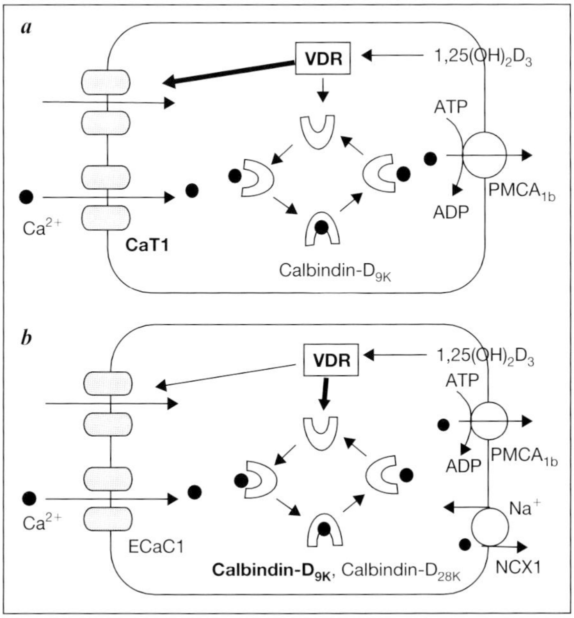

Fig. 2. Gene targets of 1,25(OH)$_2$D$_3$ action in the enterocyte (***a***) and renal tubular cell (***b***). ***a*** In the enterocyte is the main effect of 1,25(OH)$_2$D$_3$ via VDR on CaT1 expression. This model is based on the findings that in the absence of functional VDR, active intestinal calcium absorption is impaired. However, only CaT1 (and ECaC1) gene expression in duodenum is severely impaired, while the decrease in calbindin-D$_{9K}$ is only modest and PMCA$_{1b}$ expression is not altered. (***b***) In the kidney inactivation of VDR results in decreased renal calcium reabsorption. Differing from gene expression in duodenum, calbindin-D$_{9K}$ expression in the kidney is highly dependent on the presence of VDR, whereas the expression of the other calcium transport genes is not consistently altered. The major targets of 1,25(OH)$_2$D$_3$ action are indicated in **bold**.

Even in mouse with a normal vitamin D status, a single pharmacological injection of vitamin D enhanced the expression of these two factors [27].

Intriguingly, PMCA$_{1b}$ expression in Leuven and Tokyo VDR null mice was comparable to WT littermates [8]. The defect in calbindin-D$_{9K}$ expression was not consistent. A decrease of calbindin-D$_{9K}$ RNA and protein level was found by different groups in duodenum of the Tokyo VDR null [6, 8], and was described in Boston VDR null mice [7, 28, 29]. However, Leuven VDR null mice presented with normal calbindin-D$_{9K}$ protein content, which consequently could not account for the HVDRR phenotype of these mice [8]. In contrast, duodenal CaT1 and to a lesser degree ECaC1 RNA levels were dramatically and consistently downregulated in the Tokyo and the Leuven VDR null mice to less than 10% of their WT littermates. Moreover, Leuven VDR null mice failed to adapt to a 0.02% calcium diet: upregulation of CaT1 expression by more than 6 fold and doubling of calbindin-D_{9K} protein content were only seen in VDR WT littermates.

Until recently, the unidentified calcium influx mechanism was not regarded primordial, as calcium entered into the enterocyte even in the absence of vitamin D [30]. Comparison of duodenal gene expression patterns in Tokyo and Leuven VDR null mice indicated that among the candidate calcium transporting genes, only CaT1 and ECaC1 are severely impaired in the absence of a functional VDR. This implies a regulatory role for the epithelial calcium channels in active calcium absorption, or a more complex regulation driven by the interaction between calcium influx and calbindin-D_{9K}. The permanent activation of the CaT1 and ECaC1 channels may indeed require the immediate intracellular uptake of each calcium molecule delivered through the channel by calbindin-D_{9K}, with subsequent mobilization of calcium towards the basolateral membrane.

Further research, including the characterization of the phenotype of ECaC1, CaT1 or calbindin-D_{9K} null mice once they are generated and when they are viable, will be necessary to support this concept.

Renal Calcium Reabsorption

In normal adult animals, a major portion (>95%) of filtered calcium in the kidney is reabsorbed. In the distal nephron, tubular calcium transport consists of passive entry of calcium across the apical membrane through the epithelial calcium channel (ECaC1), cytosolic diffusion of calcium bound to calbindin (calbindin-D_{28K} and calbindin-D_{9K}), and active extrusion of calcium across the opposite basolateral membrane by the Na^+/Ca^{2+} exchanger (NCX1) and the plasma membrane Ca^{2+}-ATPase ($PMCA_{1b}$) (fig. 2b). Although urinary calcium excretion in VDR null mice was similar to WT mice under a normal diet, it is inappropriately high given the hypocalcemia in these mice [9, 29]. Normalization of serum calcium levels by the rescue diet resulted in a manifest increase of calcium excretion suggesting that renal tubular calcium reabsorption is impaired in VDR null mice. The parameter that correlated best herewith was the expression of calbindin-D_{9K} which was found to be decreased in all strains of VDR null mice both on the normal and the rescue diet [6, 8, 9, 28, 29]. Gene expression of calbindin-D_{28K} and of $PMCA_{1b}$ was not influenced by the absence of VDR, while NCX and ECaC1 RNA levels were inconsistent in the different strains. These data suggest that calbindin-D_{9K} may be an important mediator of calcium transport in the distal tubule and that its expression is highly dependent on the presence of VDR.

Deficiency in 1,25(OH)$_2$D Production (Vitamin D-Dependent Rickets Type I)

Generation of 1α(OH)ase Null Mice

The engineering of 1α(OH)ase null mice was reported by two different groups. The 1α(OH)ase gene was ablated by targeting part of exon 7 and 8 [31], or exons 6 to 9 [32]. In both cases the heme-binding domain and part of or complete hormone-binding domain were knocked out. No exact data are available on life expectancy in these mice but both strains demonstrate failure to thrive.

Mineral Homeostasis in 1α(OH)ase Null Mice

Regarding calcium homeostasis both 1α(OH)ase null models are identical. They demonstrate hypocalcemia, severe secondary hyperparathyroidism, hypophosphatemia, elevated serum alkaline phosphatase and increased phosphaturia, analogous to the phenotype of the VDR null mice. However 1α(OH)ase null mice genuinely lack the capacity to synthesize 1,25(OH)$_2$D$_3$: circulating levels of 1,25(OH)$_2$D$_3$ were undetectable, whereas circulating levels of 25(OH)D$_3$ doubled. This emphasizes the nonredundant role played by the renal 1α(OH)ase in producing the hormonally active metabolite of vitamin D. Furthermore, this confirms that the phenotype of the 1α(OH)ase null mice matches the clinical manifestations of VDDR-I [33].

Typical features of advanced rickets are observed histologically in bone of 1α(OH)ase null mice: disorganization and widening of the columnar alignment of hypertrophic chondrocytes, resulting in increased width of the growth plate, impaired calcification of the hypertrophic cartilage and accumulation of osteoid in trabecular and cortical bone. Panda et al. [32] also mentioned reduced osteoclasts in the 1α(OH)ase null mutant bone. Such a decrease was not observed in VDR null mice and the reason for this discrepancy is unclear at the moment. Further studies will be required to assess the role of calcium per se in the genesis of skeletal dysfunction in the 1α(OH)ase null mice. At this moment, it is only known that a calcium enriched diet normalizes serum calcium levels [34] but whether this will completely rescue the growth plate disorganization and skeletal defects remains questionable as a VDR-independent effect of 1,25(OH)$_2$D$_3$ on skeletal homeostasis has been suggested [35].

The treatment of choice for VDRR-I is long-term replacement therapy with 1,25(OH)$_2$D$_3$. The use of the monohydroxylated analogue 1α(OH)D$_3$, which is activated by the liver enzymes is another possibility. The comparison of pharmacological strategies in this animal model is eagerly anticipated.

Calcium Absorption and Reabsorption in 1α(OH)ase Null Mice

At present, data on calcium absorption are limited to assessment of calbindin-D_{9K} in duodenum: comparable to northern analysis of duodenum of Tokyo and Boston VDR null mice, RNA levels are clearly downregulated in both models of 1α(OH)ase null mice [31, 32]. However, functional analysis of calcium absorption and data on gene expression of the epithelial calcium channels and PMCA are lacking. In kidney, gene expression of ECaC1, Calbindin-D_{9K}, Calbindin-D_{28K} and NCX1 were significantly decreased in 1α(OH)ase null mice [32, 34]. Feeding these mice a rescue diet normalized the expression of calcium transport proteins except for calbindin-D_{9K}, suggesting that high dietary calcium intake is an important regulator of renal calcium transport proteins in a still undefined manner.

Conclusion

Both the VDR null mice and the 1α(OH)ase null mice provide mouse models for the human diseases VDDR-II and VDDR-I, respectively. These mice are useful models to decipher whether some effects can be substituted by the calcium ion, whether the effects of $1,25(OH)_2D_3$ occur exclusively via the VDR, whether other vitamin D metabolites or other products of the 1α(OH)ase exist and how they function and finally to investigate the mechanisms of non-genomic effects. Both mouse models lack not only $1,25(OH)_2D_3$ but also $24,25(OH)_2D$ as 24-hydroxylase expression is extremely dependent on $1,25(OH)_2D_3$. The contribution of $24,25(OH)_2D$ on the rachitic phenotype of the VDR and 1α(OH)ase null mice therefore requires further study.

Phosphopenic Rickets

Phosphorus and phosphate ions play an important role in the control of cellular metabolism and bone integrity. Phosphate is required for the formation of hydroxyapatite – an essential component of bone mineral. When phosphate concentrations in the extracellular fluid and serum are low, inadequate mineralization of osteoid occurs resulting in rickets or osteomalacia, depending on the skeletal age. The kidney is a major regulator of phosphate homeostasis. The bulk of filtered phosphate is reabsorbed in the proximal tubule through the Na-phosphate cotransporter type IIa (NPT2a) which mediates the rate-limiting step [36]. Although NPT2a null mice exhibit decreased renal phosphate reabsorption and hypophosphatemia, rickets do not occur [37].

However two inherited defects of renal phosphate-wasting disorders that produce hypophosphatemia are a cause of defective mineralization, including the X-linked hypophosphatemic rickets [38] and the autosomal-dominant hypophosphatemic rickets (ADHR) [39] (fig. 3).

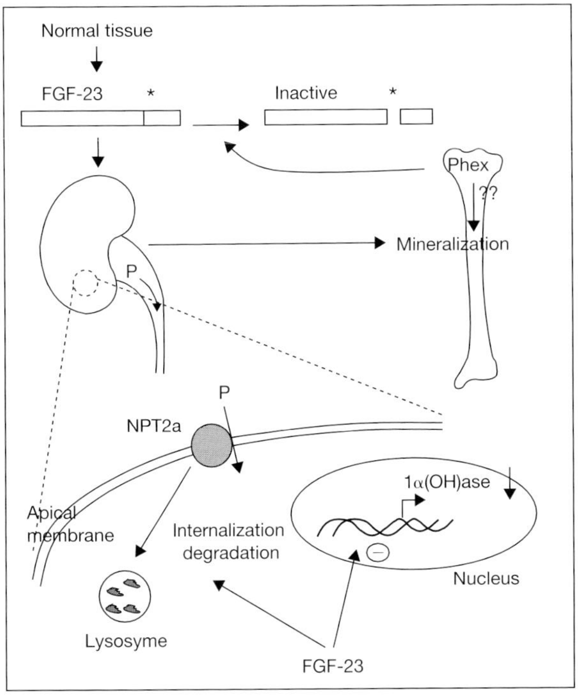

Fig. 3. Proposed model of pathogenesis of phosphopenic rickets. FGF-23 is normally metabolized through the actions of Phex endopeptidase and is protected from metabolism by mutations found in patients with ADHR. FGF-23 leads to rapid internalization and subsequent lysosomal degradation of NPT2a in renal tubular cells and decreases gene expression of 1α(OH)ase. FGF-23 levels can also be increased by mutations in Phex, a protease expressed in bone tissue, which cleaves and inactivates FGF-23. Mutations in Phex are found in X-linked dominant hypophosphatemic rickets.

X-Linked Hypophosphatemic Rickets

The primary defects in X-linked hypophosphatemic rickets (XLH) are mutations that inactivate PHEX, predicted to encode a membrane-associated metalloendopeptidase.

Mouse Models of XLH

In two mouse models of hypophosphatemic rickets (HYP and Gy) deletions in the murine PHEX gene were discovered at the 3′ and 5′ ends, respectively [40–43]. These mice exhibit the same phenotypic features that characterize patients with XLH showing growth retardation, rickets and osteomalacia, hypophosphatemia, renal phosphate wasting and inappropriately low $1,25(OH)_2D_3$ levels.

Phex is predominantly expressed in bone and teeth, but not in kidney [44]. This localization pattern of Phex together with other lines of evidence (parabiosis and cross-kidney transplantation experiments) indicates that XLH and Hyp are caused by a humoral mechanism. The current model hypotheses that the endopeptidase Phex degrades a novel phosphaturic hormone, also called phosphatonin, with fibroblast growth factor-23 (FGF-23) being a good candidate [45, 46].

Molecular Features in Kidney and Bone

Both renal phosphate handling and vitamin D metabolism are impaired in these mice [47]. Studies demonstrated that the renal phosphate transport defect can mainly be ascribed to a decrease in the number of high-affinity NPT2a. The inappropriately low $1,25(OH)_2D_3$ level for the degree of hypophosphatemia can be attributed to a decrease in the activity of renal $1\alpha(OH)$ase and increase in the abundance and activity of renal 24(OH)ase [44].

Several studies have suggested that the bone phenotype in Hyp mice is not only determined by the hypophosphatemic environment [47]. Phex is expressed at high levels in normal osteoblasts where its expression is temporally associated with the formation of mineralized extracellular matrix. Cultured osteoblasts from Hyp mice display an apparently intrinsic mineralization defect [44, 48]. Although targeted overexpression of Phex to osteoblasts in Hyp mice using the mouse osteocalcin promoter could normalize Phex endopeptidase activity in bone, it failed to correct the mineralization defect of bone and the systemic hypophosphatemia [49]. These data indicate that expression of Phex in osteoblasts is not sufficient to rescue the Hyp phenotype and that other sites of Phex expression and/or additional factors are likely to be important in the pathogenesis of XLH. A possible explanation may be that phosphate transport is defective in osteoblasts from Hyp mice which is shown to be Phex independent [50].

Autosomal-Dominant Hypophosphatemic Rickets

The responsible gene for ADHR has recently been identified and named FGF-23 [39]. Missense mutations in the consensus proteolytic cleavage sequence of the FGF-23 gene product cause this disorder. It is suggested that the mutations confer a gain of function on FGF-23 by blocking its degradation. FGF-23 expression is barely detectable in normal tissues and the lack of expression in kidney indicates that ADHR is caused by a humoral mechanism.

Mouse Studies

Several approaches were undertaken to assess the function of FGF-23. Both the effect of an excess of FGF-23 [51] as well as gene inactivation of FGF-23 were investigated [52].

When injected into mice, recombinant full-length FGF-23 produced mild phosphaturia and hypophosphatemia, while the N-terminal and C-terminal fragments of wild-type FGF-23 did not affect serum phosphate levels. These data indicate that the processing abolishes the activity of the FGF-23 protein to induce phosphaturia and hypophosphatemia. Mutant FGF-23 that is resistant to the cleavage also retained the activity to induce hypophosphatemia [53]. In addition, CHO cells stably expressing the wild-type or mutant FGF-23, when grown as tumors in nude mice, fully reproduced the human syndrome of severe hypophosphatemia, with increased renal phosphate clearance and a decrease of bone mineral content, increase of osteoid and widening of growth plate.

Investigating the underlying molecular mechanisms, it was observed that administration of FGF-23 induced a rapid decrease in renal 1α(OH)ase expression and increase in 24(OH)ase expression resulting in diminished serum 1,25$(OH)_2D_3$ levels [54]. This was followed by reduced expression of NPT2a and hypophosphatemia. These results indicate that FGF-23 is a regulator of mineral homeostasis with unique properties controlling vitamin D metabolism and phosphate reabsorption.

FGF-23 null mice were recently generated [52] and body size was not different from WT mice at birth. However, progressive growth retardation was observed and life span was decreased. At 10 days only serum phosphate was increased, but at 9 weeks serum phosphate as well as calcium and 1,25$(OH)_2D_3$ were increased. These results indicate that FGF-23 is not necessary during fetal development, but required for normal growth after birth and that it plays a role in mineral homeostasis and vitamin D metabolism.

Conclusion

The PHEX gene and FGF-23 were identified as responsible genes for XLH and ADHR, respectively. It is tempting to propose a simplified model invoking a common metabolic pathway. The model suggests that FGF-23 is phosphaturic, that FGF-23 and/or its processed N-terminal and C-terminal fragments are degraded by PHEX, and that some mutations in FGF-23 can abolish the degradation by PHEX and therefore FGF-23 retains its phosphaturic action. It is clear that FGF-23 plays a central role in the pathophysiology of these disorders; however, its role in normal physiology and the mechanism by which it regulates renal phosphate handling or vitamin D metabolism are not fully understood.

Normal Mineral Rickets

Hypophosphatasia is a rare inherited disorder characterized by deficient activity of the tissue-nonspecific isoenzyme of alkaline phosphatase (TNAP) and skeletal disease due to impaired mineralization of cartilage and bone matrix [55]. Several forms of this disease exist. In the infantile form, patients seem well as neonates, but then present with failure to thrive and rachitic disease before 6 months of age. Skeletal deterioration is common thereafter and it has been estimated that 50% of these infants die several months later.

In this disorder 3 phosphocompounds (phosphoethanolamine, inorganic pyrophosphate (PP_i) and pyridoxal 5′-phosphate) accumulate endogenously and seem therefore to be natural substrates for TNAP [56].

Generation of Alkaline Phosphatase Null Mice as a Model for Infantile Hypophosphatasia

Two laboratories independently disrupted the mouse TNAP gene generating null mutant strains [57–58]. Phenotypic differences exist between the two strains, but both represent a good model for infantile hypophosphatasia.

Mice homozygous for the TNAP mutation appear normal at birth, but show already growth retardation after 4–6 days. TNAP null mice develop epileptic seizures and die before weaning, often after a prolonged seizure attack. Survival of TNAP null mice requires parenteral administration of pyridoxal to prevent these lethal seizures. Abnormalities in pyridoxal 5′-phosphate explain the seizures, apnea, increased apoptosis in thymus and abnormal myelinization of lumbar nerve roots found in the TNAP null mice, but the mineralization abnormalities in these mice appear unrelated to this substrate's metabolism.

Bone Metabolism

Despite their skeletal disease and profound deficiency of ALP activity, plasma and urine calcium and phosphate levels are similar in null mice and wild type mice, which exclude essentially other causes of rickets. Although null mice appear normal at 6 days of age on radiographic analysis, delayed appearance of epiphyses or secondary ossification centers, fractures, osteopenia and bone deformities are noted with aging [59]. Thus rachitic disease (that is complicated by gradual generalized skeletal demineralization) develops in a pattern that is typical of patients with the infantile form of hypophosphatasia.

Histopathology of bone revealed a widening of the osteoid seams with large islands of osteoid within the mineralized bone. This resulted from defective skeletal matrix mineralization but without features of secondary hyperparathyroidism. Moreover, the zone of hypertrophic chondrocytes was diminished suggesting a developmental arrest of chondrocyte differentiation in growth plates. This observation documents that TNAP itself plays a critical role in mineralization of the mouse as well as the human skeleton.

Osteoblastic Dysfunction in TNAP Null Mice

Bone resorbing activity of TNAP null osteoclasts, as assessed in a bone organ culture, is comparable to WT osteoclasts [60]. Also, the gene expression of several proteins that are typical for certain stages of osteoblast development were similar in the different genotypes. However, although cultures of primary TNAP osteoblasts were able to form cellular nodules as well as WT osteoblasts do, they lacked the ability to mineralize these nodules in vitro. Mineralization was also delayed in TNAP +/− cultures. This fact that even heterozygous osteoblasts show delayed mineralization provides a rationale for the presence of bone disease in carriers of hypophosphatasia.

Incubation with media supplemented with recombinant TNAP or with conditioned media from WT osteoblasts, but not with enzymatically inactive TNAP restored mineralization in TNAP null osteoblast cultures. Moreover precipitation was restricted to the nodular structures suggesting a regulated process. These data indicate that osteoblasts in TNAP null mice differentiate normally but are unable to initiate mineralization in vitro.

TNAP Is a Regulator of Bone Mineralization

The model has been proposed that TNAP functions by hydrolyzing PP_i generating hereby the P_i needed for hydroxyapatite crystallization. However, it has also been hypothesized that the ability of TNAP to hydrolyze PP_i is important to promote calcification by hydrolyzing this potent inhibitor of mineralization. PP_i is produced by the nucleoside triphosphate pyrophosphohydrolase activity of a family of isozymes, with plasma cell membrane glycoprotein-1 (PC-1) being the only member present in matrix vesicles. It was recently shown that normal bone mineralization occurs in knockout mice null for both TNAP and PC-1 [61]. These data indicate that the primary function of TNAP in mineralizing tissue is to control PP_i concentrations adequate for controlled mineralization and that the P_i-generating role for TNAP seems to be secondary.

Conclusion

These transgenic mice provide models for several types of mineralization defects in human pathology. When the defect is present during bone development and bone growth it will affect the organization of the growth plate and interferes with the mineralization of osteoid, the matrix formed by the osteoblasts. This will result in the typical features of rickets. When the mineralization defect occurs later in life it will only affect osteoblastic function leading to the clinical picture of osteomalacia.

Three major pathways are mainly coordinating the process of bone mineralization: calcium and phosphate homeostasis which are dependent on an intact vitamin D axis or phosphate transport axis respectively and at the other hand proteins regulating the mineralization process in which alkaline phosphatase is the best known player. Mutations in one of these proteins will lead to rickets and/or osteomalacia. However, it is not unlikely that other genes are also involved.

References

1 Haussler MR, Whitfield K, Haussler CA, Hsieh JC, Thompson PD, Selznick SH, Dominguez CE, Jurutka PW: The nuclear vitamin D receptor: Biological and molecular regulatory properties revealed. J Bone Miner Res 1998;13:325–349.

2 Rosen H, Reshef A, Maeda N, Lippoldt A, Shpizen S, Triger L, Eggertsen G, Bjorkhem I, Leitersdorf E: Markedly reduced bile acid synthesis but maintained levels of cholesterol and vitamin D metabolites in mice with disrupted sterol 27-hydroxylase gene. J Biol Chem 1998;273: 14805–14812.

3 Kato S, Yanagisawa J, Murayama A, Kitanaka S, Takeyama K: The importance of 25-hydroxyvitamin D_3 1α-hydroxylase gene in vitamin D-dependent rickets. Curr Opin Nephrol Hypertens 1998;7: 377–383.

4 Malloy PJ, Pike JW, Feldman D: The vitamin D receptor and the syndrome of hereditary 1,25-dihydroxyvitamin D-resistant rickets. Endocrine Rev 1999;20:156–188.

5 St-Arnaud R, Arabian A, Travers R, Barletta F, Raval-Pandya M, Chapin K, Depovere J, Mathieu C, Christakos S, Demay MB, Glorieux F: Deficient mineralization of intramembranous bone in vitamin D-24-hydroxylase-ablated mice is due to elevated 1,25-dihydroxyvitamin D and not to the absence of 24,25-dihydroxyvitamin D. Endocrinology 2000;141:2658–2666.

6 Yoshizawa T, Handa Y, Uematsu Y, Takeda S, Sekine K, Yoshihara Y, Kawakami T, Arioka K, Sato H, Uchiyama Y, Masushige S, Fukamizu A, Matsumoto T, Kato S: Mice lacking the vitamin D receptor exhibit impaired bone formation, uterine hypoplasia and growth retardation after weaning. Nat Genet 1997;16:391–396.

7 Li YC, Pirro AE, Amling M, Delling G, Baron R, Bronson R, Demay MB: Targeted ablation of the vitamin D receptor: An animal model of vitamin D-dependent rickets type II with alopecia. Proc Natl Acad Sci USA 1997;94:9831–9835.

8 Van Cromphaut SJ, Dewerchin M, Hoenderop JGJ, Stockmans I, Van Herck E, Kato S, Bindels RJM, Collen D, Carmeliet P, Bouillon R, Carmeliet G: Duodenal calcium absorption in vitamin D receptor-knockout mice: Functional and molecular aspects. Proc Natl Acad Sci USA 2001;98:13324–13329.

9 Erben RG, Soegiarto DW, Weber K, Zeitz U, Lieberherr M, Gniadecki R, Moller G, Adamski J, Balling R: Deletion of deoxyribonucleic acid binding domain of the vitamin D receptor abrogates genomic and nongenomic functions of vitamin D. Mol Endocrinol 2002;16:1524–1537.

10 Murayama A, Takeyama K, Kitanaka S, Kodera Y, Hosoya T, Kato S: The promoter of the human 25-hydroxyvitamin D_3 1α-hydroxylase gene confers positive and negative responsiveness to PTH, calcitonin, and 1α, 25$(OH)_2D_3$. Biochem Biophys Res Commun 1998;249:11–16.
11 Omdahl J, May B: The 25-hydroxyvitamin D 24-hydroxylase; in Feldman D, Glorieux FH, Pike JW (eds): Vitamin D. San Diego, Academic Press, 1997, pp 69–85.
12 Dostal LA, Toverud SU: Effect of vitamin D_3 on duodenal calcium absorption in vivo during early development. Am J Physiol 1984;246:G528–G534.
13 Amling M, Priemel MHT, Chapin K, Rueger JM, Baron R, Demay MB: Rescue of the skeletal phenotype of vitamin D receptor ablated mice in the setting of normal mineral ion homeostasis: Formal histomorphometric and biomechanical analyses. Endocrinology 1999;140:4982–4987.
14 Li YC, Amling M, Pirro AE, Priemel M, Meuse J, Baron R, Delling G, Demay MB: Normalization of mineral ion homeostasis by dietary means prevents hyperparathyroidism, rickets, and osteomalacia, but not alopecia in vitamin D receptor-ablated mice. Endocrinology 1998;139: 4391–4396.
15 Yasuda H, Shima N, Nakagawa N, Yamaguchi K, Kinosaki M, Mochizuki S, Tomoyasu A, Yano K, Goto M, Murakami A, Tsuda E, Morinaga T, Higashio K, Udagawa N, Takahashi N, Suda T: Osteoclast differentiation factor is a ligand for osteoprotegerin/osteoclastogenesis-inhibitory factor and is identical to TRANCE/RANKL. Proc Natl Acad Sci USA 1998;95:3597–3602.
16 Takeda S, Yoshizawa T, Nagai Y, Yamato H, Fukumoto S, Sekine K, Kato S, Matsumoto T, Fujita T: Stimulation of osteoclast formation by 1,25-dihydroxyvitamin D requires its binding to vitamin D receptor (VDR) in osteoblastic cell: Studies using VDR knockout mice. Endocrinology 1999; 140:1005–1008.
17 Donohue MM, Demay MB: Rickets in VDR null mice is secondary to decreased apoptosis of hypertrophic chondrocytes. Endocrinology 2002;143:3691–3694.
18 Amling M, Neff L, Tanaka S, Inoue D, Kuida K, Weir E, Philbrick WM, Broadus AE, Baron R: Bcl-2 lies downstream of parathyroid hormone-related peptide in a signaling pathway that regulates chondrocyte maturation during skeletal development. J Cell Biol 1997;136:205–213.
19 Yagishita N, Yamamoto Y, Yoshizawa T, Sekine K, Uematsu Y, Murayama H, Nagai Y, Krezel W, Chambon P, Matsumoto T, Kato S: Aberrant growth plate development in VDR/RXRγ double null mutant mice. Endocrinology 2001;142:5332–5341.
20 Bronner F, Pansu D: Nutritional aspects of calcium absorption. J Nutr 1999;129:9–12.
21 Norman AW: Intestinal calcium absorption: A vitamin D-hormone-mediated adaptive response. Am J Clin Nutr 1990;51:290–300.
22 Hoenderop JG, van der Kemp AW, Hartog A, van de Graaf SF, van Os CH, Willems PH, Bindels RJ: Molecular identification of the apical Ca^{2+} channel in 1,25-dihydroxyvitamin D_3 responsive epithelia. J Biol Chem 1999;274:8375–8378.
23 Peng JB, Chen XZ, Berger UV, Vassilev PM, Tsukaguchi H, Brown EM, Hediger MA: Molecular cloning and characterization of a channel-like transporter mediating intestinal absorption. J Biol Chem 1999;274:22739–22746.
24 Christakos S, Gabrielides C, Rhoten WB: Vitamin D-dependent calcium binding proteins: Chemistry, distribution, functional considerations, and molecular biology. Endocr Rev 1989;10: 3–26.
25 Freeman TC, Howard A, Bentsen BS, Legon S, Walters JRF: Cellular and regional expression of transcripts of the plasma membrane calcium pump PMCA1 in rabbit intestine. Am J Physiol 1995;269:G126–G131.
26 Matkovits T, Christakos S: Variable in vivo regulation of rat vitamin D-dependent genes (osteopontin, Ca, Mg-adenosine triphosphatase, and 25-hydroxyvitamin D_3 24-hydroxylase): Implications for differing mechanisms of regulation and involvement of multiple factors. Endocrinology 1995;136:3971–3982.
27 Cai Q, Chandler JS, Wasserman RH, Kumar R, Penniston JT: Vitamin D and adaptation to dietary calcium and phosphate increase intestinal plasma membrane calcium pump gene expression. Proc Natl Acad Sci USA 1993;90:1345–1349.
28 Li YC, Pirro AE, Demay MB: Analysis of vitamin D-dependent calcium-binding protein messenger ribonucleic acid expression in mice lacking the vitamin D receptor. Endocrinology 1998;139: 847–851.

29 Li YC, Bolt MJG, Cao LP, Sitrin MD: Effects of vitamin D receptor inactivation on the expression of calbindins and calcium metabolism. Am J Physiol Endocrinol Metab 2001;281:E558–E564.
30 Fullmer CS, Chandra S, Smith CA, Morrison GH, Wasserman RH: Ion microscopic imaging of calcium during 1,25-dihydroxyvitamin D-mediated intestinal absorption. Histochem Cell Biol 1996;106:215–222.
31 Dardenne O, Prud'homme J, Arabian A, Glorieux FH, St-Arnaud R: Targeted inactivation of the 25-hydroxyvitamin D_3–1_α-hydroxylase gene (CYP27B1) creates an animal model of pseudovitamin D-deficiency rickets. Endocrinology 2001;142:3135–3141.
32 Panda DK, Miao D, Tremblay ML, Sirois J, Farookhi R, Hendy GN, Goltzman D: Targeted ablation of the 25-hydroxyvitamin D 1α-hydroxylase enzyme: Evidence for skeletal, reproductive, and immune dysfunction. Proc Natl Acad Sci USA 2001;98:7498–7503.
33 Bouillon R: The many faces of rickets. N Engl J Med 1998;338:653–661.
34 Hoenderop JGJ, Dardenne O, Van Abel M, Van Der Kemp AWCM, Van Os CH, St.-Arnaud R, Bindels RJM: Modulation of renal Ca^{2+} transport protein genes by dietary Ca^{2+} and 1,25-dihydroxyvitamin D_3 in 25-hydroxyvitamin D_3–1α-hydroxylase knockout mice. FASEB J 2002; 16:1398–1406.
35 Panda DK, Miao D, Huo R, Hendy GN, Goltzman D: Comparison of mice with deletions of the 25OHvitamin D_3–1α hydroxylase [1αOHase], of the vitamin D receptor (VDR), and of both, suggest an in vivo role for VDR-dependent and independent regulation of calcium and skeletal homeostasis. J Bone Miner Res 2002;17(suppl 1):S132.
36 Murer H, Hernando N, Forster I, Biber J: Proximal tubular phosphate reabsorption: molecular mechanisms. Physiol Rev 2000;80:1373–1409.
37 Beck L, Karaplis AC, Amizuka N, Hewson AS, Ozawa H, Tenenhouse HS: Targeted inactivation of Npt2 in mice leads to severe renal phosphate wasting, hypercalciuria, and skeletal abnormalities. Proc Natl Acad Sci USA 1998;95:5372–5377.
38 HYP Consortium: A gene (PEX) with homologies to endopeptidases is mutated in patients with X-linked hypophosphatemic rickets. Nat Genet 1995;11:130–136.
39 The ADHR Consortium: Autosomal dominant hypophosphatemic rickets I associated with mutations in FGF-23. Nat Genet 2000;26:345–348.
40 Eicher EM, Southard JL, Scriver CR, Glorieux FH: Hypophosphatemia. Mouse model for human familial hypophosphatemic (vitamin D-resistant) rickets. Proc Natl Acad Sci USA 1976;73: 4667–4671.
41 Lyon MF, Scriver CR, Baker LRI, Tenenhouse HS, Kronick J, Mandla S: The Gy mutation: Another cause of X-linked hypophosphatemia in mouse. Proc Natl Acad Sci USA 1986;83:4899–4903.
42 Beck L, Soumounou Y, Martel J, Krishnamurthy G, Gauthier C, Goodyer C, Tenenhouse HS: Pex/PEX tissue distribution and evidence for a deletion in the 3' region of the Pex gene in X-linked hypophosphatemic mice. J Clin Invest 1997;99:1200–1209.
43 Strom TM, Francis F, Lorenz B, Böddrich A, Econs MJ, Lehrach H, Meitinger T: Pex gene deletions in Gy and Hyp mice provide mouse models for X-linked hypophosphatemia. Hum Mol Genet 1997;6:165–171.
44 Tenenhouse HS: X-linked hypophosphataemia: a homologous disorder in humans and mice. Nephrol Dial Transplant 1999;14:333–341.
45 Tenenhouse HS, Sabbagh Y: Novel phosphate-regulating genes in the pathogenesis of renal phosphate wasting disorders. Pflügers Arch 2002;444:317–326.
46 Jonsson KB, Zahradnik R, Larsson T, White KE, Hampson G, Miyauchi A, Ljunggren O, Koshiyama H, Sugimoto T, Oba K, Yamamoto T, Imanishi Y, Econs M, Lavigne J, Jueppner H: FGF-23 is a circulating factor that is elevated in oncogenic osteomalacia and X-linked hypophosphatemic rickets. J Bone Miner Res 2002;17(suppl 1):S158.
47 Jan de Beur SM, Levine MA: Molecular pathogenesis of hypophosphatemic rickets. J Clin Endocrinol Metab 2002;87:2467–2473.
48 Xiao ZS, Crenshaw M, Guo R, Nesbitt T, Drezner MK, Quarles LD: Intrinsic mineralization defect in hyp-mouse osteoblasts. Am J Physiol 1998;275:E700–E708.
49 Liu S, Guo R, Tu Q, Quarles LD: Overexpression of Phex in osteoblasts fails to rescue the Hyp mouse phenotype. J. Biol Chem 2002;277:3686–3697.

50 Bhargava A, Aravindan R, Drezner MK: Abnormal phosphate transport in Hyp-mouse osteoblasts may underlie the inability to rescue the HYP phenotype. J Bone Miner Res 2002;17(suppl 1):S278.

51 Shimada T, Mizutani S, Muto T, Yoneya T, Hino R, Takeda S, Takeuchi Y, Fujita T, Fukumoto S, Yamahita T: Cloning and characterization of FGF-23 as a causative factor of tumor-induced osteomalacia. Proc Natl Acad Sci USA 2001;98:6500–6505.

52 Shimida T, Kakitani M, Hasegawa H, Yamazaki Y, Ohguma A, Takeuchi Y, Fujita T, Fukumoto S, Tomizuka K, Yamashita T: Targeted ablation of FGF-23 causes hyperphosphatemia, increased 1,25-dihydroxyvitamin D level and severe growth retardation. J Bone Miner Res 2002;17(suppl 1):S168.

53 Shimada T, Takanori M, Urakawa I, Yoneya T, Yamazaki Y, Okawa K, Takeuchi Y, Fujita T, Fukumoto S, Yamashita T: Mutant FGF-23 responsible for autosomal dominant hypophosphatemic rickets is resistant to proteolytic cleavage and causes hypophosphatemia in vivo. Endocrinology 2002;143:3179–3182.

54 Shimada T, Muto T, Hasegawa H, Yamazaki Y, Takeuchi Y, Fujita T, Fukumoto S, Yamashita T: FGF-23 is a novel regulator of mineral homeostasis with unique properties controlling vitamin D metabolism and phosphate reabsorption. J Bone Miner Res 2002;17(suppl 1):S425.

55 Whyte MP: Hypophosphatasia: Nature's window on alkaline phosphatase function in man; in Bilezikian JP, Raisz LG, Rodan GA (eds): Principles of Bone Biology. San Diego, Academic Press, 1996, pp 951–968.

56 Whyte MP: Hypophosphatasia and the role of alkaline phosphatase in skeletal mineralization. Endocr Rev 1994;15:439–461.

57 Waymire KG, Mahuren JD, Jaje JM, Guilarte TR, Coburn SP, MacGregor GR: Mice lacking tissue non-specific alkaline phosphatase die from seizures due to defective metabolism of vitamin B_6. Nat Genet 1995;11:45–51.

58 Narisawa S, Fröhlander N, Millan JL: Inactivation of two mouse alkaline phosphatase genes and establishment of a model of infantile hypophosphatasia. Dev Dyn 1997;208:432–446.

59 Fedde KN, Blair L, Silverstein J, Coburn SP, Ryan LM, Weinstein RS, Waymire K, Narisawa S, Millan JL, Macgregor GR, Whyte MP: Alkaline phosphatase knock-out mice recapitulate the metabolic and skeletal defects of infantile hypophosphatasia. J Bone Miner Res 1999;14:2015–2026.

60 Wennberg C, Hessle L, Lundberg P, Mauro S, Narisawa S, Lerner UH, Millan JL: Functional characterization of osteoblasts and osteoclasts from alkaline phosphatase knockout mice. J Bone Miner Res 2000;15:1879–1888.

61 Hessle L, Johnson KA, Anderson HC, Narisawa S, Sali A, Goding JW, Terkeltaub R, Millan JL: Tissue-nonspecific alkaline phosphatase and plasma cell membrane glycoprotein-1 are central antagonistic regulators of bone mineralization. Proc Natl Acad Sci USA 2002;14:9445–9449.

Roger Bouillon, MD
Laboratory for Experimental Medicine and Endocrinology
Gasthuisberg, Herestraat 49, B–3000 Leuven (Belgium)
Tel. +32 16 34 60 23, Fax +32 16 34 59 34, E-Mail Roger.Bouillon@med.kuleuven.ac.be

Hochberg Z (ed): Vitamin D and Rickets.
Endocr Dev. Basel, Karger, 2003, vol 6, pp 220–232

Rickets in Developing Countries

Abdullah Bereket

Department of Pediatrics, Division of Pediatric Endocrinology,
Marmara University, School of Medicine, Istanbul, Turkey

Contents

Outline

Nutritional rickets remains prevalent in developing regions of the world such as Africa, the Indian subcontinent, Asia, Latin America and the Middle East. Rickets causes considerable childhood morbidity and disability, and constitutes a significant public health problem in developing countries. Current knowledge regarding the extent of the problem, etiology, risk factors, clinical issues and prevention of rickets in developing countries will be presented.

The Scope of the Problem

The prevalence of rickets is highly variable among developing countries and even within different regions of the same country (table 1). Lack of

Country	Prevalence, %	Reference
Algeria	18	2
Argentina	0.2	17
China	40.7	15
India	4–27	12–14
Nigeria	2.4–14.9	1
Turkey	1.67–19	11

Table 1. Prevalence of nutritional rickets in various developing countries

large-scale, epidemiologic studies and heterogeneity in respect to genetic, nutritional, lifestyle and socioeconomic status accounts for this variability. Furthermore, figures undergo alterations over the time due to changing socio-economic conditions, migration and new feeding practices. Nevertheless, in these parts of the world, rickets is still among the five most common diseases in children. In Nigeria, 2.4% of children under five had overt rickets, 14.9% had findings suggestive of rickets. There is still a higher prevalence of rickets among hospitalized children among whom, up to 41% had evidence of rickets [1]. A study in an urban area of Algeria revealed a prevalence of 35–45% among children in 1963, 1973 and 1974 which was reduced to 18% in 1984–85 following a prophylaxis programme [2]. However, in some countries such as Sudan, incidence of rickets seems to be increasing due to changing socio-economic conditions [3]. Hospital and community-based studies from Tunisia, Libya and Egypt confirm that rickets is still prevalent in all North African countries [4, 5]. In the Middle-East, high prevalence of rickets have been reported from Northern Yemen where 27% of children under age 5 had rickets [6]. Rickets occurs in newborns, young infants, toddlers and even in adolescent girls from Saudi Arabia [7]. Vitamin D deficiency is significant in mothers and their newborns as well [8]. In Kuwait and Iran, nutritional rickets has been identified as a preventable health problem among infants and children [9, 10]. In Turkey, rickets was detected in 6% of 8,631 children under age 3 who presented to an outpatient clinic for various reasons [11]. The prevalance of rickets in India varies in different regions of the country due to ethnic, socio-cultural and economic diversity. Prevalence rates varying between 4 and 27% have been reported from Delhi, 20% in central India and 3.3% among pre-school children in Calcutta [12–14]. Rickets is a significant public health problem in China. In a survey of 184,902 children under age 3, prevalence of rickets was found to be 40.7% between 1977 and 1983. The prevalence rate was higher in the Northern (49.1%) part of the country compared to central and southern China (3.1 and 24.6%, respectively) [15]. Congenital rickets is prevalent in North China and the incidence has been reported to be 5–30% higher in infants born late in the cold season [16]. In Argentina, the overall incidence of rickets is relatively low (0.3 cases per 1,000 hospital admissions) but an incidence of 2.04/1,000 has been reported in Patagonia in the south of the country, and 2.6/1,000 among inner-city dwellers in Buenos Aires province [17].

Epidemiology

In developing countries, rickets occurs most commonly in the 4 months to 3 years age group. However, congenital rickets and rickets in early months of life have been reported among offspring of vitamin D-deficient mothers [8]. Late rickets in older children seen in Africa may be a feature of calcium deficiency. The incidence of rickets is slightly higher in boys for reasons yet unknown. However, rickets in adolescent ages more commonly seen in teenage girls who lack adequate sunlight during rapid growth period [7]. In general, rickets is more commonly seen in winter and early spring due to less sunlight available for infants and mothers during these months [11].

Etiology

It is incompletely understood why rickets occurs so frequently in tropical countries with abundant sunlight which should prevent vitamin D deficiency. Various reasons have been advocated to explain its occurrence including [18–20] (fig. 1):

- Inadequate dietary vitamin D intake.
- Darkly pigmented skin which reduces vitamin D production.
- Inadequate exposure to sunlight due to excessive clothing and remaining indoors due to seasonal, cultural or religious reasons (housing conditions and air pollution are also factors limiting sunlight exposure in urban children and mothers in the Middle East, Asia and Latin America [21–23]).
- Dietary Ca deficiency is a major factor contributing to development of rickets in Africa [24, 25]. The typical African diet is rich in grains and leaves that contain inhibitors of Ca absorption such as phytates, oxalate, tannates and phosphates. In a placebo-controlled trial, Nigerian children with rickets found to have low intake of calcium and better response to calcium or calcium plus vitamin D than to vitamin D alone [21]. Rickets due to dietary calcium deficiency has also been described in South Africa and Bangladesh [26, 27].

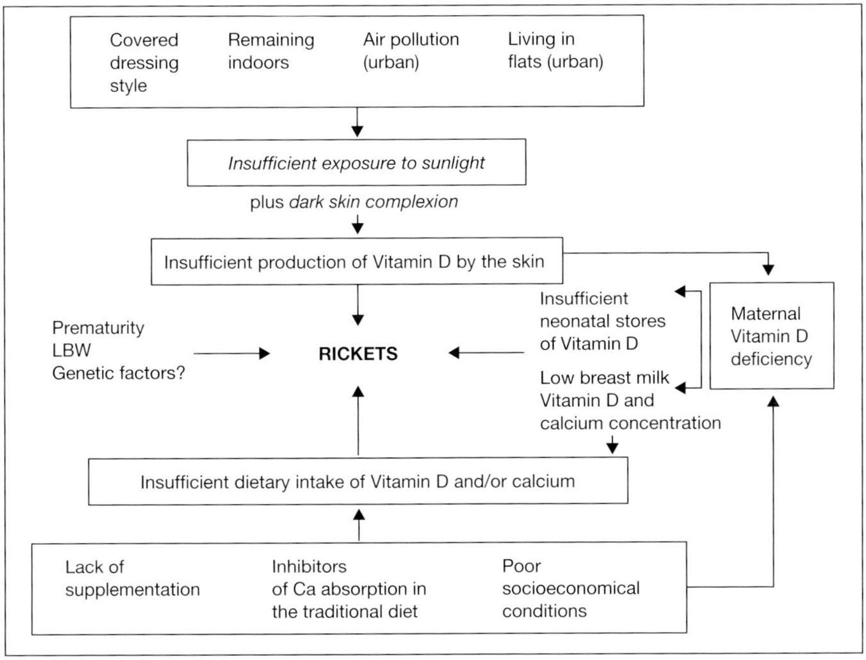

Fig. 1. Etiopathogenesis and risk factors for nutritional rickets in developing countries.

Risk Factors

Different studies have investigated the risk factors for rickets in developing countries [3, 9, 11, 23, 28–32]:

In Nigeria, although the rachitic children were moderately malnourished, their protein nutritional status and growth being better than those of severely malnourished children who grew slower and developed rickets less often [31]. This observation is consistent with the fundamental basis of rickets, being a disease of the growth plate and actively growing children are more likely to develop rickets than are children whose linear growth is impeded.

Additional risk factors that predispose to rickets in developing countries include insufficient exposure to sunlight, prolonged breast-feeding without supplementation, inadequate weaning practices, prematurity, marasmus, type of residence (flats) and lower socioeconomic status. Maternal education level was found to be important in some but not all studies.

Premature and low-birthweight (LBW) babies are at higher risk for development of rickets. Hospital-based studies in Kenya demonstrated that 58.8% of premature infants had rickets by 6 months [33]. Likewise, 33% of

Table 2. Effect of dressing style on serum vitamin D levels in Turkish women

	Noncovered	Traditional	Strict religious
25(OH)vitamin D, nmol/l	56 ± 41	32 ± 24	9 ± 6

very-low-birthweight (VLBW) infants in Tanzania had metabolic bone disease by 6–12 weeks of age [34].

Air pollution and housing conditions are other important factors in urban children. A study done in nonsupplemented 9- to 24-month-old infants from India showed that 25(OH)vitamin D levels were 12.6 nmol/l in infants that live in polluted areas whereas they were 28.2 nmol/l in those from nonpolluted areas [21]. Alkaline phosphatase and PTH levels were also higher in children who live in polluted compared with nonpolluted areas (663 vs. 404 IU/l and 42.9 vs. 14.7 pg/ml, respectively). Likewise, serum 25(OH)vitamin D levels were lower in children who live in a house that does not receive direct sunlight compared to those who live in a house that receives adequate sunlight (67 vs. 87 nmol/l, respectively) [35].

Maternal Vitamin D Deficiency

Maternal vitamin D deficiency is also common in developing countries, that is another factor for predisposing development of rickets in infants (Pakistan, Saudi Arabia, Turkey) [8, 35–40]. Congenital rickets has been described from Kuwait, China and other countries. Severe vitamin D deficiency (<25 nmol/l) has been detected in 46–80% of pregnant women and nursing mothers in different regions of Turkey [35–37]. Their dietary vitamin D intake was far below the RDA (185 ± 117/day) [35, 41].

Low socioeconomic status, covered clothing style and low educational level were factors associated with maternal vitamin D deficiency. The most important risk factor for low serum 25(OH)vitamin D level in the newborn was the maternal level of 25(OH)vitamin D lower than 25 nmol/l (OR = 15.2, p = 0.002). Bone mineral density revealed osteopenia in 40% of the women with a low vitamin D level. All women with osteopenia were from the low socioeconomic class and 80% of them were dressed in the traditional covered style [36]. Study of 48 premenopausal women also showed that, serum 25(OH)vitamin D levels changed significantly according to type of dressing [40] (table 2).

Other Susceptible Groups

In many developing countries, rickets is not limited to infants. Recently, 21 adolescents (20 females, 1 male) with symptomatic rickets were reported from Saudi Arabia with a prevalence rate of 68 per 100,000 children years (10–15 years) [7]. All adolescents had an inadequate dietary calcium and vitamin D intake. All but two drank daily at least one can of carbonated soft drink and half drank more than two cans daily. The median daily sun exposure was estimated at 15 min. Moreover, traditional clothing style of women which covers the entire body and face prevents exposure of the skin to sunlight and explains why more females developed rickets.

Children of immigrants who live in developed countries are also at increased risk for rickets. Vitamin D status in 8-year-old Turkish and Moroccan children living in the Hague, Netherlands, showed that 42% of Turkish and 23% of Moroccan children had low 25(OH)vitamin D level compared to an indigenous reference population [42]. Likewise, in the United States, clinical rickets has been described from children who are adopted from the former Soviet Union [43]. Of 65 children with nutritional rickets diagnosed in Norway between 1998 and 1999, 54 were children of immigrants [44]. Immigration to a Northern country may further increase the risk of rickets especially when traditional nutritional and dressing habits are kept since exposure to sunlight will be more limited in that new country.

Presenting Symptoms and Morbidity

Congenital and early rickets often present with hypocalcemic seizure. Rachitic rosary is a common finding in newborns with congenital rickets. Hypotonia, sweating, irritability, craniotabes, enlarged wrists, occipital flattening, Harrison's groove and frequent respiratory tract infections are other features of rickets in infancy. In older infants, common presenting symptoms include delayed walking, bowing of the legs, abnormal gait and delayed dentition. Rickets not only causes skeletal system problems but also leads to significant morbidity by affecting other systems. Respiratory system problems associated with rickets have long been known as 'rachitic pneumopathy'. Children with rickets are 13 times more likely to get pneumonia and almost twice as likely to die of it after adjustment for family size, birth order, crowding and months of exclusive breastfeeding [45]. A recent study from Yemen showed, in 529 children hospitalized with severe pneumonia, that rickets was detected in 50% [46]. A community-based study from Uruguay indicates that prevention and treatment of rickets is important in the prevention of morbidity and mortality from pneumonia [47].

Table 3. Comparison of different treatment modalities in vitamin D-deficiency rickets [50]: change is seen in parameters before and 4 weeks after the treatment

	300,000 IU po	300,000 IU i.m.	600,000 IU p.o.
ΔBMD, mg/cm^3	27.4 ± 22.0	34.3 ± 26	51.9 ± 18.0
ΔAlkP, U/l	166 ± 131	239 ± 123	378 ± 354
ΔCa, mg/dl	1.7 ± 1.6	2.1 ± 2.0	3.3 ± 2.6
Δ25(OH)D	18.0 ± 5.1	20.2 ± 6.2	24.8 ± 10.4
ΔPTH, pg/ml	30.1 ± 18.2	34.4 ± 14.4	36.8 ± 20.8
Hypercalcemia	none	none	3/10

Investigations

Serum calcium, phosphorus and alkaline phosphatase concentrations and radiography are available in most developing countries. Measurement of PTH and 25(OH)vitamin D is costly which limits their routine use.

Serum calcium levels may be normal or reduced. Hypocalcemia is more evident in neonatal rickets and in younger infants. The serum phosphorus level is low or normal depending on biochemical stage of rickets. Alkaline phosphatase is elevated. In malnourished children, the alkaline phosphatase may be low even in florid rickets and tends to rise with improvement of the general nutritional status. Since alkaline phosphatase is a zinc-dependent enzyme, this may be explained partly by zinc deficiency in protein energy malnutrition [10, 22, 48].

The commonest radiological findings include osteoporosis, cupping, spreading, fraying, irregularity, stippling and widening of the cartilage shaft junctions of long bones. The typical radiological signs might be absent in spite of gross demineralization in children with severe malnutrition [22].

Treatment of Rickets

Treatment of vitamin D deficiency rickets can be achieved by vitamin D 2,000–5,000 IU/day orally for 4–8 weeks. In practice, mothers' compliance with regular daily doses tends to be difficult, and regular follow-up visits might be costly to parents or even not affordable. Stosstherapy with 150,000 or 300,000 IU given orally in fractionated doses of 100,000 IU every hour is an effective, safe and practical therapeutic method [49, 50]. Hypercalcemia was reported in 30% of patients given 600,000 IU [50] (table 3). Parenteral treatment is not necessary unless diarrhea or malabsorption is present. Calcium supplementation should also be provided for the first 2 weeks of therapy to prevent so-called 'hungry bone syndrome'. Biochemical response is seen within 7 days, and radiographic evidence of healing starts after 10–14 days. A repeat stosstherapy can be considered when biochemical and radiological improvement is insufficient at 4 weeks of therapy. Stosstherapy must be supervised.

In calcium-deficiency rickets, 1,000 mg of elemental calcium/day orally for 6 months is needed in addition to vitamin D which can be given as stosstherapy [24].

Regardless of the type of rickets, siblings of a patient with rickets should also be screened since they share similar genetic and environmental risk factors with their siblings.

Prevention

Total vitamin D concentration in human milk is 15–50 IU/l. Although, sun exposure and an appropriate diet may increase vitamin D levels in breast milk by up to 100 IU/l, it is still far below the daily amount of 200–400 IU recommended for infants. Thus, routine vitamin D supplementation is necessary during the first year of life to prevent vitamin D-deficiency rickets and is implemented in many countries [51–57].

Noncompliance with routine prophylactic vitamin D administration is an important factor for development of rickets in some countries. Siklar et al. [53] detected 28 cases of rickets out of 551 (5%) children aged 0–3 years in an outpatient setting in Ankara Hospital. 18 never had vitamin D supplementation. Only 5 of them had received vitamin D supplementation. This observation emphasizes the importance of monitoring compliance in prophylaxis programs.

Breast milk calcium concentration is 340 mg/l compared to cow's milk calcium concentration of 1,339 mg/dl. However, 55% of breast milk calcium is absorbed whereas only 38% of cow's milk or formula calcium is absorbed. Thus, breast milk is considered a good source of calcium. Nevertheless, studies in Gambia have shown that breast milk of black mothers contains 22% less calcium than breast milk of white mothers [58]. Dietary calcium supplementation may influence gestational milk calcium content, but not during lactation [59]. Therefore, ensuring adequate dietary intake of calcium and vitamin D of pregnant women is essential.

In industrialized countries, fortification of food with vitamin D and calcium has been a common measure for the prevention of rickets [60, 61]. Formulas, milk, cereals and flour are widely used in fortification. However, after resurgence of exclusive breast-feeding in these countries, incidence of vitamin D-deficiency rickets increased especially in the black population [62]. The content of vitamin D in fortified milk is highly variable. No more than 20% of milk or its products contains the required 400–600 IU of vitamin D per quart and 10–15% of sampled milk does not contain any detectable levels. Several cases of vitamin D intoxication have been reported that apparently resulted from drinking milk that had been fortified with excess amounts of vitamin D [63]. Lastly, the expense of fortification of food should be considered.

Vitamin D intoxication has also been reported from overzealous recommendations of prophylactic vitamin D or inadequate recommendations of stosstherapy for delayed dentition or delayed walking not associated with rickets [64]. Therefore, education of both healthcare providers and the public is of utmost importance to avoid such problems during implementation of prevention programs.

Conclusions

In the light of the above-mentioned facts, the following summary of recommendations can be made for prevention of rickets in developing countries [65, 66]:

1. All pregnant women should have adequate sunshine and dairy products. Vitamin D 1,000 U daily or 100,000 U as a single dose should be given at the last trimester of pregnancy to women with insufficient dietary vitamin D and calcium intake.
2. Breast-feeding should be encouraged up to 18 months especially in calcium-deficiency areas to provide enough calcium.
3. In areas of calcium-deficiency rickets, adequate calcium intake with inexpensive, locally acceptable food sources of calcium should be provided (preferably from fortified dairy products) during the weaning period and afterwards.
4. All infants should have supplemental vitamin D 400 IU/day during the first year of life regardless of the type of feeding.
5. All infants, children and adolescents should have adequate sunshine (30 min/week naked, or 2 h/week clothed but no hat).
6. Dietary calcium and vitamin D intake of children and adolescents should be raised to suggested guidelines [66] by consuming fortified food or supplements (table 4).
7. Education of parents about dietary sources of vitamin D and suggestion of acceptable alternatives to cultural and social factors which limit exposure to sunlight should be implemented.

Table 4. ESPE-bone Club recommendations for daily requirements of calcium, phosporus and vitamin D in childhood and adolescence [66]

	Caclium, mg	Phosphorus, mg	Vitamin D, U
3rd trimester pregnancy + lactation	1,500	1,500[3]	400–1,000[1]
Premature infants	180/kg	140/kg	200–400[1]
Term – 1st year	400	300[3]	200–800[1]
Childhood	800	800[3]	0–400[2]
Adolescence	1,200	1,200[3]	0–1000[2]
Chronic disease	800–1,200	800–1,200[3]	400[2,4]
Drug therapy	800–1,200	800–1,200[3]	0–1,000[2]

[1]The higher dose is recommended for dark skin complexion and when sun exposure is limited.

[2]During childhood and adolescence, vitamin D requirement change with physical activity, geographical and cultural sun exposure and skin complexion. In all ages, stosstherapy, using the right dose, is an option.

[3]Phosphate is present in all food composed of plant or animal cells. In a normal diet there is no need for supplementation.

[4]An initial dose of 1,200 U is recommended for malabsorption, to be monitored by serum 25(OH)D levels.

8. Larger population-based studies are needed in each developing country to establish:
   a. True prevalence and scope of rickets.
   b. Etiology and specific local risk factors of rickets.
   c. RDA of dietary vitamin D and calcium to prevent rickets for that specific population.
   d. Easy, safe and inexpensive ways of supplementing vitamin D and calcium in that population.

References

1 Akpede GO, Omotara BA, Ambe JP: Rickets and deprivation: A Nigerian study. J R Soc Health 1999;119:216–222.

2 Parent MA, Khadraui S, de Schampheliere I: Early clinical rickets and its asociation with malnutrition. J Trop Pediatr 1987;1:13–15.

3 elHag A, Karrar ZA: Nutritional vitamin D deficiency rickets in Sudanese children. Ann Trop Paediatr 1995;15:69–76.

4 Jalal OM, El Nabawy M, Hassan A: Incidence of rickets in two children populations in Egypt. Aimn Shams Med J 1970;21:133–137.

5 Nagi NA: Vitamin D deficiency rickets in malnourished children. J Trop Med Hyg 1972;75: 251–254.
6 Underwood P, Margetts B: High levels of childhood rickets in rural north Yemen. Soc Sci Med 1987;24:37–41.
7 Narchi H, El Jamil M, Kulaylat N: Symptomatic rickets in adolescence. Arch Dis Child 2001;84: 501–503.
8 Taha SA, Dost SM, Sedrani SH: 25-Hydroxyvitamin D and total calcium: Extraordinarily low plasma concentrations in Saudi mothers and their neonates. Pediatr Res 1984;8:73941.
9 Lubani MM, al-Shab TS, al-Saleh QA, et al: Vitamin-D-deficiency rickets in Kuwait: The prevalence of a preventable disease. Ann Trop Paediatr 1989;9:134–139.
10 Salimpoor R: Rickets in Tehran: Study of 200 cases. Arch Dis Child 1975;1:63–66.
11 Ozkan B, Buyukavcı M, Aksoy H, Tan H, Akdağ R: Incidence of rickets among 0- to 3-year-old children in Erzurum. Çocuk Sağlığı Hastalıkları Dergisi 1999;42:389–396.
12 Banik ND, Nayar S, Krishna R, Raj L: A study of epidemiological basis of malnutrition in preschool children in slum areas in Delhi. Indian Pediatr 1973;1:19–25.
13 Ghosh S, Sarin S, Seghal SK: A study of rickets. J Indian Pediatr Soc 1962;1:253.
14 Choudhary MK: Nutritional profile of Calcutta preschool children. II. Clinical observations. Indian J Med Res 1975;63:185–199.
15 Ma XC: Epidemiology of rickets in China. J Pract Paediatr 1986;1:323.
16 Zhao HZ, Guo HC: Congenital rickets in children. J Prac Pediatr 1986;1:284–285.
17 Karrar ZA: Vitamin D deficiency rickets in developing countries. Ann Trop Paediatr 1998;18: S89.
18 Mimouni F: Etiology of nutritional rickets: Geographic variations. J Pediatr 1996;128:600–601.
19 Walker AR: Etiology of nutritional rickets: Geographic variations. J Pediatr 1998;132:187–189.
20 Walker AR: Etiology of nutritional rickets: Geographic variations. J Pediatr 1997;130:501–503.
21 Pulliyel JM, Agarwal K, Upadhyay P, Mawer EB, Berry JL, Mughal Z: The impact of atmospheric pollution related haze on vitamin D status in two-year-olds in Delhi, India. Bone Research Society Annual Meeting, Montreal, 2000.
22 Coulter JBS: Nutritional rickets. Africa Hlth 1998;20:27–28.
23 Ekanem EE, Bassey DE, Eyong M: Nutritional rickets in Calabar, Nigeria. Ann Trop Paediatr 1995;15:303–306.
24 Thacher TD, Fischer PR, Pettifor JM, Lawson JO, Isichei CO, Reading JC, Chan GM: A comparison of calcium, vitamin D, or both for nutritional rickets in Nigerian children. N Engl J Med 1999;19:563–568.
25 Thacher TD, Fischer PR, Pettifor JM, Lawson JO, Isichei CO, Chan GM: Case-control study of factors associated with nutritional rickets in Nigerian children. J Pediatr 2000;137:367–373.
26 Fischer Pr, Rahman A, Cimma JP, Kyaw-Myint TO: Nutritional rickets without vitamin D deficiency in Bangladesh. J Trop Paediatr 1999;45:291–293.
27 Bhimma R, Pettifor JM, Coovadia HM, Moodley M, Adhikari M: Rickets in black children beyond infancy in Natal. S Afr Med J 1995;85:668–672.
28 Lulseged S, Fitwi G: Vitamin D deficiency rickets: Socio-demographic and clinical risk factors in children seen at a referral hospital in Addis Ababa. East Afr Med J 1999;76:457–461.
29 Nyakundi PM, Kinuthia DW, Orinda DA: Clinical aspects and causes of rickets in a Kenyan population. East Afr Med J 1994;71:536–542.
30 Majid Molla A, Badawi MH, al Yaish S, Sharma P, el Salaam RS, Molla AM: Risk factors for nutritional rickets among children in Kuwait. Pediatr Int 2000;42:280–284.
31 Walter EA, Scariano JK, Easington CR, Polaco AM, et al: Rickets and protein malnutrition in Northern Nigeria. J Trop Pediatr 1997;43:98.
32 Bishop N: Rickets today – Children still need milk and sunshine. N Engl J Med 1999;341: 602–603.
33 Oyatsi DP, Musoke RN, Wasunna AO: Incidence of rickets of prematurity at Kenyatta National Hospital, Nairobi. East Afr Med J 1999;76:63–66.
34 Msomekela M, Manji K, Mbise RL, Kazema R, Makwaya C: A high prevalence of metabolic bone disease in exclusively breast-fed very low birthweight infants in dar-es-Salam, Tanzania. Ann Trop Paediatr 1999;19:337–344.

35 Pehlivan İ, Hatun Ş, Aydoğan M, Babaoğlu K, Türker G, Gökalp AS: Factors effecting 25(OH)D_3 levels in the last trimester of pregnancy. Vth National Congress of Pediatric Endocrinology, Istanbul, 2000.
36 Andiran N, Yordam N, Özön A: The risk factors for vitamin D deficiency in breast-fed newborns and their mothers. ESPE 39th Annual Meeting, Brussels, 2000, pp 3–425.
37 Gullu S, Erdogan MF, Uysal AR, Baskal N, Kamel AN, Erdogan G: A potential risk for osteomalacia due to sociocultural lifestyle in Turkish women. Endocr J 1998;45:675–678.
38 el-Sonbaty MR, Abdul-Ghaffar NU: Vitamin D deficiency in veiled Kuwaiti women. Eur J Clin Nutr 1996;50:315–318.
39 Atiq M, Suria A, Nizami SQ, Ahmed I: Maternal vitamin deficiency in Pakistan. Acta Obstet Gynecol Scand 1998;77:970–973.
40 Alagol F, Shihadeh Y, Boztepe H, Tanakol R, Yarman S, Azizlerli H, Sandalci O: Sunlight exposure and vitamin D deficiency in Turkish women. J Endocrinol Invest 2000;23:173–177.
41 American Academy of Pediatrics Committee on Nutrition: Calcium requirements of infants, children, and adolescents. Pediatrics 1999;104:1152–1157.
42 Meulmeester JF, van den Berg H, Wedel M, et al: Vitamin D status, parathyroid hormone and sunlight in Turkish, Moroccan and Caucasian children in The Netherlands. Eur J Clin Nutr 1990; 44:461–470.
43 Reeves GD, Bachrach S, Carpenter TO, Mackenzie WG: Vitamin D deficiency rickets in adopted children from the former Soviet union: An uncommon problem with unusual clinical and biochemical features. Pediatrics 2000;106:1484–1488.
44 Brunvand L, Brunvate R: Health problems among immigrant children in Norway. Tidsskr Nor Laegeforen 2001;28(suppl 121):715–718.
45 Muhe L, Lulseged S, Mason KE, Simoes EA: Case control study of the role of nutritional rickets in the risk of developing pneumonia in Ethiopian children. Lancet 1997;349:1801–1804.
46 Banajeh SM, al-Sunbali NN, al-Sanahani SH: Clinical characteristics and outcome of children aged 5 years hospitalized with severe pneumonia in Yemen. Ann Trop Paediatr 1997;17:321–326.
47 Hortal M, Benitez A, Contera M, Etorena A, Meny M: A community-based study of acute respiratory tract infection in children in Uruguay. Rev Infect Dis 1990;12(suppl 8):96673.
48 Reddy V, Srikantia SG: Serum alkaline phosphatase in malnourished children with rickets. J Pediatr 1967;71:595–597.
49 Shah B, Finberg L: Single-day therapy for nutritional vitamin D deficiency rickets: A preferred method. J Pediatr 1994;125:487–490.
50 Ozkan B, Buyukavcı M, Energin M, Dirican ME, Alp H, Akdağ R: Nutritional rickets: Comparison of three different therapeutic approaches (300,000 U p.o., 300,000 U i.m., and 600,000 U p.o.). Çocuk Sağlığı Hastalıkları Dergisi 2000;43:30–35.
51 Specker BL, Tsang RC, Hollis BW: Effect of race and diet on human milk vitamin D and 25-hydroxyvitamin D. Am J Dis Child 1985;139:1134–1137.
52 Specker BL: Do North American women need supplemental vitamin D during pregnancy or lactation? Am J Clin Nutr 1994;59(suppl):484S–491S.
53 Şıklar Z, Tasar A, Tene H, Tanyer G, Dallar Y, Tuygan N: 0–3 yas arası çocuklarda raşitizm sıklığı ve özellikler. Klinik Bilimler Doktor 2002;8:613–615.
54 Pitkin RM: Calcium metabolism in pregnancy and the perinatal period: A review. Am J Obstet Gynecol 1985;151:99–101.
55 Cross NA, Hillman LS, Allen SH, Krause GF, Vieira NE: Calcium homeostasis and bone metabolism during pregnancy, lactation, and pot weaning: A longitudinal study. Am J Clin Nutr 1995;61: 514–523.
56 Ritchie LD, Fung EB, Halloran BP, Turnlund JR,Van Loan MD, Cann CE, King JC: A longitudinal study of calcium homeostasis during human pregnancy and lactation and after resumption of menses. Am J Clin Nutr 1998;67:693–701.
57 Salle BL, Delvin EE, Lapillonne A, Bishop JN, Glorieux FH: Perinatal metabolism of vitamin D. Am J Clin Nutr 2000;71(suppl):1317S–1324S.
58 Prentice A, Jarjou LMA, Cole TJ, Stirling DM, et al: Calcium requirements of lactating Gambian mothers: Effects of a calcium supplement on breastmilk calcium concentration maternal bone mineral content, and urinary calcium excretion. Am J Clin Nutr 1995;62:58–67.

59 Feeley RM; Etienmiller RR, Benton-Jones J, Barnhart H: Calcium, phosphorus and magnesium contents of human milk during early lactation. J Pediatr Gastroenterol Nutr 1983;2:262–267.
60 Pietrek J, Preece MA, Windo J, O'Riordan JL, Dunnigan MG, McIntosh WB, Ford JA: Prevention of vitamin D deficiency in Asian infants. Lancet 1976;7970:1145–1148.
61 Singleton N, Tucker SM: Vitamin D status of Asian infants. Br Med J 1978;6113:607–610.
62 Kreiter SR, Schwartz RP, Kirkman HN, Charlton P, Calikoglu AS, Davenport ML: Nutritional rickets in African American breast-fed infants. J Pediatr 2000;137:153–157.
63 Jacobus CH, Holick MF, Shao Q, Chen TC, Holm IA, Kolodny JM, Fuleihan GE, Seely EV: Hypervitaminosis D associated with drinking milk. N Engl J Med 1992;326:1213–1215.
64 Bereket A, Erdogan T: Oral alendronate therapy for vitamin D intoxication of the infant. Pediatrics 2002;in press.
65 Brooks DG, Brown IRF, Bone CDM: Vitamin D supplements in pregnant asian women: Effects on calcium status and fetal growth. Br Med J 1980;280:751–754.
66 Hochberg Z, Bereket A, Davenport M, Delemarre-Van de Waal H, De Schepper J, Levine MA, Shaw N, Shoenau E, Weisman Y, Zadik Z: Consensus development for the supplementation of vitamin D in childhood and adolescence. Horm Res 2002;58:39–51.

Abdullah Bereket, MD
Bozkir Sokak No: 4/7
Selamicesme-Istanbul (Turkey)
Tel. +90 216 327 10 10, ext 577, Fax +90 216 325 60 79, E-Mail abereket@e-kolay.net

Hochberg Z (ed): Vitamin D and Rickets.
Endocr Dev. Basel, Karger, 2003, vol 6, pp 233–258

Prophylactic Vitamin D Supplementation

Ali S. Calikoglu, Marsha L. Davenport

University of North Carolina at Chapel Hill, Chapel Hill., N.C., USA

Contents

The value of prophylactic vitamin D supplementation was established more than one hundred years ago. Since then, public health policies and physician practices have differed from country to country based on latitude, numbers of women breast-feeding, numbers of new cases of rickets ascertained, perceived health risk, economic and social forces. In this chapter, the rationale for prophylactic vitamin D supplementation in breast-fed infants and other children at risk will be presented along with discussions of dosing regimens and potential risks of supplementation.

While a role for sunlight exposure in preventing and treating rickets was suggested as early as 1822, the first evidence that dietary vitamin D supplementation was effective in preventing rickets provided by Mellanby in 1919. He was inspired by a common folklore practice in Britain and Scandinavian countries in which fish liver oils were used to prevent and treat rickets. He showed that adding cod liver oil to the diet could cure experimentally-produced rickets in dogs. Shortly after this observation, Steenbock and Hess independently demonstrated that food exposed to radiation from a mercury arc lamp could develop antirachitic properties [1, 2]. This concept was later used to establish the practice of supplementing evaporated milk with irradiated ergosterol, an inexpensive source of vitamin D. Supplementation of milk and infant formulas derived from cow's milk with vitamin D was nearly universal in Western countries by the 1930s and eliminated rickets as a major health problem there. In 1966, Harrison [3] declared that 'rickets is a medical curiosity in children'. Vitamin D deficiency and its consequences are problems that both developed and developing countries struggle with in the 21st century and rickets remains a problem for many otherwise healthy individuals.

Vitamin D is required to maintain normal blood levels of calcium and phosphate. These minerals are needed for the normal mineralization of bone as well as muscle contraction, nerve conduction and general cellular function of all cells of the body. Vitamin D modulates the transcript of cell cycle proteins that decrease cell proliferation and increase cell differentiation of several specialized cells of the body such as enterocytes and osteoclastic precursors. The active form of vitamin D, 1,25-dihydroxyvitamin D (1,25$(OH)_2$D), restores blood levels of calcium and phosphate to normal when concentrations are low by increasing the intestinal absorption of dietary calcium and phosphate and releasing calcium and phosphate from bone. Vitamin D deficiency results in low 25-hydroxyvitamin D (25(OH)D) and $1,25(OH)_2D$ synthesis, a reduction in serum calcium levels, and a secondary increase in PTH. As a result, bone turnover is increased and more phosphorus is wasted by the kidneys [4, 5].

Sources of Vitamin D

Sunlight

The major source of vitamin D for most humans is exposure to sunlight. When human skin is exposed to sunlight, ultraviolet B photons with energies between 290 and 315 nm convert 7-dehydrocholesterol (7-DHC) to previtamin D_3 [6]. Exposure of an individual's whole body to one minimal erythema dose (MED) of sunlight is equivalent to ingesting about 250 μg (10,000 IU) of vitamin D, which is 17–50 times the daily adequate intake (AI) for vitamin D. The AI for vitamin D, the daily intake established as sufficient to maintain healthy blood levels of vitamin D from dietary sources, was set as 5–15 μg (200–600 IU) by the Institute of Medicine in 1997 [7].

When sunlight is insufficient to meet daily needs, nutritional vitamin D becomes essential. Vitamin D is very rare in unfortified foods. Vitamin D is naturally present in the flesh of fatty fish such as salmon, and oils of fish including cod and tuna liver. In some countries such as the United States and Canada, milk, some cereals and some breads are fortified with vitamin D.

In order to maintain a vitamin D-sufficient status, adequate sunlight exposure should be obtained. However, the amount of vitamin D that any given individual produces upon exposure to sunlight is subject to numerous personal and environmental variables including latitude, season, pollution, skin pigmentation, clothing [8], use of sunscreens [9, 10], and the length and timing of exposures.

Geographic and Seasonal Factors

The latitude, season and time of day influence vitamin D synthesis in skin. The further a person lives from the equator, the more ultraviolet radiation is blocked by the atmosphere. One study demonstrated that serum 25(OH)D levels in blacks who had moved from Zaire to Belgium was three times lower than that of blacks in Zaire [11].

At certain latitudes, little or no vitamin D is produced by sunshine for several months during the winter. Using a model to determine the effect of season and latitude on vitamin D production, Webb and colleagues demonstrated that most cutaneous production of vitamin D in Boston (42.2°N) occurred during the summer months of June and July. There was a gradual decline in the production of previtamin D_3 after August, and there was essentially no previtamin D_3 formed in skin from November through February [12]. The cutaneous production of previtamin D_3 is also influenced by the time of the day that sunlight exposure occurs. In Boston, sunlight was capable of producing vitamin D_3 in the skin from 07.00 to as late as 17.00 h in summer, while previtamin D_3 photosynthesis in the skin began at 09.00 and ceased at 16.00 h in the spring and autumn due to the increase in the zenith angle of the sun. No previtamin D_3 could be produced by skin in Edmonton, Canada (52°N) for 6 months (mid-October to mid-April). In contrast, the production of previtamin D_3 occurred throughout the year in Los Angeles, USA (34°N) and San Juan, Puerto Rico (18°N) [12].

Similarly, in the Southern hemisphere, the photoconversion of 7-DHC to previtamin D_3 was compared in Ushuaia (latitude 55°S) and Buenos Aires (34°S), the former of which is known to have an incidence of nutritional rickets 8–12 times higher than in the rest of Argentina. Ampules containing 7-DHC were exposed to sunlight one day in the middle of each month. Previtamin D_3 + vitamin D_3 formed in Buenos Aires were 2–5 times higher than those in Ushuaia ($p < 0.02$) for the four seasons [13]. Climatic variations from year to year also contribute to differences in vitamin D production [14].

Skin Pigmentation

Skin pigmentation is a very important factor in production of vitamin D. Melanin absorbs ultraviolet B and prevents the formation of previtamin D_3. Thus, increased melanin pigmentation will reduce the efficiency of the sun-mediated vitamin D synthesis. Although the amount of sunlight exposure needed for Caucasians in summertime is surprisingly short, the increased amount needed for dark-skinned infants is unknown. To achieve a serum 25(OH)D concentration >27.5 nmol/l (11 ng/ml) in the infant, Specker and colleagues [15] estimate that the infants of mothers with *low* serum 25(OH)D [<87.5 nmol/l (35 ng/ml)] would need to be in the sunlight 10–30 min per week wearing only a diaper or 30 min to 2 h per week fully clothed with no hat. Infants of mothers with a *high* serum 25(OH)D [>87.5 nmol/l (35 ng/ml)] would require <10 min per week wearing only a diaper or 30 min per week fully clothed with no hat. Adopting conservative estimates, the authors suggest that infants would need to be outdoors for either 30 minutes per week (diaper only) or 2 h per week (fully clothed, no hat). All of the black infants in this study had no sunshine exposure and their mothers had low vitamin D status. Therefore, it was not possible to determine the amount of sunshine exposure needed to maintain adequate vitamin D for black infants. In an adult study, however, Clemens et al. [16] demonstrated that an African American may need to be exposed to sunlight ten times longer than a Caucasian to achieve the same vitamin D production.

Cultural, Social and Ethnic Factors

In addition to these environmental factors, the cultural, social, and ethnic factors affect the vitamin D synthesis in the skin [17, 18]. The amount of vitamin D produced correlates with one's time spent outdoors in circumstances (time and place) where ultraviolet photons are available to the skin. Differences in job requirements, leisure activities, concern about skin cancer, sunscreen use and clothing styles are all factors. Sunscreen, if used correctly, reduces the absorption of solar ultraviolet B on the surface of the skin before it penetrates into the deeper viable layers, thereby diminishing or completely blocking the number of ultraviolet B photons that can reach the 7-DHC stores. The application of sunscreen with a sun protection factor (SPF) of 8 before whole-body exposure to 1 MED of simulated sunlight reduces vitamin D production by 97.5%, and SPF 15 reduces vitamin D production by 99% [9, 10]. Clothing also absorbs ultraviolet B radiation and prevents the cutaneous production of vitamin D within covered surfaces [8]. Muslims who are covered from head to toe present a major problem in terms of vitamin D synthesis. Their vitamin D production is almost 0, and all will need vitamin D supplementation [19].

In summary, skin production via sunlight exposure is the main physiological source for vitamin D. Many factors including latitude, season, the duration and the timing of exposure, clothing, use of sunscreen and degree of skin pigmentation influence vitamin D synthesis. Individuals with deeply pigmented skin, particularly those living in more northern latitude or those using complete body coverage have increased risk for vitamin D deficiency.

Fortified Milk and Food

In the USA and Canada, fortified milk is considered to be the major food source of vitamin D. However, in several studies few of their milk samples tested contained the amount of Vitamin D listed on the label (10 μg or 400 IU per quart) [20, 21]. In a 1992 study of fortified milk and infant formulas in the United States, <30% of the 52 samples contained 80–120% of the amount stated. 62% of the milk samples contained <80% of the amount stated while 70% of the formula samples contained >200% of the amount stated [22]. Contrary to popular belief, ice cream, yogurt, and cheese do not have vitamin D.

Placental Transfer

Vitamin D and 25(OH)D, which cross the placenta during the last months of gestation [23], furnish the main vitamin D requirement of the newborn. Maternal vitamin D status is important in determining the amount of vitamin D transported across the placenta during fetal life and, therefore, the quantity of vitamin D reserves at birth. Following birth the vitamin D status of the average term infant is 60–70% of measured maternal vitamin D levels. Maternal and infant serum 25(OH)D concentrations continue to correlate through the first 8 weeks of life [15]. Indeed, vitamin D deficiency rickets in early infancy is most prevalent in those infants whose mothers have poor vitamin D reserves due to inadequate diet, dark skin pigmentation, or religious dress codes that limit/prevent skin exposure. Because the length of gestation is also important in determining Vitamin D stores at birth, prematurity is another risk factor for Vitamin D deficiency.

Breast Milk

After several weeks of life, even normal infants can no longer support their vitamin D needs from fetal stores. Breast-fed infants rely primarily on endogenous synthesis to maintain a normal vitamin D status because the amount of vitamin D obtained through breast milk is insufficient. The total vitamin D and 25(OH)D in human milk equals approximately 12–60 IU/l [21, 24], and thus will not provide the recommended AI of 200 IU per day for infants [25]. Breast-fed infants who have vitamin D-deficient mothers or who are premature are at high risk for vitamin D deficiency in the first weeks of life and those who receive inadequate sunlight exposure are at risk for vitamin D deficiency until they are weaned.

Prevalence of Vitamin D Deficiency Rickets in Infants and Toddlers

Developing Countries

Nutritional rickets remains prevalent in developing regions of the world such as Africa, the Indian subcontinent, Asia and the Middle East, and ranks among the five most common diseases in children. In Nigeria, 2.4% of children under five had overt rickets and 14.9% had findings suggestive of rickets [26]. In Turkey, rickets was detected in 6% of children under age 3 who presented to an outpatient clinic for various reasons [27]. Surprisingly, rickets also occurs frequently in tropical countries with abundant sunlight [28]. Whereas a genetic predisposition may be a contributing factor, life style and environmental factors have also been implicated. These include inadequate dietary vitamin D and/or calcium intake, darkly pigmented skin, inadequate exposure to sunlight due to excessive clothing, remaining indoors for seasonal, cultural or religious reasons and air pollution.

The most important risk factor for low serum 25(OH)D level in the newborn is a low maternal level of 25(OH)D. Maternal vitamin D deficiency is common in developing countries [29–31]. Severe vitamin D deficiency was identified in 46–80% of pregnant women and nursing mothers in different regions of Turkey [32]. The dietary vitamin D intake of these women was far below AI for the USA and was associated with low socioeconomic status, covered clothing style and a low educational level. Measurements of bone mineral density revealed osteopenia in 40% of the women with a low serum 25(OH)D level. These women were from low socioeconomic class and 80% of them dressed in traditional attire that covered nearly all the skin. As anticipated, concentrations of serum 25(OH)D were significantly related to the type of clothing [33].

Dietary calcium deficiency is a major factor contributing to the development of rickets in Africa [34]. The typical African diet is rich in grains that contain inhibitors of calcium absorption such as phytates, oxalate, tannates and phosphates. In a placebo-controlled trial, Nigerian children with rickets were found to have low intake of calcium and responded better to calcium or calcium plus Vitamin D than to Vitamin D alone [35]. Rickets due to dietary calcium deficiency has also been described in South Africa and Bangladesh [36–38].

Immigrants in Developed Countries

Children of immigrants who live in developed countries are also at increased risk for rickets. 42% of Turkish and 23% of Moroccan children living in The Hague, Netherlands, had low serum levels of 25(OH)D, as compared to an indigenous reference population [39]. Rickets has been common problem in US children adopted from Russia and in immigrants to Canada. Of 17 cases of rickets referred to a children's hospital in Toronto between 1988 and 1993, twelve involved children born to parents who were recent immigrants. All were of Asian or African origin with dark skin, had been exclusively breast-fed with no vitamin D supplementation, and had had little or no sunlight exposure [40]. In 2002, 50% of 160 pregnant women from non-European ethnic minorities in South Wales were vitamin D deficient (vitamin D level <8 ng/ml) [41].

Most interesting, is the high prevalence of vitamin D deficiency in Asians, whose ethnic origin is from India, Pakistan or Bangladesh, and who immigrated to the United Kingdom. Vitamin D deficiency in this population began to be reported in the early 1960s [42–44] and continues to be a common problem for Asian pregnant mothers [41, 45] as well as their infants and young children [46].

A survey of nonpregnant subjects in the UK revealed that up to 88% of asymptomatic female Asians were vitamin D-deficient (<8 ng/ml) throughout the year compared with 2.3% of non-Asian residents [47].

Although increased skin pigmentation, diminished exposure to sunlight in more northern climates and reduced dietary intake of vitamin D may be factors in the high prevalence of vitamin D deficiency in these Asians, another important factor may be increased 25(OH)D-24-hydroxylase activity. Awumey et al. [48] found lower levels of vitamin D, 25(OH)D, urinary calcium and urinary phosphorus, and higher levels of PTH and $1,25(OH)_2D$ in Asian Indians than in Caucasians living in the southern USA. In cultured fibroblasts, 25(OH)D-24-hydroxylase activity was markedly increased and only partially reversed by 25(OH)D.

Developed Countries

Vitamin D deficiency rickets appears to be quite common, even in developed countries. In fact, there is evidence to suggest that the prevalence of vitamin D deficiency rickets in developed countries is increasing. More than 100 cases of rickets in infants and toddlers living in the United States have been reported over the past decade, of which all were breast-fed and more than 90% were dark-skinned [49–59]. In the past several years, groups have described from 1 to 30 cases of rickets from different geographical areas in the United States [60–64]. The age at diagnosis for the children described in these and other reports ranged from 3 to 25 months. All were breast-fed and most were dark-skinned. Of the few Caucasians that developed rickets, one was kept exclusively indoors [55], one had 'an unusual' diet [58], one had been switched to unfortified goats' milk [52], and another child received no milk after discontinuation of breast-feeding at 2 months of age [49].

The largest study described 30 children with nutritional rickets who had been evaluated during the 1990s at two academic institutions in North Carolina [59]. All had X-ray signs of rickets and high serum alkaline phosphatase levels. Low serum calcium levels were found in 60% while low serum phosphorus levels were present in 97%. All children were African-American and had been breast-fed (average duration = 12.5 months). Most had poor intake of dairy products after 1 year of age. The majority was diagnosed on the basis of skeletal abnormalities (bowed legs, flared wrists, rachitic rosary, fractures) and/or failure to thrive. Others were diagnosed incidentally or during evaluations for seizures and developmental delays. Growth retardation at the time of diagnosis was often profound. Length was <5th percentile in 65% and <2nd percentile in 42%. Weight was <5th percentile in 43% and <2nd percentile in 23%.

Vitamin D deficiency is not restricted to infants and toddlers, but is common in older children, young adults, and the elderly. In a 2002 study, the prevalence and determinants of hypovitaminosis D among African-American and white women of reproductive age in the USA were studied [65]. Data from 1,546 African-American women and 1,426 white women aged 15–49 years who were not pregnant and who participated in the third National Health and Nutrition Examination Survey (1988–1994) were used. The prevalence of hypovitaminosis D (serum 25(OH)D $\leq$37.5 nmol/l) was 42.4 $\pm$ 3.1% ($\pm$ SE) among African-Americans and 4.2 $\pm$ 0.7% among whites. Among African-Americans, hypovitaminosis D was independently associated with consumption of milk or breakfast cereal $<$3 times/week, no use of vitamin D supplements, season, urban residence, low body mass index, and no use of oral contraceptives.

Potential Factors for Increasing Rickets in Developed Countries

Several factors are likely involved in what appears to be a resurgence in rickets including decreased sun exposure for the population as a whole, increase in the number of women breast-feeding, and a decrease in the number of physicians routinely prescribing vitamin D supplementation for breast-fed infants.

Decreased Sun Exposure

Decreased sun exposure is likely to be a factor in the low vitamin D levels ascertained in individuals of all ages. Increasing air pollution is a factor in some areas and changes in lifestyle have reduced the opportunities for casual sunlight exposure for both mothers and infants. People in general are spending more time indoors in the comfort of a controlled temperature and are pursuing more indoor activities such as watching TV and using computers. In summer, a time when ultraviolet B radiation is usually abundant, more clothes are worn to accommodate air-conditioning, decreasing the possibility of casual sun exposure. There is also an increase in public awareness that sunlight exposure increases the risk for skin cancers [66, 67]. The American Academy of Pediatrics (AAP) Committee on Environmental Health recommended that infants younger than 6 months should be kept out of direct sunlight and that others use sunscreen when physical protection is not adequate [68]. There has been an increased use of sunscreens [69] and avoidance of direct sunlight to reduce the risk of skin cancer.

Increased Breast-Feeding

Breast-fed infants with limited sunlight exposure are at higher risk for vitamin D deficiency than formula-fed infants because breast milk contains only 12–60 IU/l vitamin D [24], an amount insufficient to prevent rickets [21]. Darkly pigmented skin requires longer sunlight exposure than light skin to maximize vitamin D formation [70, 71], therefore dark-skinned mothers are at increased risk of being vitamin D deficient. Their infants are more likely to have low vitamin D stores at birth, receive less vitamin D in breast milk [72] and produce less vitamin D themselves from sunlight.

There is a recent increase in the proportion of women who breast-feed their infants in the USA [73]. In the most recent Ross Laboratories Mothers' Survey, the percentage of mothers in the USA who initiated breast-feeding increased from 52.2 to 59.7% (14% change) between 1989 and 1995 and the percentage who continued breast-feeding until 6 months of age increased from 18.1 to 21.6% (19.3% change). More importantly, the proportion of minority women breast-feeding increased at an even greater rate than that of the general population [5, 59, 73]. The percentage of African-American women breast-feeding at 6 months increased from 6.4 to 11.2%. Although the overall percentage remained small, this represented a 75% change. The increase in rate of breast-feeding is very encouraging. However, as the number of African-American women who breast-feed increases [63], the number of infants at risk for vitamin D deficiency also increases.

Decreased Vitamin D Supplementation

Another potential factor contributing to the rise in nutritional rickets is that the number of pediatricians that prescribe vitamin supplementation for breast-fed infants is declining. In a survey of pediatricians in San Diego, California in 1995, only 41% routinely recommended vitamins before 5 months of age to exclusively breast-feeding infants [74]. A 1999 survey of pediatricians in North Carolina showed that only 44.6% of pediatricians recommended vitamin supplementation for all breast-fed infants and 13% never recommended vitamins for infants. Also, the more recently a pediatrician had begun practicing medicine, the less likely he/she was to recommend vitamin supplementation for breast-fed infants [75]. Sixty-two percent of pediatricians graduated before 1970 prescribed vitamins for all breast-fed infants. This percentage fell to 50% for those graduated in the 1970s, to 38% for those graduated in the 1980s and to 33.8% for those graduated in the 1990s. These prescription patterns appear to reflect changes in the AAP policies on vitamin D supplementation in infancy and childhood. In 1963, the AAP Committee on Nutrition recommended that all infants receive 10 μg (400 IU) of vitamin D per day. They emphasized the higher incidence of vitamin D deficiency in individuals with deeply-pigmented skin and that sunlight exposure could not be relied on to improve vitamin D status. Subsequent policy statements from 1978 until the present have been weaker, for example, recommending vitamin D as a possible supplement for breast-fed infants whose mothers are vitamin D deficient or for infants that are not exposed to adequate sunlight. A new policy statement recommending vitamin D supplementation for all breast-fed infants is expected to be released in 2003.

Prophylactic Vitamin D Supplementation in Healthy Infants

Rationale

To Prevent Rickets

The primary metabolic abnormality in rickets occurs at the zone of provisional calcification. Diminished calcification of cartilage cell columns, continued osteoid production by osteoblasts, and diminished resorption of osteoid and calcium because of impaired osteoclast function result in a widened, irregularly calcified physis. The contiguous metaphysis is also affected with metaphyseal broadening or 'cupping' likely caused by stress at sites of ligament attachment, splaying of cartilage cells peripherally, and microfracturing of the primary spongiosa by herniation of cartilage into this area.

In cases of ongoing, untreated rickets, deformities caused by softening of bone occur in the face of normal stress on the skeleton. Depending upon the child weight-bearing pattern, physical examination may reveal enlargement of the wrists, knees and costochondral junctions. Bowing of the lower extremities is typically seen in the newly ambulating child and can be the first clinical finding alerting the physician to the possibility of rickets. Neuromuscular manifestations of vitamin D deficiency such as hypotonia, weakness and retardation or regression in motor milestones may also be evident, and can precede the skeletal abnormalities [64]. Other skeletal abnormalities can include a Harrison's groove where the diaphragm attaches to the lower ribs, an hourglass shaped thorax, coxa vara, genu valgum, delayed closure of the fontanelles, frontal bossing and postural molding of the skull [76].

It can be assumed that most diagnosed cases of vitamin D deficiency with significant skeletal deformities, failure to thrive and/or seizures are the 'tip of the iceberg'. Mild vitamin D deficiency does not manifest itself as clinical rickets but rather as undetected malabsorption of calcium, elevated parathyroid hormone levels and rapid bone remodeling. Therefore, the majority of children with vitamin D deficiency are expected to have a subtler phenotype that may be clinically significant, but not identified.

Vitamin D deficiency and even modest growth retardation in early life are likely to decrease peak bone mass. Bone mass increases throughout childhood and accrues most rapidly during early to midpuberty, with the majority of bone mass having been acquired by the end of puberty. Decreased bone mass increases the rate of fracture in children and the risk of osteoporosis and fracture in adulthood [77].

To Prevent Disorders Such as Cancer and Type I Diabetes

The long-term consequences of vitamin D deficiency may be more far reaching than previously appreciated. Vitamin D exerts most of its action by binding its active metabolite, $1,25(OH)_2D$ to the vitamin D receptor (VDR). The receptor-ligand complex binds to its response elements on its target genes to modify the transcription of those genes. As expected, the antirachitic effect of $1,25(OH)_2D$ is achieved by the action of the $1,25(OH)_2D$-VDR complex on the intestinal enterocyte, which leads to absorption of calcium and phosphorous.

VDRs are located in virtually every tissue and the number of genes whose expression is known to be regulated by vitamin D has multiplied recently. Vitamin D regulates the differentiation, growth and function of a broad range of cells with functions beyond that calcium and phosphorus metabolism, including keratinocytes, islet cells of the pancreas, and cells of the immune system [78, 79]. Based on epidemiology and in vitro and animal experiments, vitamin D has now been linked to multiple sclerosis, certain cancers (prostate, breast and colorectal), schizophrenia and type I diabetes mellitus.

The relationship between prostate cancer and vitamin D was suggested over a decade ago. It is known that individuals with vitamin D deficiency, dark skin and/or decreased ultraviolet light exposure are at higher risk for prostate cancer and that the highest death rates from colon cancer are in areas that historically had a high prevalence of rickets. In vitro experiments have shown a growth inhibitory effect of vitamin D on cancer cell lines and animal models have demonstrated tumor shrinkage in xenografts. Clinical trials of vitamin D and vitamin D analogues in cancer patients are currently being conducted.

$1,25(OH)_2D$ has an immunomodulatory effect and can either prevent or markedly suppress experimental autoimmune encephalomyelitis, rheumatoid arthritis, systemic lupus erythematosus, inflammatory bowel disease and type I diabetes. Most pertinent to the decision whether or not vitamin D supplementation is desirable in infants and toddlers, is a birth-cohort study in Finland that links low intake of vitamin D and signs of rickets during the first year of life with the development of type I diabetes in adolescence [80]. In this study, children who regularly took the recommended dose of vitamin D (2,000 IU daily) had a relative risk (RR) of developing type I diabetes of 0.22 compared with those who received less than the recommended dose. Furthermore, children suspected of having rickets during the first year of life had a RR of 3.0 compared with those who did not.

This study advances the hypothesis that low pre- and perinatal vitamin D levels imprint on the functional characteristics of tissues throughout the body.

It appears likely that vitamin D deficiency in infancy increases the risk of developing a wide range of adult-onset disorders.

Issues Critical to the Development of Rational Vitamin D Supplementation Policies

Vitamin D supplementation must not be regarded as only preventive therapy for symptomatic rickets. The goal of a vitamin D supplementation policy should be to achieve vitamin D sufficiency in all children. Infants who are fed formula exclusively generally do not need supplementation. For those who are not formula-fed, vitamin D supplementation should provide a minimum of 5 μg (200 IU) a day to meet the AI recommended by the National Academy of Sciences and Food and Nutrition Board [7]. It should be started within the first weeks of life and continued until vitamin D is adequately derived from food. The ideal preparation should contain vitamin D only and should be safe to have in the home. Vitamin D supplementation should not cause any harm and it should not interfere with breast-feeding. Although no ethnic or minority group should be singled out for supplementation, awareness campaigns should focus on populations at greatest risk. Supplementation should begin with the pregnant mother, and the mother's vitamin D status should be taken into account when assessing infant vitamin D needs. Finally, supplementation should be cost-effective. In such analyses, costs should include those of long-term sequelae (such as cancer risk) in addition to the more immediate costs of rickets, growth failure, and seizures.

Concerns

Opponents to prophylactic vitamin D supplementation have raised several legitimate concerns. Women who hear that infants fed formula do not need supplements might conclude that breast milk is inferior, or might cut short their breast-feeding when they learn a supplement is necessary. Formula manufacturers may use a policy change for supplementing breast-fed infants with vitamin D as a tool for marketing formula, discouraging breast-feeding even more. There is also the possibility that a policy to supplement breast-fed infants in developed countries could erode exclusive breast-feeding in developing countries, where widespread supplementation may not be economically feasible.

Dosing and Administration of Vitamin D Supplementation

The amount of vitamin D required to maintain adequate calcium metabolism and healthy bone development for all ages is very difficult to determine due to many confounding factors. Studies that estimate vitamin D requirements suffer from problems with one or more of these variables, particularly exposure to sunlight. Therefore, the vitamin D requirements for children and adults have not been precisely defined. Historically, the daily recommended dose of vitamin D was based on the vitamin D content in a teaspoon of fish oil, a quantity shown to be sufficient to prevent rickets.

The recommended dietary allowance (RDA) is the average daily dietary intake level that is sufficient to meet the nutrient requirements of nearly all (97–98%) healthy individuals in each life-stage and gender group. There is insufficient evidence to establish a RDA for vitamin D. Instead, an Adequate Intake (AI), a level of intake sufficient to maintain healthy blood levels of vitamin D, has been established. In 1998, The Food and Nutrition Board of the Commission on Life Sciences of the National Research Council proposed an AI of 200 IU/day from birth to the age of 50, 400 IU/day from age 51 to 70 and 600 IU/day over age 70 [7].

Recommendations for vitamin D intake do not take into account potential ethnic differences in metabolism of vitamin D. 24-Hydroxylation of 25(OH)D, which inactivates it, appears to be more active in South Asians [48] and African Americans [81] than in Caucasians. In one study, adult Caucasian subjects given 2.5 mg (100,000 IU) of vitamin D_2 for 4 days raised their serum 25(OH)D concentrations from 65 nmol/l (26 ng/ml) to 167.5 nmol/l (67 ng/ml), while African-Americans given the same dose only increased from 20 nmol/l (8 ng/ml) to 75 nmol/l (30 ng/ml). Therefore, South-Asian and African-American children may require higher doses of prophylactic vitamin D supplements than the suggested AI. Higher levels of supplementation may also be needed for those living at extreme latitudes.

Vitamin D Supplementation to Lactating Mothers

It has been suggested that supplementation of lactating mothers with vitamin D would eliminate the concern for infant vitamin D deficiency. Several studies have shown that the vitamin D content of breast milk can be raised by supplementing the mothers' vitamin D levels, but sufficient vitamin D levels cannot be achieved in human milk without doses exceeding the current AIs for mothers. Maternal ultraviolet B exposure greatly alters the vitamin D content of human milk, but the concentrations quickly fall without further exposure. A Finnish study by Ala-Houhala et al. [82] looked at three groups of healthy, well nourished mothers: Group 1: 17 mothers given 50 μg (2,000 IU) of vitamin D a day, infants not supplemented. Group 2: 16 mothers given 25 μg (1,000 IU) of vitamin D a day, infants not supplemented. Group 3: 16 mothers not supplemented, breast-fed infants given 10 μg (400 IU) of vitamin D a day. At birth, serum concentrations of all three vitamin D metabolites were comparable in all groups. At 8 weeks, the 25(OH)D concentrations in infants in groups 1 and 3 were similar, but in group 2 they were significantly lower, with three infants at or below the risk limit for rickets. At 15 weeks, the infant 25(OH)D concentrations were significantly lower for group 2 than for groups 1 and 3. The following conclusions were made: (1) breast milk does not have enough antirachitic activity by itself or when mothers are supplemented with 25 μg (1,000 IU) of vitamin D per day; (2) vitamin D supplementation of 10 μg (400 IU) per day to breast-fed infants is adequate to prevent rickets during winter in northern latitudes; (3) an adequate supply of vitamin D to breast-fed infants is achieved only by increasing maternal supplementation to 50 μg (2,000 IU) per day, the safety of which is unknown.

Daily Dosing to Infants and Children

Although the AI for vitamin D for infants and children has been set at 200 IU, the dose, schedule, and duration of vitamin D supplementation as well as the target population remain controversial due to the lack of well-designed clinical studies on these matters. Nevertheless, daily oral vitamin D supplementation at doses between 200 and 400 IU is the most widely used regimen to prevent vitamin D deficiency. Most of the studies evaluating the efficacy of various amounts of vitamin D in preventing rickets were conducted before the 1950s. While many of these early studies are now questionable from the standpoint of modern experimental design, they did provide evidence that intakes of 300–500 IU of vitamin D per day healed severe rickets and therefore these doses should be effective in preventing rickets. Estimations of vitamin D requirements ranged from 100 to 400 IU/day. Doses of vitamin D greater than 400 IU/day did not appear to result in a greater degree of protection against rickets.

More recent and better-designed studies have confirmed these observations. Fomon et al. [83] explored the effects of vitamin D intake on linear growth in infancy. Three groups of infants received daily vitamin D doses of 7.5, 8.75–13.75, or 34.5–54.25 μg (300, 350–550 or 1,380–2,170 IU) during the first year of life. While the study was not placebo-controlled and the sample size was small, the groups had no differences in length, weight, or serum calcium concentrations suggesting that a vitamin D dose as small as 300 IU/day is sufficient to maintain normal linear growth and a dose as high as 2,000 IU/day is safe.

In 1991, Pittard et al. [84] compared the efficacy and safety two doses of vitamin D in 52 low-birth-weight or full-term infants. Infants were randomly assigned to receive either 10 μg (400 IU) or 20 μg (800 IU) of vitamin D daily from birth to 16 weeks of age. Normal calcium, phosphorus, PTH, and 25(OH)D concentrations were maintained at all doses and no hypercalcemia was observed.

Specker et al. [85] confirmed that both latitude and vitamin D intake affect vitamin D status in infancy. Two hundred and fifty-six term infants from two northern and two southern cities in China were studied in a randomized trial of vitamin D supplementation at three doses (100, 200, or 400 IU/day) during the first 6 months of life. Serum 25(OH)D concentrations were lower in infants living in northern than southern China. Serum concentrations increased as the vitamin D dose increased in infants from northern China, but there was no dose effect among infants in southern China. Among infants in northern China supplemented daily with 100 IU or 200 IU of vitamin D, 36 and 30%, respectively, had serum 25(OH)D concentrations below the lower limit of normal [27.5 nmol/l (11 ng/ml)], while only 2 of 33 (6%) infants supplemented with 400 IU were vitamin D deficient. No cases of rickets were observed in the 280 infants who completed the 6-month study. These data suggest that a dose of at least 400 IU is necessary to maintain optimal vitamin D levels in infants, particularly those in northern latitudes.

In conclusion, although The Food and Nutrition Board of the Commission on Life Sciences of the National Research Council [7] has proposed 200 IU/day as the AI for vitamin D, this dose may be too low. Since there is no known risk of toxicity at doses ≤2,000 IU (<1,000 IU per The Food and Nutrition Board [7]), the authors propose that vitamin D supplementation at a daily dose of 400 IU will provide adequate prevention of vitamin D deficiency without significantly increasing risk.

Intermittent Dosing to Infants and Children

Intermittent high oral or parenteral doses of vitamin D have been used in populations in which compliance is an issue or when a systematic survey of high-risk infants is difficult to organize. In some countries, therefore, the custom of giving daily vitamin supplements to infants has never been established. Instead, infants, usually under direct medical supervision, are administered single large (100,000–300,000 IU) oral or intramuscular doses of vitamin at intervals of 6 weeks to 3 months. While this approach is cheaper and practical in implementation, it has resulted in vitamin D intoxication in some cases.

In a study by Zeghoud et al. [86], 30 infants were given a single dose of 15 mg (600,000 IU) of cholecalciferol. Two weeks after ingestion, all but two had 25(OH)D levels over 120 nmol/l. Although no hypercalcemia was observed, serum calcium concentrations two weeks after administration were significantly elevated. Six months after the dose, 25(OH)D levels remained elevated in half of the infants.

In a study from Germany, 43 infants were supplemented with an oral dose of 15 mg (600,000 IU) of ergocalciferol repeatedly at ages of 1, 4, 7, 11, 15 and 20 months. This treatment was effective in preventing vitamin D deficiency. 25(OH)D levels were elevated well above the normal range but returned to it before each subsequent dose. All infants had normal calcium levels before the first dose but 14 infants (34%) had hypercalcemia at one or more points during study. In this study, hypercalciuria was not assessed and follow-up for long-term consequences of reported hypercalcemia was not provided [87]. The potential toxicity of this dosing regimen was made evident by a retrospective survey in which 13 of 152 patients with nephrocalcinosis had received bolus vitamin D prophylaxis in infancy [15 mg (600,000 IU) of ergocalciferol every 3 months] [88].

More modest doses of intermittent vitamin D have also been used. The oral administration of 5 mg (200,000 IU) cholecalciferol at birth produced a modest but sufficient increase in 25(OH)D concentrations 2 weeks later. Fifty eight percent had 25(OH)D levels over 120 nmol/l at 2 weeks, which fell to less than 120 nmol/l by 6 months [89].

Oliveri et al. reported that a single oral dose of 3.75 mg (150,000 IU) ergocalciferol was sufficient to maintain normal 25(OH)D levels in children between 5 and 11 years of age without causing hypercalcemia or hypercalciuria when it is administered at the beginning of autumn [90]. Since the study was performed in older children and the winter increment of PTH was not inhibited with this treatment, its efficacy in preventing rickets and its safety in infants remain unclear.

Oral doses of 2.5 mg (100,000 IU) cholecalciferol given every 3 months enabled infants to maintain serum 25(OH)D concentrations >15 nmol/l throughout the 9-month follow-up. However, 23% of infants who received 2.5 mg (100,000 IU) of cholecalciferol had high 25(OH)D levels (>120 nmol/l) 2 weeks after ingestion [89].

In conclusion, intermittent high dose vitamin D supplementation is also an effective way to prevent vitamin D deficiency. While the efficacy and safety of smaller doses have yet to be studied, the use of the doses of 100,000 IU or greater carries the risk of hypervitaminosis D.

Duration of Vitamin D Supplementation

There is no consensus on the optimal duration of vitamin D supplementation. Since breast milk fails to provide a sufficient amount of vitamin D to infants, vitamin D supplementation should be given at least during the period when infant is exclusively breast-fed. When formula, which contains 400 IU/l vitamin D, or vitamin D fortified food is introduced to diet, the amount of vitamin D that is supplemented could be reduced proportionally. Vitamin D supplementation can be discontinued when the infant consistently consumes enough formula, vitamin D fortified food, or vitamin D fortified milk (standard in a few countries such as the USA) to provide the AI. In the United Kingdom where milk is not fortified, vitamin supplementation is recommended to continue until 3 years of life [91].

Risks Associated with Vitamin D Supplementation

Vitamin D supplementation during infancy may cause hypervitaminosis D as well as an excess of other vitamins and minerals when vitamin D is given in a multivitamin form. Hypervitaminosis D is rarely fatal but it can cause significant morbidity due to the complications of hypercalcemia and hypercalciuria. Complications include general symptoms, such as muscle weakness and fatigue; central nervous system symptoms; gastrointestinal problems; cardiac rhythm abnormalities; urinary system complications such as kidney stones and nephrocalcinosis; and soft tissue calcifications.

The risks associated with vitamin D supplementation depend on the following factors: the type of vitamin D given, the dosage and duration of supplementation, and the vitamin preparation. Vitamins D_2 and D_3 are similar in terms of toxicity, although vitamin D_2 has poorer stability and purity. While vitamin D_3 is used for food fortification, vitamin D_2 is generally used as the oral supplement in the United States and Europe. The half-lives of vitamins D_2 and D_3 are 20 days to months. Therefore, hypercalcemia secondary to hypervitaminosis of parent vitamin D preparations can last as long as 18 months. Other preparations of vitamin D including 25(OH)D and $1,25(OH)_2D$ are not routinely used for vitamin D supplementation. The half-life of 25(OH)D is shorter (15 days). The half-life of $1,25(OH)_2D$, which is water-soluble and cannot be stored, is very brief. Therefore, hypercalcemia associated with this therapy can be corrected quickly.

As previously established, hypervitaminosis D is a substantial risk when vitamin D is given in high intermittent doses. Repeated doses of vitamin D exceeding 100,000 IU may result in hypercalcemia and nephrocalcinosis may develop. However, concerns that daily vitamin D doses of 50 μg (2,000 IU) or less may cause hypervitaminosis D are not well-substantiated. In the 1950s, milk and cereals were enriched with vitamin D [45–50 μg (1,800–2,000 IU)] in the United Kingdom. An epidemic of hypercalcemia was observed in the following years and the number of children with hypercalcemia declined when the amount of vitamin D enrichment was lowered to 10–15 μg (400–600 IU). This observation led to the conclusion that even a modest amount of vitamin D can cause vitamin D intoxication [92]. However, this conclusion was probably in error. First, only a small group of children among the thousands who ingested 100 μg (4,000 IU) or more of vitamin D per day developed hypervitaminosis. Of these, most had distinct phenotypic features consistent with Williams syndrome. No data are available to suggest that 2,000 IU or less of vitamin D daily is harmful.

Taken together, existing data are inadequate for quantitative risk assessments. Studies are needed to determine the 'no observed adverse effect' level for vitamin D intake in infancy. For now, daily vitamin D supplementation for infants in doses as high as 25 μg (1,000 IU) appears to be safe.

Other potential risks for vitamin D supplementation include the toxicity of other vitamins and minerals when vitamin D is supplemented in a multivitamin form (as in the USA). The amounts of the various vitamins vary greatly amongst the preparations, thus increasing the probability of vitamin toxicity. Adverse effects of vitamin A have been observed at doses as low as 25,000 IU daily and include skin lesions, alopecia, pseudotumor cerebri, hepatotoxicity, and death. There is no evidence that vitamin A supplements <10,000 IU daily are toxic but as little as 10,000 IU in pregnant women may be teratogenic. Vitamin C toxicity includes oxalate kidney stones, excessive iron absorption, and gastrointestinal distress. Adverse effects are observed at 1–1.5 g daily. There is no evidence that vitamin C supplements <250 mg daily are harmful. 100–800 IU of vitamin E given daily for 3 years had no apparent toxicity. Thiamin, riboflavin, niacin, vitamin B_6, and vitamin B_{12} have no toxicity. Therefore, toxicity of concomitant vitamins is extremely unlikely when vitamin D is supplemented as a multivitamin preparation at 200–400 IU daily.

Vitamin D Supplementation for Prematurity, Illness and Drug Therapies

Prematurity

The length of gestation is important in determining vitamin D stores at birth. Because 80% of the calcium and phosphorus deposited in the fetus occurs during the last trimester of pregnancy, infants born prematurely begin life with very hypomineralized bones compared with full-term infants. This poor mineralization may be exacerbated by prolonged total parenteral nutrition, decreased sun exposure due to prolonged hospitalization, and use of steroids and diuretics that interfere vitamin D action or calcium metabolism. Osteopenia and/or rickets in early infancy appear to be primarily related to calcium/phosphorus deficiency in low birth weight infants. However, vitamin D is necessary to obtain catch-up of bone mass in the first years of life. Although premature infants are born with normal circulating concentrations of 25(OH)D, it is unlikely that their stores of vitamin D or 25(OH)D are extensive because of their shortened gestation and lack of adipose tissue for storage [81, 93].

Chronic Illness

Although the focus of this chapter has been on the supplementation of vitamin D for otherwise healthy children with insufficient sunlight exposure or

Table 1. Causes of vitamin D deficiency

Deficient vitamin D synthesis or absorption	impaired cutaneous production low dietary intake malabsorption
Accelerated loss of vitamin D	increased metabolism (phenobarbital, primidone, phenytoin, rifampin) impaired enterohepatic recirculation
Impaired 25-hydroxylation	liver disease isoniazid
Impaired 1α-hydroxylation	renal failure ketoconazole vitamin D-dependent rickets type I (1α-hydroxylase mutation) oncogenic osteomalacia X-linked hypophosphatemic rickets
Target organ resistance	phenytoin vitamin D-dependent rickets type II (receptor mutation)

oral intake of vitamin D-supplemented foods, vitamin D supplementation is also commonly needed in certain disease states. Once vitamin D_3 is made in the skin or vitamin D_2 and/or vitamin D_3 are ingested from the diet, they are transported to the liver where they are metabolized to their major circulating form, 25(OH)D. 25(OH)D is biologically inert on calcium metabolism at physiological concentrations and requires a further hydroxylation in the kidney to form its biologically active metabolite, $1,25(OH)_2D$ [6].

Because several organs including the skin, intestines, liver, kidney and fat are involved in the synthesis, absorption, activation and storage of vitamin D, many diseases and/or their therapies are associated with vitamin D deficiency [94]. Children with chronic diseases involving other organ systems may also be at increased risk of vitamin D deficiency due to poor dietary intake, limited sunlight exposure, and decreased fat reserves. The prevalence of vitamin D deficiency reported for children with chronic diseases such as cystic fibrosis vary widely. Important variables to consider in addition to skin pigmentation, season, etc. are severity of disease, nutrition, and vitamin D supplementation patterns. Causes of vitamin D deficiency can be categorized as resulting from deficient vitamin D synthesis or absorption, accelerated metabolism of vitamin D, impaired vitamin D activation or resistance to the biologic effects of 1,25(OH)2D (table 1) [5]. Individuals with chronic disease often require supplementation with vitamin D, 25(OH)D or $1,25(OH)_2D$, at relatively high doses.

Drug Therapies

Vitamin D therapy may also be needed to prevent or ameliorate the skeletal effects of drugs on bone metabolism, the most important of these being glucocorticoids and chemotherapeutic agents [95]. The mechanism of glucocorticoid action on bone turnover is complex. The most significant effect of glucocorticoids on bone is inhibition of bone formation by decreasing osteoblastic cell replication and differentiation, and increasing apoptosis of mature osteoblasts. Glucocorticoids also increase bone resorption, inhibit 1-hydroxylase in macrophages, and inhibit calcium transport in the intestine [96].

Chemotherapy as well as the underlying disease being treated diminishes bone mineral density. Vitamin D levels are reduced in some individuals and may result, in part, from accelerated rate of cell turnover or impaired vitamin D synthesis [95]. Serum levels of osteocalcin, a marker for bone formation, are frequently low in children with cancer at the beginning of chemotherapy, and increase into the normal range after several months of therapy. Levels of carboxy-terminal telopeptide of type I collagen (1CTP), a marker of bone resorption, also increase significantly. In addition to decreased bone mineral density in childhood cancer survivors, there is an increased incidence of fractures and osteonecrosis. Risk factors include increased age at time of exposure, estrogen deficiency, female gender, corticosteroids use, and cranial radiation.

Although overt rachitic bone disease or symptomatic hypocalcemia is seldom reported in children with chronic diseases, clinical findings related to mild defects in mineral metabolism such as muscle weakness, bone pain and impaired mobility, may be present but not recognized. Nonambulatory patients with neurological diseases and patients with fat malabsorption appear at highest risk.

Conclusion

The prevalence of rickets in the world including developed countries appears to be rising. The majority of rickets cases in developed countries over the past decade have occurred in breast-fed infants and children with dark skin or those who remain fully clothed for religious or social reasons; that is those at greatest risk for inadequate vitamin D production from sun exposure. Not only do these children often produce inadequate amounts of vitamin D, but many begin life with small stores as a result of maternal vitamin D deficiency. Unlike baby formula which is enriched with vitamin D, breast milk does not contain adequate vitamin D, therefore these breast-fed infants require supplemental vitamin D. Occasional cases of rickets are reported in children consuming milk or other fluids that do not contain vitamin D supplementation and in special populations, such as immigrant South Asians, who appear to metabolize vitamin D quickly.

Multiple factors have converged to cause the prevalence of rickets to rise. These include decreased sunlight exposure, a decrease in the number of physicians recommending supplementation and a much desired increase in the number of minorities breast-feeding. The consequences of rickets on skeletal growth and development can be profound. Even more disturbing, however, are other potential consequences of vitamin D deficiency such as the development of osteoporosis, type I diabetes and cancer.

Many questions about vitamin D action, metabolism, and requirements remain to be answered. However, rickets can easily be prevented by daily or intermittent vitamin D supplementation. Vitamin D preparations that are palatable, inexpensive and easily attainable should be made available. In the UK, the Department of Health's committee on Medical Aspects of Food Policy recommends vitamin D supplements for all children up to 3 years, and up to 5 years in those at high risk of developing vitamin D deficiency [91]. Minimally, vitamin D supplementation should be recommended for infants and toddlers with risk factors for decreased vitamin D stores and/or vitamin D production. Because the skin synthesis of vitamin D is very difficult to estimate because of changes in variables such as age, season, latitude, time of day, skin exposure, and sunscreen, a policy that recommends supplementation for children of all ethnicities appears most reasonable. Vitamin D supplementation of formulas with 400 IU vitamin D/l is standard, providing adequate vitamin D intake to most formula-fed infants. Until more data is available, it is reasonable that all breast-fed infants and toddlers be supplemented with 400 IU of vitamin D daily until they are receiving adequate vitamin D from other sources (such as milk or food supplemented with vitamin D). Higher doses may need to be considered for special populations such as those who metabolize vitamin D quickly. There is little or no evidence for toxicity of doses up to 1,000 IU per day, and these doses are sufficient to prevent rickets and other potentially serious sequelae in otherwise healthy populations.

Studies to determine the prevalence of vitamin D deficiency rickets and vitamin insufficiency in various populations are needed. Further research is necessary to determine which populations should be targeted for supplementation as well as its most effective dosing and timing. Public health policies should be developed to assure understanding and compliance with recommendations. These recommendations should be modified based on geographic, environmental, ethnic, and cultural factors in each country.

References

1 Gibbs D: Rickets and the crippled child: An historical perspective. J R Soc Med 1994;87:729–732.
2 DeLuca H: Historical overview; in Feldman D, Glorieux FH, Pike JW (eds): Vitamin D. San Diego, Academic Press, 1997, pp 3–11.
3 Harrison HE: The disappearance of rickets. Am J Publ Hlth 1966;56:734–737.
4 Joint FAO/WHO Expert Consultation: Vitamin D; Human Vitamin and Mineral Requirements. Bangkok, Thailand, FAO/WHO, 2001, pp 109–120.
5 Thomas MK, Demay MB: Vitamin D deficiency and disorders of vitamin D metabolism. Endocrinol Metab Clin N Am 2000;29:611–627, viii.
6 Holick MF: Vitamin D and bone health. J Nutr 1996;126:1159S–1164S.
7 Standing Committee on the Scientific Evaluation of Dietary Reference Intakes: National Academy of Sciences and Food and Nutrition Board. Washington, National Academy Press, 1997.
8 Matsuoka LY, Wortsman J, Dannenberg MJ, Hollis BW, Lu Z, Holick MF: Clothing prevents ultraviolet-B radiation-dependent photosynthesis of vitamin D_3. J Clin Endocrinol Metab 1992; 75:1099–1103.
9 Matsuoka LY, Ide L, Wortsman J, MacLaughlin J, Holick MF: Sunscreens suppress cutaneous vitamin D_3 synthesis. J Clin Endocrinol Metab 1987;64:1165–1168.
10 Matsuoka LY, Wortsman J, Hanifan N, Holick MF: Chronic sunscreen use decreases circulating concentrations of 25-hydroxyvitamin D: A preliminary study. Arch Dermatol 1988;124:1802–1804.
11 M'Buyamba-Kabangu JR, Fagard R, Lijnen P, Bouillon R, Lissens W, Amery A: Calcium, vitamin D-endocrine system, and parathyroid hormone in black and white males. Calcif Tissue Int 1987; 41:70–74.
12 Webb AR, Kline L, Holick MF: Influence of season and latitude on the cutaneous synthesis of vitamin D_3: Exposure to winter sunlight in Boston and Edmonton will not promote vitamin D_3 synthesis in human skin. J Clin Endocrinol Metab 1988;67:373–378.
13 Ladizesky M, Lu Z, Oliveri B, San Roman N, Diaz S, Holick MF, Mautalen C: Solar ultraviolet B radiation and photoproduction of vitamin D_3 in central and southern areas of Argentina. J Bone Miner Res 1995;10:545–549.
14 Devgun MS, Johnson BE, Paterson CR: Ultraviolet radiation, weather and the blood levels of 25-hydroxyvitamin D. Clin Physiol Biochem 1983;1:300–304.
15 Specker BL, Valanis B, Hertzberg V, Edwards N, Tsang RC: Sunshine exposure and serum 25-hydroxyvitamin D concentrations in exclusively breast-fed infants. J Pediatr 1985;107:372–376.
16 Clemens TL, Adams JS, Henderson SL, Holick MF: Increased skin pigment reduces the capacity of skin to synthesize vitamin D_3. Lancet 1982;1:74–76.
17 Seeler RA: Religious/cultural causes of vitamin D deficiency in infants. J Pediatr 2001;138:954.
18 Holick MF: Environmental factors that influence the cutaneous production of vitamin D. Am J Clin Nutr 1995;61:638S–645S.
19 Holick MF: Photobiology of vitamin D; in Feldman DF, Glorieux HH, Pike J (eds): Vitamin D. San Diego, Academic Press, 1997, pp 33–39.
20 Leerbeck E, Sondergaard H: The total content of vitamin D in human milk and cow's milk. Br J Nutr 1982;44:7–12.
21 Hollis BW, Roos BA, Draper HH, Lambert PW: Vitamin D and its metabolites in human and bovine milk. J Nutr 1981;111:1240–1248.
22 Holick MF, Shao Q, Liu WW, Chen TC: The vitamin D content of fortified milk and infant formula. N Engl J Med 1992;326:1178–1181.
23 David L: Common Vitamin D-Deficiency Rickets; in Glorieux FH (ed): Rickets. New York, Vevey/Raven Press, 1991, pp 107–122.
24 Specker BL, Tsang RC, Hollis BW: Effect of race and diet on human-milk vitamin D and 25-hydroxyvitamin D. Am J Dis Child 1985;139:1134–1137.
25 Lammi-Keefe CJ: Vitamins D and E in human milk; in Jensen RG (ed): Handbook of Milk Composition. San Diego, Academic Press, 1995, pp 706–717.
26 Akpede GO, Omotara BA, Ambe JP: Rickets and deprivation: A Nigerian study. J R Soc Health 1999;119:216–222.

27 Ozkan B, Buyukavci M, Aksoy H, Tan H, Akdag R: Incidence of rickets among 0 to 3 year old children in Erzurum. Cocuk Sagligi Hastaliklari Dergisi 1999;42:389–396.
28 Walker AR: Etiology of nutritional rickets: Geographic variations. J Pediatr 1998;132:187–189.
29 Gullu S, Erdogan MF, Uysal AR, Baskal N, Kamel AN, Erdogan G: A potential risk for osteomalacia due to sociocultural lifestyle in Turkish women. Endocr J 1998;45:675–678.
30 el Sonbaty MR, Abdul-Ghaffar NU: Vitamin D deficiency in veiled Kuwaiti women. Eur J Clin Nutr 1996;50:315–318.
31 Alagol F, Shihadeh Y, Boztepe H, Tanakol R, Yarman S, Azizlerli H, Sandalci O: Sunlight exposure and vitamin D deficiency in Turkish women. J Endocrinol Invest 2000;23:173–177.
32 Andiran N, Yordam N, Ozon A: Risk factors for vitamin D deficiency in breast-fed newborns and their mothers. Nutrition 2002;18:47–50.
33 Ozkan B, Buyukavci M, Energin M, Dirican ME, Alp H, Akdag R: Nutritional rickets: Comparison of three different therapeutic approaches. Cocuk Sagligi Hastaliklari Dergisi 2000; 43:30–35.
34 Thacher TD, Fischer PR, Pettifor JM, Lawson JO, Isichei CO, Chan GM: Case-control study of factors associated with nutritional rickets in Nigerian children. J Pediatr 2000;137:367–373.
35 Thacher TD, Fischer PR, Pettifor JM, Lawson JO, Isichei CO, Reading JC, Chan GM: A comparison of calcium, vitamin D, or both for nutritional rickets in Nigerian children. N Engl J Med 1999;341: 563–568.
36 Fischer PR, Rahman A, Cimma JP, Kyaw-myint TO, Kabir AR, Talukder K, Hassan N, Manaster BJ, Staab DB, Duxbury JM: Nutritional rickets without vitamin D deficiency in Bangladesh. J Trop Pediatr 1999;45:291–293.
37 Bhimma R, Pettifor JM, Coovadia HM, Moodley M, Adhikari M: Rickets in black children beyond infancy in Natal. S Afr Med J 1995;85:668–672.
38 Bishop N: Rickets today – children still need milk and sunshine. N Engl J Med 1999;341: 602–604.
39 Meulmeester JF, van den BH, Wedel M, Boshuis PG, Hulshof KF, Luyken R: Vitamin D status, parathyroid hormone and sunlight in Turkish, Moroccan and Caucasian children in The Netherlands. Eur J Clin Nutr 1990;44:461–470.
40 Binet A, Kooh SW: Persistence of vitamin D-deficiency rickets in Toronto in the 1990s. Can J Publ Hlth 1996;87:227–230.
41 Datta S, Alfaham M, Davies DP, Dunstan F, Woodhead S, Evans J, Richards B: Vitamin D deficiency in pregnant women from a non-European ethnic minority population: An interventional study. BJOG 2002;109:905–908.
42 Isaia G, Giorgino R, Adami S: High prevalence of hypovitaminosis D in female type 2 diabetic population. Diabetes Care 2001;24:1496.
43 Ford JA: Rickets and osteomalacia: High risk for Asian immigrants in Britain. Nurs Mirror 1979;149:36–37.
44 Iqbal SJ, Kaddam I, Wassif W, Nichol F, Walls J: Continuing clinically severe vitamin D deficiency in Asians in the UK (Leicester). Postgrad Med J 1994;70:708–714.
45 Alfaham M, Woodhead S, Pask G, Davies D: Vitamin D deficiency: A concern in pregnant Asian women. Br J Nutr 1995;73:881–887.
46 Lawson M, Thomas M: Vitamin D concentrations in Asian children aged 2 years living in England: population survey. BMJ 1999;318:28.
47 Pal BR, Shaw NJ: Rickets resurgence in the United Kingdom: Improving antenatal management in Asians. J Pediatr 2001;139:337–338.
48 Awumey EM, Mitra DA, Hollis BW, Kumar R, Bell NH: Vitamin D metabolism is altered in Asian Indians in the southern United States: A clinical research center study. J Clin Endocrinol Metab 1998;83:169–173.
49 Feldman KW, Marcuse EK, Springer DA: Nutritional rickets. Am Fam Physcn 1990;42: 1311–1318.
50 Bhowmick SK, Johnson KR, Rettig KR: Rickets caused by vitamin D deficiency in breast-fed infants in the southern United States. Am J Dis Child 1991;145:127–130.
51 Chang YT, Germain-Lee EL, Doran TF, Migeon CJ, Levine MA, Berkovitz GD: Hypocalcemia in nonwhite breast-fed infants: Vitamin D deficiency revisited. Clin Pediatr (Philadelphia) 1992;31:695–698.

52 Eugster EA, Sane KS, Brown DM: Minnesota rickets: Need for a policy change to support vitamin D supplementation. Minn Med 1996;79:29–32.

53 Gessner BD, de Schweinitz E, Petersen KM, Lewandowski C: Nutritional rickets among breast-fed black and Alaska Native children. Alaska Med 1997;39:72–74, 87.

54 Menking FW: Vitamin D deficiency in two breast-fed infants. Kans Med 1997;97:10–12.

55 Pugliese MT, Blumberg DL, Hludzinski J, Kay S: Nutritional rickets in suburbia. J Am Coll Nutr 1998;17:637–641.

56 Duplechin RY, Nadkarni M, Schwartz RP: Hypocalcemic tetany in a toddler with undiagnosed rickets. Ann Emerg Med 1999;34:399–402.

57 Herman MJ, Bulthuis DB: Incidental diagnosis of nutritional rickets after clavicle fracture. Orthopedics 1999;22:254–255.

58 Kaper BP, Romness MJ, Urbanek PJ: Nutritional rickets: Report of four cases diagnosed at orthopaedic evaluation. Am J Orthop 2000;29:214–218.

59 Kreiter SR, Schwartz RP, Kirkman HN Jr, Charlton PA, Calikoglu AS, Davenport ML: Nutritional rickets in African-American breast-fed infants. J Pediatr 2000;137:153–157.

60 Shah M, Salhab N, Patterson D, Seikaly MG: Nutritional rickets still afflict children in north Texas. Tex Med 2000;96:64–68.

61 Carvalho NF, Kenney RD, Carrington PH, Hall DE: Severe nutritional deficiencies in toddlers resulting from health food milk alternatives. Pediatrics 2001;107:E46.

62 Welch TR, Bergstrom WH, Tsang RC: Vitamin D-deficient rickets: The reemergence of a once-conquered disease. J Pediatr 2000;137:143–145.

63 Wright A, Schanler R: The resurgence of breast-feeding at the end of the second millennium. J Nutr 2001;131:421S–425S.

64 Tomashek KM, Nesby S, Scanlon KS, Cogswell ME, Powell KE, Parashar UD, Mellinger-Birdsong A, Grummer-Strawn LM, Dietz WH: Nutritional rickets in Georgia. Pediatrics 2001;107:E45.

65 Nesby-O'Dell S, Scanlon KS, Cogswell ME, Gillespie C, Hollis BW, Looker AC, Allen C, Doughertly C, Gunter EW, Bowman BA: Hypovitaminosis D prevalence and determinants among African American and white women of reproductive age: Third National Health and Nutrition Examination Survey, 1988–1994. Am J Clin Nutr 2002;76:187–192.

66 National Coalition for Skin Cancer Prevention: The National Forum for Skin Cancer Prevention in Health, Physical Education, Recreation and Youth Sports. American Association for Health Education, 1900 Association Drive, Reston, VA, 20191:1988.

67 Fuller KE, Casparian JM: Vitamin D: balancing cutaneous and systemic considerations. South Med J 2001;94:58–64.

68 American Academy of Pediatrics: Committee on Environmental Health: Ultraviolet light: a hazard to children. Pediatrics 1999;104:328–333.

69 Holick MF, Matsuoka LY, Wortsman J: Regular use of sunscreen on vitamin D levels. Arch Dermatol 1995;131:1337–1339.

70 Mimouni F: Vitamin D Functions and Requirements in the First Year of Life; in Tsang RC, Mimouni F (eds): Calcium Nutriture for Mothers and Children. New York, Glendale/Raven Press, 1992, pp 39–51.

71 Matsuoka LY, Wortsman J, Haddad JG, Kolm P, Hollis BW: Racial pigmentation and the cutaneous synthesis of vitamin D. Arch Dermatol 1991;127:536–538.

72 Gertner JM, Glassman MS, Coustan DR: Feto-maternal vitamin D relationship at term. J Pediatr 1989;97:637–640.

73 Ryan AS: The resurgence of breast-feeding in the United States. Pediatrics 1997;99:E12.

74 Schanler RJ, O'Connor KG, Lawrence RA: Pediatricians' practices and attitudes regarding breast-feeding promotion. Pediatrics 1999;103:E35.

75 Davenport ML, Uckun A, Calikoglu AS. Pediatrician patterns of prescribing vitamin supplementation for infants: Do they contribute to rickets? Pediatr Res 2002;51:663.

76 States LJ: Imaging of metabolic bone disease and marrow disorders in children. Radiol Clin N Am 2001;39:749–772.

77 Cooper C, Fall C, Egger P, Hobbs R, Eastell R, Barker D: Growth in infancy and bone mass in later life. Ann Rheum Dis 1997;56:17–21.

78 Piemonti L, Monti P, Sironi M, Fraticelli P, Leone BE, Dal Cin E, Allavena P, Di CV: Vitamin D_3 affects differentiation, maturation, and function of human monocyte-derived dendritic cells. J Immunol 2000;164:4443–4451.
79 Cantorna MT: Vitamin D and autoimmunity: Is vitamin D status an environmental factor affecting autoimmune disease prevalence? Proc Soc Exp Biol Med 2000;223:230–233.
80 Hypponen E, Laara E, Reunanen A, Jarvelin MR, Virtanen SM: Intake of vitamin D and risk of type 1 diabetes: A birth-cohort study. Lancet 2001;358:1500–1503.
81 Scanlon KS (ed): Vitamin D Expert Panel Meeting. 1–43. Atlanta, Centers for Disease Control and Prevention, 2001.
82 Ala-Houhala M, Koskinen T, Terho A, Koivula T, Visakorpi J: Maternal compared with infant vitamin D supplementation. Arch Dis Child 1986;61:1159–1163.
83 Fomon SJ, Younoszai MK, Thomas LN: Influence of vitamin D on linear growth of normal full-term infants. J Nutr 1966;88:345–350.
84 Pittard WB III, Geddes KM, Hulsey TC, Hollis BW: How much vitamin D for neonates? Am J Dis Child 1991;145:1147–1149.
85 Specker BL, Ho ML, Oestreich A, Yin TA, Shui QM, Chen XC, Tsang RC: Prospective study of vitamin D supplementation and rickets in China. J Pediatr 1992;120:733–739.
86 Zeghoud F, Ben Mekhbi H, Djeghri N, Garabedian M: Vitamin D prophylaxis during infancy: comparison of the long-term effects of three intermittent doses (15, 5, or 2.5 mg) on 25-hydroxyvitamin D concentrations. Am J Clin Nutr 1994;60:393–396.
87 Markestad T, Hesse V, Siebenhuner M, Jahreis G, Aksnes L, Plenert W, Aarskog D: Intermittent high-dose vitamin D prophylaxis during infancy: effect on vitamin D metabolites, calcium, and phosphorus. Am J Clin Nutr 1987;46:652–658.
88 Ronnefarth G, Misselwitz J: Nephrocalcinosis in children: A retrospective survey. Members of the Arbeitsgemeinschaft fur padiatrische Nephrologie. Pediatr Nephrol 2000;14:1016–1021.
89 Holick MF: Sunlight 'D'ilemma: Risk of skin cancer or bone disease and muscle weakness. Lancet 2001;357:4–6.
90 Oliveri B, Cassinelli H, Mautalen C, Ayala M: Vitamin D prophylaxis in children with a single dose of 150,000 IU of vitamin D. Eur J Clin Nutr 1996;50:807–810.
91 Dietary reference values for food energy and nutrients for the United Kingdom. London, HMSO, Report on Health and Social Subjects 41, Department of Health, 1991.
92 Holmes RP, Kummerow FA: The relationship of adequate and excessive intake of vitamin D to health and disease. J Am Coll Nutr 1983;2:173–199.
93 Care D: Vitamin D in pregnancy, the fetoplacental unit and lactation; in Feldman D, Glorieux FH, Pike JW (eds): Vitamin D. San Diego, Academic Press, 1997, pp 437–446.
94 Chesney RW: Vitamin D deficiency and rickets. Rev Endocr Metab Disord 2001;2:145–151.
95 Hochberg Z, Bereket A, Davenport M, Delemarre-Van De Waal HA, De Schepper J, Levine MA, Shaw N, Schoenau E, Van Coeverden SC, Weisman Y, Zadik Z: Consensus development for the supplementation of vitamin D in childhood and adolescence. Horm Res 2002;58:39–51.
96 Raisz LG, Lukert BP: Glucocorticoid and vitamin D Interactions; in Feldman DF (ed): Vitamin D. San Diego, Academic Press, 1997, pp 789–796.

Marsha L. Davenport, MD
Associate Professor of Pediatrics
Department of Pediatrics
Division of Endocrinology, CB#7220, 361 MSRB
University of North Carolina at Chapel Hill
Chapel Hill, NC 27599–7220 (USA)
Tel. +1 919 966 4435, Fax +1 919 966 2423, E-Mail mld@med.unc.edu

Hochberg Z (ed): Vitamin D and Rickets.
Endocr Dev. Basel, Karger, 2003, vol 6, pp 259–281

Consensus Development for the Supplementation of Vitamin D in Childhood and Adolescence

Ze'ev Hochberg[a], *Abdullah Bereket*[b], *Marsha Davenport*[c], *Henriette A. Delemarre-Van de Waal*[d], *Jean De Schepper*[e], *Michael A. Levine*[f], *Nicolas Shawg Eckhard Schoenau*[h], *Silvia C. van Coeverden*[d], *Yosef Weismani Zvi Zadik*[j], *on behalf of the European Society for Paediatric Endocrinology (ESPE) Bone Club*

[a]Meyer Children Hospital, Haifa, Israel; [b]Marmara University, Istanbul, Turkey; [c]University of North Carolina, Chapel Hill, N.C., USA; [d]Vrije Universiteit, Amsterdam, The Netherlands; [e]Academic Hospital V.V.B., Brussels, Belgium; [f]Johns Hopkins University, Baltimore, Md., USA; [g]Birmingham Children's Hospital, Birmingham, UK; [h]Universitätskinderklinik, Cologne, Germany; [i]Dana Children's Hospital, Tel Aviv, Israel; [j]Kaplan Hospital Rehovot, Israel

Contents

This article has previously been published in Horm Res 2002;58:39–58.

The need for dietary supplementation of vitamin D during infancy has been widely accepted, yet rickets remains common even in the most affluent societies [1]. Several studies have suggested a relationship between childhood calcium and vitamin D intake and bone mineralization, fractures in adolescents, and osteoporosis in adulthood; but nutritional requirements and recommendations for supplementation are controversial. To insure that risk factors for vitamin D deficiency are well understood and that daily requirements for calcium and vitamin D for children are recognized, the Bone Club of the European Society for Paediatric Endocrinology (ESPE) convened a consensus development symposium on July 6, 2001.

The Consensus Process

The consensus development panel included pediatric endocrinologists from ten universities in Europe and the USA. Each of the participants reviewed the literature on a topic related to pediatric and adolescent vitamin D supplementation, and these reviews were presented at the consensus symposium. The reviews were then discussed by the panel and the symposium audience. The discussion was added to the reviews and the second draft was distributed to the panel members for comments. The final draft was presented as a consensus statement, and was approved by all panel members and the Board of the ESPE Bone Club. This statement is a consensus by the panel on the recommendations for prevention and treatment of vitamin D deficiency in the healthy pediatric population as well as at-risk pediatric populations such as infants and children during accelerated growth (puberty and catch-up from disease), with chronic diseases, on drug therapy, in developing countries, of a dark-skinned race and/or living away from the equator.

Definitions

Vitamin D is not a vitamin in the strict definition because it can be produced by exposure of the skin to sunlight. As such, humans do not have a dietary requirement for vitamin D when sufficient sunlight is available. However, nutritional vitamin D becomes essential when sunlight is insufficient to meet daily needs. This has become particularly acute as more people reside in urban centers where they are exposed to suboptimal levels of sunlight. Ultraviolet light from the sun is blocked by air pollution, clothes, tall buildings, indoor dwelling, and sunscreens, and these factors all reduce the ability of the skin to synthesize vitamin D_3. Moreover, people living far north (or south) of the equator obtain little purposeful ultraviolet radiation during the winter months. Under these conditions, vitamin D (and its hormone derivative calcitriol) can be considered a bona fide vitamin in that it must be supplied in the diet [2].

The World Health Organization has defined the 'international unit' of vitamin D_3 as the activity of 0.025 μg of the international standard preparation of crystalline vitamin D_3. Thus, 1 IU of vitamin D_3 is 0.025 μg, or 65 pmol. The unit definition of the active metabolite calcitriol was set to be equivalent in molar terms to that of the parent vitamin D_3. Thus, 1 unit is 65 pmol of calcitriol, but as only a small fraction (<1/1,000) of vitamin D is converted to the active metabolite, a unit of calcitriol is over 1,000-fold more active than vitamin D itself. The vitamin D requirements for children or adults have not been precisely defined. Historically, it was defined on the basis of the vitamin D content in a teaspoon of fish oil, a quantity shown to be sufficient to prevent rickets. A more rigorous scientific definition is unavailable. The recommended dietary allowance (RDA) is the average daily dietary intake level that is sufficient to meet the nutrient requirements of nearly all (97–98%) healthy individuals in each life stage and gender group. There is insufficient evidence to establish a RDA for vitamin D. Instead, an adequate intake (AI), a level of intake sufficient to maintain healthy blood levels of calcitriol, has been established. The 1998 AI's proposed by the Food and Nutrition Board of the Commission on Life Sciences of the National Research Council are 400 IU/day for infants, 200 IU/day up to the age of 50, 400 IU/day from age 51 to 70 and 600 IU/day over age 70 [3]. As vitamin D is endogenously produced and stored in adipose tissue for long periods of time, it is difficult to determine with exactness the dietary requirements. The daily requirement is also dependent on the dietary levels of calcium and phosphorus, age, sex and skin pigmentation, and exposure to sunshine (table 1).

Nutritional Rickets and Treatment: An Overview

Nutritional rickets can be classified according to the primary metabolic abnormality into disorders resulting from a decreased availability of vitamin D, calcium or phosphorus. Vitamin D deficiency rickets occurs most commonly during two periods in infancy, in the early months of life and during the toddler period. Vitamin D and 25-hydroxyvitamin D (25(OH)D), which cross the placenta during the last months of gestation, furnish the main vitamin D requirement of the newborn in its first months of life. Indeed, vitamin D deficiency rickets in early infancy is most prevalent in those infants whose mothers have poor vitamin D reserves due to inadequate diet, dark skin pigmentation, or religious dress codes that limit/prevent skin exposure. Vitamin D supplementation of 400 IU/day (10 μg) should be given to all pregnant women who are at high risk for vitamin D deficiency. It remains to be determined whether vitamin D

Table 1. Previous recommendations for calcium, phosphorus and vitamin D supplementation in premature infants

a European Society of Pediatric Gastroenterology and Nutrition

	Breast-fed	Formula-fed (total amount per day)
Calcium, mg/kg	up to 180 (milk + supplement)	80–180
Phosphorus, mg/kg	up to 17 (added to milk)	up to 120
Vitamin D, IU	800–1,600	800–1,600

b American Academy of Pediatrics

	Weight 800–1,200 g	1,200–1,800 g
Calcium, mg/kg	210	185
Phosphorus, mg/kg	140	75–120
Vitamin D, IU	500	500

c Canadian Pediatric Society

	0–7 days	7 days – discharge from NICU	Discharge from NICU to 1 year of age
Calcium, mg/kg	60–80	160–240	250 (breast-fed)/day 370 (formula-fed)/day
Phosphorus, mg/kg	30–45	75–120	105 (breast-fed)/day 270 (formula-fed)/day
Vitamin D, IU	40–120 (birth weight <1,000 g) 40–260 (>1,000 g)	400 (800 for Blacks and Asians)	400

supplementation should be given to all pregnant women or only to high-risk subgroups. Thus, measurement of serum 25(OH)D levels during the last trimester of pregnancy is recommended in at-risk mothers.

Human milk is an inadequate source of vitamin D [4]. The total vitamin D and 25(OH)D in human milk equals approximately 12–60 IU/l, and thus will not provide the recommended AI of 400 IU/day for infants. To prevent postnatal rickets in breast-fed infants, especially those of high-risk mothers, vitamin D supplementation should be started in the neonatal period with a daily intake of 400 IU/day and continued at least until the age of 1 year. Whether supplemental of vitamin D is required beyond infancy and in older children is still controversial. It is complicated by the fact that mild vitamin D deficiency does not manifest itself as clinical rickets but rather as undetected malabsorption of calcium, elevated parathyroid hormone levels and rapid bone remodeling. Thus, for at-risk children, the currently recommended dose of 200 IU/day would be less than half the estimated daily requirement to prevent vitamin D deficiency.

Overt vitamin D deficiency rickets can be safely and effectively treated by daily administration of 2,000–4,000 IU of vitamin D. Radiological signs of healing will usually be evident within 2–4 weeks, whereupon the vitamin D dose can be reduced to 400 IU/day. Another treatment approach to vitamin D deficiency rickets has been to administer vitamin D as a single, large dose, so-called 'stoss therapy'. The European method in which a single or divided dose of up to 300,000 IU is administered orally or intramuscularly has been in use since the 1930s. Higher dose, or stoss therapy in well-nourished children, may be excessive and result in hypercalciuria and nephrocalcinosis [5].

Nutritional Rickets in Developing Countries

Nutritional rickets remains prevalent in developing regions of the world such as Africa, the Indian subcontinent, Asia and the Middle East. The prevalence of rickets is highly variable among these nations and even within different regions of the same country. Lack of large-scale, epidemiologic studies and heterogeneity with respect to genetic, nutritional, lifestyle and socioeconomical status accounts for this variability. Nevertheless, in these parts of the world, rickets is among the five most common diseases in children. In Nigeria, 2.4% of children under 5 had overt rickets and 14.9% had findings suggestive of rickets [6]. In Turkey, rickets was detected in 6% of children under age 3 who presented to an outpatient clinic for various reasons [7].

Rickets not only causes skeletal system problems but also leads to significant morbidity through affects on other systems. Children with rickets are 13 times more likely to get pneumonia ('rachitic pneumopathy') and almost twice as likely to die of it even after adjustment for family size, birth order, crowding and length of exclusive breast-feeding [8, 9].

It is unclear why rickets occurs so frequently in tropical countries with abundant sunlight [10]. Whereas genetic predisposition may contribute, lifestyle and the environment have been implicated to explain its occurrence. These include inadequate dietary vitamin D or calcium intake, darkly pigmented skin, inadequate exposure to sunlight due to excessive clothing, remaining indoors due to seasonal, cultural or religious reasons and air pollution.

Dietary calcium deficiency is a major factor contributing to development of rickets in Africa [11, 12] (table 2). The typical African diet is rich in grains that contain inhibitors of calcium absorption such as phytates, oxalate, tannates and

Table 2. Dietary calcium intake (mg/day): recommendations in the USA

Age	1997 NAS	1994 NIH
0–6 months	210	400
6 months to 1 year	270	600
1–3 years	500	800
4–8 years	800	800 (4–5 years) 800–1,200 (6–8 years)
9–13 years	1,300	800–1,200 (9–10 years) 1,200–1,500 (11–18 years)

phosphates. In a placebo-controlled trial, Nigerian children with rickets were found to have low intake of calcium and responded better to calcium or calcium plus vitamin D than to vitamin D alone [8]. Rickets due to dietary calcium deficiency has also been described in South Africa and Bangladesh [13–15].

In Nigeria, most rachitic children were moderately malnourished; their protein nutritional status and growth being better than those of severely malnourished children who grew slower and developed rickets less often [11]. This is consistent with the fundamental basis of rickets, being a disease of the growth plate and actively growing children are more likely to develop rickets than are children whose linear growth is impeded.

Additional risk factors that predispose to rickets in developing countries include insufficient exposure to sunlight, marasmus, prematurity, prolonged breast-feeding, no access to nutritional supplementation, type of residence and lower socioeconomic status. Maternal education level was found to be important in some but not all studies [16–19].

In many developing countries, rickets is not limited to infants. In Saudi Arabia the prevalence of symptomatic rickets is 68/100,000 children years at age 10–15 years [20] and all adolescents have an inadequate dietary calcium and vitamin D intake [21]. The median daily sun exposure was estimated at 15 min. Moreover, traditional clothing for women, which covers the entire body and the face, prevents exposure of the skin to sunlight and explains why more females develop vitamin D deficiency.

Maternal vitamin D deficiency is also more common in developing countries [22–24]. Severe vitamin D deficiency has been identified in 46–80% of pregnant women and nursing mothers in different regions of Turkey [25].

The dietary vitamin D intake of these women was far below the US AI and was associated with low socioeconomic status, covered clothing style and a low educational level. The most important risk factor for low serum 25(OH)D level in the newborn was low maternal level of 25(OH)D. Measurements of bone mineral density revealed osteopenia in 40% of the women with a low serum 25(OH)D level. Women with osteopenia were from low socioeconomic class and 80% of them dressed in traditional attire that covered nearly all the skin. Concentrations of serum 25(OH)D were significantly related to the type of clothing [26].

Prevention of vitamin D deficiency, particularly in breast-fed infants, requires vitamin D supplementation during the first year of life, and calcium supplementation may also be necessary to achieve the recommended daily intake in certain children [27–30].

Breast milk calcium concentration is 340 mg/l compared to cow's milk calcium concentration of 1,339 mg/l. However, an average 55% of breast milk calcium is absorbed whereas only 38% of calcium in cow's milk or formula is absorbed. Thus, in general, breast milk is a good source of absorbable calcium. However, studies in Gambia have shown that breast milk of black mothers contains 22% less calcium than breast milk of white mothers [28]. Dietary calcium supplementation may influence gestational milk calcium content, but not during lactation [31]. Therefore, ensuring adequate dietary intake of calcium and vitamin D of pregnant women is essential.

Treatment of nutritional rickets in developing countries is essentially the same as that in developed countries [32]. Parenteral administration of vitamin D is also effective but is recommended only when diarrhea or malabsorption is present. Calcium supplementation should also be provided for the first 2 weeks of therapy to prevent hypocalcemia that can result from rapid skeletal mineralization, the so-called 'hungry bone syndrome'. Biochemical response, typically an elevation in serum phosphorus concentration, may be seen as early as 7 days and radiographic evidence of healing can be noted in 10–14 days.

In calcium deficiency rickets, 1,000 mg of oral elemental calcium is to be given daily for 6 months, in addition to vitamin D, which can be given as stoss therapy [11]. Regardless of the type of rickets, siblings of a patient with rickets should also be evaluated for the presence of subclinical vitamin D deficiency. Larger population-based studies are needed in each developing country to establish: (i) the true prevalence of rickets, hence the extent of the problem; (ii) specific local risk factors for rickets; (iii) the local intake of dietary vitamin D and calcium to prevent rickets, and (iv) easy, safe and inexpensive ways of providing adequate vitamin D and calcium.

Nutritional Rickets in Developed Countries: Racial and Ethnic Considerations

Children of immigrants who live in developed countries are also at increased risk for rickets [33]. 42% of Turkish and 23% of Moroccan children living in

The Hague, The Netherlands, had low serum levels of 25(OH)D, as compared to an indigenous reference population [34]. Likewise, in the USA, clinical rickets is common in children who are adopted from the former Soviet Union [35]. Vitamin D deficiency in Asians, whose ethnic origin is from India, Pakistan or Bangladesh, living in the UK was first reported nearly 30 years ago [36, 37]. Programs to improve life and social conditions, as well as public health initiatives to provide free vitamin D supplements, have led to declines in the prevalence of vitamin D deficiency in these ethnic groups [38]. To prevent vitamin D deficiency, the UK Committee on Medical Aspects of Food Policy (COMA) has recommended that all infants receive 400 IU of vitamin D daily either as part of a multivitamin preparation or contained in fortified infant formula milk. Furthermore, it recommends that all pregnant and lactating mothers should receive 400 IU of vitamin D daily [6, 39]. It also advises that Asian children should be encouraged to take vitamin D supplements throughout the first 5 years of life. In recent years there has been a resurgence of vitamin D deficiency in the UK among Asian children, however. In addition to skeletal rickets during the first 6–9 months of life, many infants also manifest symptomatic hypocalcemia, including seizures. Unlike other reports, which have implicated prolonged and exclusive breast-feeding [40], many of these infants have been formula fed and several have been receiving multivitamin supplements. These infants have evidence of severe vitamin D deficiency (serum concentrations of 25(OH)D <8 ng/ml), as have the majority of the mothers who have been tested. Most of these infants were born to mothers who were themselves born in the UK. These experiences have been mirrored by reports of severe vitamin D deficiency in infants [41], adults [42] and pregnant women [43]. The presentation of such cases and others [44] highlights the importance of maternal vitamin D stores to the developing fetus, as following birth the vitamin D status of an infant is 60–70% of measured maternal vitamin D levels [45].

A study of 25(OH)D levels in a resident nonpregnant adult population in the UK shows that in winter, 85% of Asians compared to 3.3% of non-Asians had 25(OH)D levels <8 ng/ml. Furthermore, even during summer 38% of the Asians had serum levels of 25(OH)D vitamin D that were <10 ng/ml; most (73%) of these vitamin-D-deficient subjects were women.

Previous studies have attributed vitamin D deficiency in Asian women to cultural and dietary habits and their infrequent use of vitamin D supplements. In these subjects, as well as others who do not use vitamin D on a routine basis, the primary source of vitamin D is skin that has been exposed to ultraviolet irradiation of the appropriate wavelength (290–310 nm). Importantly, this wavelength is not present in sunlight in Great Britain (and many other northern countries) from the end of October to the end of March.

Although inadequate sunlight exposure is not refuted, this is probably not the only factor. An interesting study undertaken in the USA [46] has shown that altered vitamin D metabolism due to markedly increased 25(OH)D, 24-hydroxylase activity may contribute to low 25(OH)D levels in Asian subjects. Thus, it appears there may be a genetic predisposition to vitamin D deficiency in Asians. This suboptimal vitamin D status facilitates the occurrence of symptomatic vitamin D deficiency when there are increased requirements as in infancy, adolescence, pregnancy and lactation.

A recent study from Denmark of veiled Moslem women indicated that in the relative absence of sunlight exposure a dietary intake of 600 IU vitamin D per day is insufficient to maintain an adequate serum level of 25(OH)D, and suggested that 1,000 IU/day might be more appropriate for that group [47]. An alternative is to give 1,000 IU/day during the third trimester of pregnancy, which has been shown to produce normal serum levels of 25(OH)D in both mothers and infants at term [48]. An alternative proposal is to employ stoss therapy with administration of a single dose of 100,000–200,000 IU vitamin D during the 6th or 7th month of pregnancy, which provides sufficient vitamin D to meet maternal and fetal needs [49].

All Asian infants should be given 400 IU vitamin D daily whether breast or formula fed. Alternatively, if daily compliance is a problem an annual stoss therapy dose of 150,000 IU vitamin D at the beginning of autumn has been shown to provide protection against vitamin D deficiency without toxicity [50]. A new public health campaign to initiate these measures and raise the awareness of the risks of vitamin D deficiency amongst Asian, African and Middle Eastern families will be required.

Nutritional Rickets in the USA

Over the past decade, reports of vitamin D deficiency rickets in infants and toddlers living in the USA have increased [51–53]. The age at diagnosis for the 96 children described in these and other reports ranged from 3 to 25 months. All were breast fed and most were dark-skinned. Ninety were African-American or other dark-skinned individuals and 6 were Caucasian. Of the 6 Caucasians that developed rickets, 1 was kept exclusively indoors [54], 1 had 'an unusual' diet [55], and 1 had been switched to unfortified goats' milk and received no vitamin D supplementation [56]. Another child received no milk after discontinuation of breast-feeding at 2 months of age [52].

The largest study described 30 children with nutritional rickets who had been evaluated during the 1990s at two academic institutions in North Carolina [57]. All children were African-American and had been breast fed (average duration = 12.5 months). The majority were diagnosed on the basis of skeletal abnormalities (bowed legs, flared wrists, rachitic rosary, fractures) and/or failure to thrive. Others were diagnosed incidentally or during evaluations for seizures and developmental delays.

A principal cause for the increasing prevalence of rickets in the USA is decreased sunlight exposure, which results from increased time spent indoors, avoidance of direct sunlight, increased use of sunscreens, and air pollution. Dark-skinned individuals (both mothers and infants) require more sun exposure (about 6 times more) than light-skinned individuals to produce the same amount of vitamin D in their skin, and therefore, are at greater risk for vitamin D deficiency. Although recent increases in the number of African-American women who are breast-feeding is encouraging in many respects [58, 59], it also means that greater numbers of dark-skinned infants will be at risk of vitamin D deficiency. Regrettably, many physicians fail to prescribe vitamins for dark-skinned infants, and in one recent study, 16% did not prescribe vitamins for any breast-feeding infants [57].

Fortification of Food with Vitamin D

Cow's milk has been fortified with vitamin D in the USA and Canada since the 1930s, but is not fortified in most European countries [60]. Although infant formula is vitamin D-fortified, the recent resurgence of exclusive breast-feeding in these countries has led to an increased incidence of vitamin D deficiency rickets, especially in Black populations [52]. The content of vitamin D in fortified milk, is highly variable, however. No more than 20% of milk or its products contains the required 400–600 IU of vitamin D per quart, and 10.15% sampled milk does not contain any detectable levels. Several cases of vitamin D intoxication have been reported that apparently resulted from drinking milk that had been fortified with excessive amounts of vitamin D [61]. Lastly, the expense of fortification of food should be considered. It is uncertain, then, if the situation in countries that provide milk fortification is significantly better than in countries that provide none at all. Fortification of cow's milk with vitamin D should be standardized and monitored to ensure appropriate compliance.

Vitamin D and Preterm Infants

The rapid postnatal growth of premature infants requires attention to prevention of the metabolic bone disease of prematurity. The daily requirements of vitamin D for the very low birth weight infant have not established by experimental approach. The main etiological factor is inadequate mineral intake rather than vitamin D deficiency [62]. Even though, a previous European recommendation prescribes a very high vitamin D dose in relation to those infant's weight [63]. The European Society of Paediatric Gastroenterology and Nutrition (ESPGAN) recommended a dose of 800–1,600 IU/day, while the American Academy of Pediatrics (AAP) and the Canadian Pediatric Society recommended 400 IU/day [64, 65]. Several studies indicate that a daily vitamin D intake of up to 400 IU maintains normal skeletal development and vitamin D status, while higher dosages may have a potential risk for hypocalcaemia and subsequent complications [66–68]. A randomized study showed that 200 up to 400 IU vitamin D per day and 960 IU/day intake (vitamin D content of used formula plus supplementation) have no different influence on bone mineral accretion in preterm infants [69].

There are no data on vitamin D supplementation in 'extreme' preterm infants (birth weight <700 g). The ideal vitamin dose is still controversial. But a total vitamin D intake of 200 up to 400 IU/day seems to be sufficient for a normal skeletal development in the premature infant, provided that calcium and phosphorus intake is adequate.

Vitamin D and Puberty

Although osteoporosis primarily affects the aging population, there is now a general agreement that failure to achieve peak bone mass at the end of adolescence can increase the risk of osteoporosis later in life. Thus, senile osteoporosis can be regarded, in part, as a paediatric disease. Moreover, bone mineral density and structural strength of bones relate to the risk for fracture at all ages, including the pediatric age [70]. The balance between the peak bone mass achieved in the first two decades of life and the subsequent bone loss that occurs later in life determines osteopenia in the elderly. More than 85% of the eventual peak skeletal mass is present by the age of 18 years, making childhood and adolescent bone growth and mineral accretion a critical process [71]. Failure to achieve an appropriate peak bone mass during this critical growth period results in increased risk of osteopenia and fractures later in life.

During puberty, the rate of longitudinal bone growth exceeds the rate of bone mass accumulation [72, 73]. This tends to produce a transient but a critical period of increased bone fragility [74–76] and the incidence of fractures, particularly in the forearm, increases sharply during puberty.

Factors that may have an effect on bone mass accumulation during puberty are nutrition, hormones and physical activity. In many studies, variations in pediatric dietary calcium intake have been shown to have a lifelong effect on bone mass [75, 77]. A positive relationship was found between milk consumption in childhood and bone mineral density of adult women [78–80]. Among other factors, the bioavailability of calcium in food products has to be taken into consideration [81, 82]. In addition, genetic polymorphisms of the vitamin D receptor may also influence the response of bone mass to calcium intake [83]. During adolescence, a 'calcium threshold' may apply, indicating that intake below this threshold affects bone accumulation, but a calcium surplus, above this threshold, does not accelerate the constant accumulation of bone [84, 85]. On the other hand, an increase of bone retention of calcium was reported for adolescent girls with a high calcium intake [86].

It is possible that the unfavorable effect of suboptimal calcium intake on bone mass during puberty is masked by the dominant effect of pubertal hormones and physical activity. A multiple regression analysis demonstrated that pubertal stage and exercise have a greater value in the regression equation than does nutritional calcium intake [87].

Vitamin D and Chronic Diseases

Because several organs are involved in the synthesis, absorption, activation and storage of vitamin D, many chronic skin, intestinal, liver and renal diseases are associated with defective vitamin D supply, activation, or action [88, 89]. Children with chronic diseases – even those that affect organs not directly involved in vitamin D metabolism – are at increased risk of functional vitamin D deficiency. Poor dietary intake, a limited sunlight exposure, and reduced adipose tissue reserves all play a role in the development of vitamin D deficiency in chronically ill children [90].

Great variability in the frequency of hypovitaminosis D has been reported in several chronic diseases, such as cystic fibrosis and anorexia nervosa [91–96]. Differences in patient characteristics (age, nutritional status, physical function and activity, severity of disease, compliance with supplementation) and differences in methodological details (season of study, the selected cut-off values and type of 25(OH)D assays), in part explain the great disparity of reported prevalence of vitamin D deficiency in chronic disease [97–99]. Beside ethnic (dark skin pigmentation, genetic) and geographical factors (northern latitude), differences in clothing, customs and food consumption (i.e. some foods may be vitamin D fortified or naturally rich in vitamin D) contribute to the differences observed between countries.

Although overt rachitic bone disease or symptomatic hypocalcemia is seldom reported in children with chronic diseases, clinical findings related to a mild defects in mineral metabolism such as muscle weakness, bone pain and impaired mobility, may be present but overlooked in chronically ill patients. Non-ambulatory patients with neurological diseases and patients with fat malabsorption origin appear at highest risk for symptomatic vitamin D deficiency, while infancy and adolescence appear the critical periods for developing symptomatic vitamin D deficiency in the chronically ill child [100, 101]. Lack of sun exposure is an important factor contributing to the development of low circulating levels of 25(OH)D. Ileal resection in children with inflammatory bowel disease, and cholestasis (rather than the parenchymal cell disease) in children with chronic liver disease, are major risk factors for hypovitaminosis D [102, 103]. Vitamin D deficiency has been reported in several other chronic diseases without malabsorption, such as type 1 diabetes, juvenile rheumatic diseases or malignancy, but the precise predisposing factors have not been identified [104–106].

Although hypovitaminosis D is a concern in children who must restrict dietary fat, such as familial hypercholesterolemia, or in adolescents with anorexia nervosa, a condition of self-imposed severe dietary restriction, low serum concentrations of 25(OH)D are not a consistent findings [107].

The biochemical profile of subclinical hypovitaminosis D in patients with chronic diseases is variable, both within and between diseases. A serum level of 25(OH)D that is $<$25 ng/ml is considered low by most experts, and levels that are $<$11 ng/ml are clearly abnormal. Serum levels of calcitriol may be normal, decreased or even increased in patients with vitamin D deficiency. PTH concentrations are generally high in patients with low 25(OH)D concentrations [108], but a 'normal' PTH level may be elevated for a specific patient.

Universal vitamin D supplementation for chronically ill children remains controversial, in part because clinical rickets is rare. Vitamin D supplementation must not be regarded as only a treatment for symptomatic rickets, but rather should be considered as a means to optimize bone mineralization during childhood and adolescence. This is particularly true for children with a variety of chronic diseases that predispose to vitamin D deficiency, in whom circulating levels of 25(OH)D remain low despite routine vitamin D supplementation. Thus, current guidelines (and compliance) for vitamin D supplementation appear to be inadequate. Nevertheless, in some studies no relationship between the vitamin D status and the degree of bone mineralization could be established [109]. These studies highlight the need to determine the relative relationships of vitamin D deficiency and other, as yet unknown factors, to the development of defective bone mineralization in children with chronic diseases.

There have been no controlled trials of vitamin D supplementation in the majority of chronic diseases associated with vitamin D deficiency to establish the efficacy and safety of a specific supplementation regimen. Furthermore, it may not be possible to develop a single, standardized vitamin D supplementation regimen for all children with chronic diseases as environmental, genetic and behavioral factors might differ widely between individuals. It is thus difficult to provide a general evidence-based management plan for most of these chronic conditions.

In children with a chronic disease that interferes with normal vitamin D absorption or synthesis, it is reasonable to provide oral vitamin D supplements at 2–3 times the locally established RDA values. This can be accomplished with 1,200 IU daily or 100,000 IU monthly, but levels of serum 25(OH)D should be monitored regularly to confirm compliance and to guide adjustment of the dose of vitamin D supplement. The optimal target level of serum 25(OH)D has not been established, and it might vary for different patients and with different medical disorders. Administration of vitamin D metabolites [e.g. 25(OH)D or parenteral vitamin D] may be appropriate for selected patients who are unable to maintain normal serum vitamin D levels with oral vitamin D [110]. The question of whether calcitriol [1,25$(OH)_2$D] supplementation has some/any advantage over vitamin D supplementation in patients with nonrenal diseases remains to be determined, The value of measuring serum bone markers in the short term or bone mineral density in the long term is for assessing the beneficial effects on bone metabolism of the vitamin D supplementation, since several factors influence bone mineralization in patients with chronic disease, Standard vitamin D supplementation (400 IU daily or 25,000 IU monthly) might be considered in the wintertime for all children with a chronic disease associated with impaired bone mineralization or treated with a medication that can interfere with vitamin D metabolism [111].

Finally, in addition to vitamin D supplementation, it is important to ensure adequate intake of calcium in order to prevent or reverse bone mineral loss (table 3).

Vitamin D and Drug Therapy

Corticosteroids impair bone formation directly through the inhibition of osteoblast activity [112] and indirectly by decreasing sex steroid secretion [113], decreasing intestinal calcium absorption [114], increasing urinary calcium excretion [115] and promoting bone resorption due to secondary hyperparathyroidism [116]. Prevention of corticosteroid-induced osteoporosis can be primary, at the onset of corticosteroid therapy, or secondary, after low bone density has developed. In adults as well as in children, there is little evidence to support the use of high-dose vitamin D in either prevention or treatment of corticosteroid-induced osteoporosis [117]. Management measures recommended by the Consensus Group for children requiring long-term corticosteroids can be summarized as follows: (i) a minimal effective dose of corticosteroids should be use; (ii) prescribe inhaled or topical steroids where possible; (iii) deflazacort is less damaging to the bone than prednisolone; (iv) assure adequate daily intake of calcium, vitamin D and proteins; (v) encourage normal physical activity, and (vi) bone damage is

Table 3. ESPE Bone Club recommendations for daily requirements of calcium, phosphorus and vitamin D in childhood and adolescence

	Calcium mg	Phosphorus mg	Vitamin D IU
Third trimester pregnancy + lactation	1,500	1,500[a]	400–1,000[b]
Premature infants	180/kg	140/kg	200–400[b]
Term – first year	400	300[a]	200–800[b]
Childhood	800	800[a]	0–400[c]
Adolescence	1,200	1,200[a]	0–1,000[c]
Chronic disease	800–1,200	800–1,200[a]	400[c,d]
Drug therapy	800–1,200	800–1,200[a]	0–1,000[c]

[a]Phosphate is present in all food composed of plant or animal cells. In a normal diet there is no need for supplementation.

[b]The higher dose is recommended for dark skin complexion and when sun exposure is limited.

[c]During childhood and adolescence, vitamin D requirement change with physical activity, geographical and cultural sun exposure and skin complexion. In all ages, stoss therapy, using the right dose, is an option.

[d]An initial dose of 1,200 IU is recommended for malabsorption, to be monitored by serum 25(OH)D levels.

worst during the initial months of corticosteroid therapy. Consider bisphosphonate treatment in cases before severe osteoporosis develops [118].

Anticonvulsants increase the rate vitamin D turnover by the liver and thereby can induce a relative deficiency of vitamin D. In one recent study of children and adolescents with cerebral palsy and epilepsy who were receiving high doses of anticonvulsants, children who were treated with 0.25 μg calcitriol and 500 mg calcium per day showed a significantly increased bone mineral density of the lumbar spine as compared to a control untreated group [119]. Recommended measures include periodic monitoring of serum 25(OH)D, initiation of vitamin D supplementation with 400 IU/day and subsequent adjustment of dosage according to serum level of 25(OH)D and provision of adequate dietary calcium.

Chemotherapy diminishes bone mineral density in some children [120]. Serum levels of osteocalcin, a marker for bone formation, are frequently below the normal range for age in children with cancer at the beginning of chemotherapy, and increase into the normal range at 6 months of therapy [121–123]. Levels of carboxy-terminal telopeptide of type 1 collagen (1CTP), a marker of bone resorption, are elevated [121], normal [122], or low [123] compared with controls at the start of chemotherapy, and increase significantly during 2 years of chemotherapy. Serum calcitriol was below the normal range at diagnosis and throughout 2 years of chemotherapy in a number of children [121–123]. Reduced serum levels of calcitriol could result from an accelerated rate of cell turnover due to chemotherapy, leading to increased utilization of vitamin D, or impaired synthesis due to corticosteroids [119, 123]. Normal osteocalcin levels in combination with a low serum calcitriol during chemotherapy indicate appropriate bone formation with ineffective mineralization, while bone resorption seems to be elevated [124].

Only one intervention study has evaluated vitamin D requirements of children treated with high doses of anticonvulsants, and it showed a positive effect of vitamin D therapy in combination with calcium. Intervention studies with calcitriol supplementation are not available in children treated with chemotherapy. Considering the reduced levels of calcitriol in those children, supplementation might seem a logical step. On the other hand, bone mineral density is not reduced in all children treated with chemotherapy, and if there is a reduction it is not always associated with a low calcitriol levels. Therefore, supplementation of vitamin D should be considered individually. Prospective controlled trials will be necessary to determine whether vitamin D supplementation can prevent disturbances in bone mineralization in children on chronic drug treatment.

Conclusions

Having entered the 21st century, there is a consensus that breast-fed infants and toddlers are at risk for vitamin D deficiency. There is also panel consensus that *all* breast-fed infants, regardless of skin color or latitude, should receive 400 IU of supplemental vitamin D per day from birth until they are receiv ing adequate formula or vitamin D-fortified cow's milk to provide 400 IU of vitamin D per day. Although nutritional rickets occurs most frequently in dark-skinned individuals, it is clear that many light-skinned individuals are also at risk of vitamin D deficiency. As it is difficult to predict whether vitamin D supplies are adequate based on complexion, lifestyle and estimated sun exposure [125], given the safety of 400 IU of vitamin D per day, it seems reasonable to recommend vitamin D supplementation to all of these children.

It is apparent that vitamin D obtained through formula feeds or given as a standard supplement of 400 IU/day is inadequate to overcome the impact of maternal vitamin D deficiency. It is important to ensure that fetal stores are optimized by supplementation of at-risk mothers with a daily dose of 400 IU vitamin D, which should theoretically result in normal maternal concentrations of 25(OH)D and calcitriol.

The following recommendations are made for prevention of nutritional rickets. (i) Pregnant women should be encouraged to use sun exposure (hands and face 15–20 min/day, at least 3 times per week) or fortified dairy products to ensure an adequate supply of vitamin D. (ii) Vitamin D 1,000 IU daily or 100,000 IU as single dose should be given at the last trimester of pregnancy to women with a history of insufficient dietary vitamin D and sunshine exposure [30, 46]. (iii) In developing countries, breast-feeding is encouraged up to 18 months especially in calcium deficiency areas to provide enough calcium. (iv) An adequate calcium intake must be ensured and inexpensive, locally acceptable food sources of calcium should be provided during weaning period and thereafter. (v) All infants should receive supplemental vitamin D 400 IU/ day during the first year of life regardless of the type of feeding. All infants, children and adolescents should have adequate sunshine (30 min/week clothed only in a diaper or 2 h/week fully clothed but no hat – dark-skinned children will require longer exposures for infants). (vi) Dietary calcium and vitamin D intake of children and adolescents should be raised to suggested guidelines by consuming fortified food or supplements. (vii) Vitamin D should be administered directly into the mouth and not added to the milk. Vitamin D is a fat-soluble vitamin and can adhere on the surface of feeding tubes and bottles.

Measurement of circulating 25(OH)D is the best biochemical parameter for vitamin D status. The target levels of 25(OH)D for starting and modifying supplementation need further study; serum levels <11 ng/ml are generally considered subnormal, but levels <25–30 ng/ml may not be adequate to ensure optimal vitamin D action.

Fortification of milk with vitamin D should be regulated and supervised to ensure that all milk products (whole milk or reduced fat milk) contains the recommended 400 IU per quart. Food fortification is not recommended, unless it can be enforced upon all producers.

Perspectives

There are many open questions regarding vitamin D deficiency. The most controversial question continues to be whether all or only selected breast-fed infants should receive supplementation. Some of the research and actions that need to take place are listed below. (1) The prevalence and scope of vitamin D deficiency in breast-fed infants and toddlers needs to be determined. It has been assumed that the cases diagnosed clinically (e.g. significant skeletal deformities, failure to thrive and/or seizures) are the 'tip of the iceberg' and that the majority of children with vitamin D deficiency have a relatively subtle phenotype and, consequently, are not identified. (2) A palatable, inexpensive liquid preparation delivering the recommended daily intake of vitamin D [126] needs to be developed. (3) The effectiveness of this daily therapy needs to be documented. (4) Health policy should be developed to make vitamin D available to all breast-feeding mothers, and to ensure analysis of its utilization. (5) Guidelines will need to be developed that directly and experimentally address the optimal vitamin D requirements for pregnant women and very low birth weight infants. (6) Finally, a public health plan to educate the public and physicians about the effects of vitamin D deficiency and the rationale for supplementation should be developed. Careful research will be needed to determine the effects of different educational initiatives on practice policies and the number of women breast-feeding.

Finally, more studies are required to understand the effect of vitamin D, not only on the skeletal mineralization and bone strength, but also on muscle strength, the immune system, gonadal function and the glucose tolerance [127–129].

References

1 Hochberg Z: Rickets: It's not just vitamin D deficiency. Curr Opinion Endocrinol Diabetes 2001; 8:23–28.

2 Utiger RD: The need for more vitamin D. N Engl J Med 1998;228:828–829.

3 Subcommittee on the Tenth Edition of the RDAs, Food & Nutrition Board, Commission on Life Sciences and National Research Council. Recommended Dietary Allowances. Washington, National Academy Press, 1989, pp 1–285.

4 Weisman Y, Bawnik JC, Eisenberg Z, Spirer Z: Vitamin D metabolites in human milk. J Pediatr 1982;100:745–748.

5 Markestad T, Hesse V, Siebenhuner M, et al: Intermittent high-dose vitamin D prophylaxis during infancy: Effect on vitamin D metabolites, calcium and phosphorus. Am J Clin Nutr 1987;46:652–658.

6 Akpede GO, Omotara BA, Ambe JP: Rickets and deprivation: A Nigerian study. J R Soc Health 1999;119:216–222.

7 Ozkan B, Buyukavcï M, Aksoy H, Tan H, Akdağ R: Incidence of rickets among 0- to 3-year-old children in Erzurum. Cocuk Sağliği ve Hastaliklari Dergisi 1999;42:389–396.

8 Muhe L, Lulseged S, Mason KE, Simoes EA: Case-control study of the role of nutritional rickets in the risk of developing pneumonia in Ethiopian children. Lancet 1997;349:1801–1804.

9 Banajeh SM, al-Sunbali NN, al-Sanahani SH: Clinical characteristics and outcome of children aged 5 years hospitalized with severe pneumonia in Yemen. Ann Trop Paediatr 1997;17:321–326.

10 Walker AR: Etiology of nutritional rickets: Geographic variations. J Pediatr 1998;132:187–189.

11 Thacher TD, Fischer PR, Pettifor JM, Lawson JO, Isïchei CO, Reading JC, Chan GM: A comparison of calcium, vitamin D, or both for nutritional rickets in Nigerian children. N Engl J Med 1999;19:563–568.

12 Thacher TD, Fischer PR, Pettifor JM, Lawson JO, Isïchei CO, Chan GM: Case-control study of factors associated with nutritional rickets in Nigerian children. J Pediatr 2000;137:367–373.

13 Fischer PR, Rahman A, Cimma JP, Kyaw-Myint TO, et al: Nutritional rickets without vitamin D deficiency in Bangladesh. J Trop Paediatr 1999;45:291–293.

14 Bhimma R, Pettifor JM, Coovadia HM, Moodley M, Adhikari M: Rickets in black children beyond infancy in Natal. S Afr Med J 1995;85:668–672.

15 Bishop N: Rickets today – Children still need milk and sunshine. N Engl J Med 1999;341:602–603.

16 Lulseged S, Fitwi G: Vitamin D deficiency rickets: Socio-demographic and clinical risk factors in children seen at a referral hospital in Addis Ababa. East Afr Med J 1999;76:457–461.

17 Ekanem EE, Bassey DE, Eyong M: Nutritional rickets in Calabar, Nigeria. Ann Trop Paediatr 1995;15:303–306.

18 Nyakundi PM, Kinuthia DW, Orinda DA: Clinical aspects and causes of rickets in a Kenyan population. East Afr Med J 1994;71:536–542.

19 el-Hag A, Karrar ZA: Nutritional vitamin D deficiency rickets in Sudanese children. Ann Trop Paediatr 1995;15:69–76.
20 Narchi H, El Jamil M, Kulaylat N: Symptomatic rickets in adolescence. Arch Dis Child 2001;84: 501–503.
21 American Academy of Pediatrics Committee on Nutrition: Calcium requirements of infants, children, and adolescents. Pediatrics 1999;104:1152–1157.
22 Gullu S, Erdogan MF, Uysal AR, Baskal N, Kamel AN, Erdogan G: A potential risk for osteomalacia due to sociocultural lifestyle in Turkish women. Endocr J 1998;45:675–678.
23 el-Sonbaty MR, Abdul-Ghaffar NU: Vitamin D deficiency in veiled Kuwaiti women. Eur J Clin Nutr 1996;50:315–318.
24 Alagol F, Shihadeh Y, Boztepe H, Tanakol R, Yarman S, Azizlerli H, Sandalci O: Sunlight exposure and vitamin D deficiency in Turkish women. J Endocrinol Invest 2000;23:173–177.
25 Andiran N, Yordam N, Ozon A: The risk factors for vitamin D deficiency in breast-fed newborns and their mothers. ESPE 39th Annual Meeting, P3–425, Brussels, 2000.
26 Ozkan B, Buyukavcï M, Energin M, Dirican ME, Alp H, Akdağ R: Nutritional rickets: Comparison of three different therapeutic approaches. Cocuk Sağliği ve Hastaliklari Dergisi 2000; 43:30–35.
27 Specker BL, Tsang RC, Hollis BW: Effect of race and diet on human milk vitamin D and 25-hydroxyvitamin D. Am J Dis Child 1985;139:1134–1137.
28 Pitkin RM: Calcium metabolism in pregnancy and the perinatal period: A review. Am J Obstet Gynecol 1985;151:99–101.
29 Cross NA, Hillman LS, Allen SH, Krause GF, Vieira NE: Calcium homeostasis and bone metabolism during pregnancy, lactation and pot weaning: A longitudinal study. Am J Clin Nutr 1995;61: 514–523.
30 Prentice A, Jarjou LMA, Cole TJ, Stirling DM, et al: Calcium requirements of lactating Gambian mothers: Effects of a calcium supplement on breast milk calcium concentration maternal bone mineral content and urinary calcium excretion. Am J Clin Nutr 1995;62:58–67.
31 Feeley RM, Etienmiller RR, Benton-Jones J, Barnhart H: Calcium, phosphorus and magnesium contents of human milk during early lactation. J Pediatr Gastroenterol Nutr 1983;2:262–267.
32 Shah B, Finberg L: Single-day therapy for nutritional vitamin D deficiency rickets: A preferred method. J Pediatr 1994;125:487–490.
33 Brunvand L, Brunvate R: Health problems among immigrant children in Norway. Tidsskr Nor Laegeforen 2001;28:121:715–718.
34 Meulmeester JF, van den Berg H, Wedel M, et al: Vitamin D status, parathyroid hormone and sunlight in Turkish, Moroccan and Caucasian children in The Netherlands. Eur J Clin Nutr 1990;44: 461–470.
35 Reeves GD, Bachrach S, Carpenter TO, Mackenzie WG: Vitamin D deficiency rickets in adopted children from the former Soviet Union: An uncommon problem with unusual clinical and biochemical features. Pediatrics 2000;106:1484–1488.
36 Ford JA, Colhoun EM, McIntosh WB, Dunnigan MG: Rickets and osteomalacia in the Glasgow Pakistani community, 1961–1971. Br Med J 1972;ii:677–680.
37 Ford JA, McIntosh WV, Butterfield R, et al: Clinical and subclinical vitamin D deficiency in Bradford children. Arch Dis Child 1976;51:939–943.
38 Dunnigan MG, Glekin BM, Henderson JB, et al: Prevention of rickets in Asian children: Assessment of the Glasgow campaign. Br Med J (Clin Res Ed) 1985;291:239–242.
39 Department of Health: Dietary reference values for food energy and nutrients for the United Kingdom. Report on Health & Social Subjects, 41. London, HMSO,1991.
40 Mughal MZ, Salama H, Greenaway T, Laing I, Mawer EB: Florid rickets associated with prolonged breast-feeding without vitamin D supplementation. BMJ 1999;318:39–40.
41 Lawson M, Thomas M: Vitamin D concentrations in Asian children aged 2 years living in England: Population survey. BMJ 1999;318:28.
42 Iqbal SJ, Kaddam I, Wassif W, Nichol F, Walls J: Continuing clinically severe vitamin D deficiency in Asians in the UK (Leicester). Postgrad Med J 1994;70:708–714.
43 Alfaham M, Woodhead S, Pask G, Davies D: Vitamin D deficiency: A concern in pregnant Asian women. Br J Nutr 1995;73:881–887.

44 Blond MH, Gold F, Pierre F, et al: Nutritional fetal rickets. A case report. J Gynecol Obstet Biol Reprod 1997;26:834–836.
45 Waiters B, Godel JC, Basu TK: Perinatal vitamin D and calcium status of northern Canadian mothers and their newborn infants. J Am Coll Nutr 1999;18:122–126.
46 Awumey EM, Mitra DA, Hollis BW, Kumar R, Bell NH: Vitamin D metabolism is altered in Asian Indians in the southern United States: A clinical research center study. J Clin Endocrinol Metab 1998;83:169–173.
47 Glerup H, Mikkelsen K, Poulsen L, et al: Commonly recommended daily intake of vitamin D is not sufficient if sunlight exposure is limited. J Intern Med 2000;247:260–268.
48 Brooke OG, Brown IR, Bone CD, et al: Vitamin D supplements in pregnant Asian women: Effects on calcium status and fetal growth. Br Med J 1980;280:751–754.
49 Hellouin de Menibus C, Mallet E, Henocq A, Lemeur H, L'Hostis C: Neonatal hypocalcemia. Results of vitamin D supplement in the mother. Study on 13,377 newborn infants. Bull Acad Natl Med 1990; 174:1051–1060.
50 Oliveri B, Cassinelli H, Mautalen C, Ayala M: Vitamin D prophylaxis in children with a single dose of 150,000 IU of vitamin D. Eur J Clin Nutr 1996;50:807–810.
51 Feldman KW, Marcuse EK, Springer DA: Nutritional rickets. Am Fam Physician 1990;42:1311–1318.
52 Bhowmick SK, Johnson KR, Rettig KR: Rickets caused by vitamin D deficiency in breastfed infants in the southern United States. Am J Dis Child 1991;145:127–130.
53 Herman MJ, Bulthuis DB: Incidental diagnosis of nutritional rickets after clavicle fracture. Orthopedics 1999;22:254–255.
54 Pugliese MT, Blumberg DL, Hludzinski J, Kay S: Nutritional rickets in suburbia. J Am Coll Nutr 1998;17:637–641.
55 Kaper BP, Romness MJ, Urbanek PJ: Nutritional rickets: Report of four cases diagnosed at orthopedic evaluation. Am J Orthop 2000;29:214–218.
56 Eugster EA, Sane KS, Brown DM: Minnesota rickets. Need for a policy change to support vitamin D supplementation. Minn Med 1996;79:29–32.
57 Kreiter SR, Schwartz RP, Kirkman HN Jr, Charlton PA, Calikoglu AS, Davenport ML: Nutritional rickets in African-American breastfed infants. J Pediatr 2000;137:153–157.
58 Wright A, Schanler R: The resurgence of breast-feeding at the end of the second millennium. J Nutr 2001;131:421S–425S.
59 Markovic V, Jelic T, Wardlaw GM, Ilich J, Goel PK, Wright JK, et al: Timing of peak bone mass in Caucasian females and its implication for the prevention of osteoporosis. J Clin Invest 1994;93: 199–208.
60 Pietrek J, Preece MA, Windo J, O'Riordan JL, Dunnigan MG, McIntosh WB, Ford JA: Prevention of vitamin D deficiency in Asian infants. Lancet 1976;7970:1145–1148.
61 Jacobus CH, Holick MF, Shao Q, Chen TC, Holm IA, Kolodny JM, Fuleihan GE, Seely EV: Hypervitaminosis D associated with drinking milk. N Engl J Med 1992;326:1213–1215.
62 Koo WW, Sherman R, Succop P, Ho M, Buckley D, Tsang RC: Serum vitamin D metabolites in very low birth weight infants with and without rickets and fractures. J Pediatr 1989;114: 1017–1022.
63 European Society of Paediatric Gastroenterology and Nutrition. Acta Paediatr Scand Suppl 1987; 336:1–14.
64 American Academy of Pediatrics: Nutritional needs of low-birth-weight infants. Pediatrics 1985; 75:976–986.
65 Canadian Pediatric Society: Nutrient needs and feeding of premature infants. Can Med Assoc J 1995;152:1765–1785.
66 Cooke R, Hollis B, Conner C, Watson D, Werkman S, Chesney R: Vitamin D and mineral metabolism in the very low birth weight infant receiving 400 IU of vitamin D. J Pediatr 1990;116: 423–428.
67 Koo WW, Krug-Wispe S, Neylan M, Succop P, Oestreich AE, Tsang RC: Effect of three levels of vitamin D intake in preterm infants receiving high mineral-containing milk. J Pediatr Gastroenterol Nutr 1995;21:182–189.
68 Pittard WB 3rd, Geddes KM, Hulsey TC, Hollis BW: How much vitamin D for neonates? Am J Dis Child 1991;145:1147–1149.

69 Backstroem MC, Maki R, Kuusela AL, et al: Randomised controlled trial of vitamin D supplementation on bone density and biochemical indices in preterm infants. Arch Dis Child Fetal Neonatal Ed 1999;80:F161–F166.
70 Goulding A, Cannan R, Williams SM, Gold EJ, Taylor RW, Lewis-Bamed NJ: Bone mineral density in girls with forearm fractures. J Bone Miner Res 1998;13:143–148.
71 Bonjour JP, Theintz G, Buchs B, Slosman D, Rizzoli R: Critical years and stages of puberty for spinal and femoral bone mass accumulation during adolescence. J Clin Endocrinol Metab 1991; 73:555–563.
72 Lappe JM, Stegman M, Davies KM, Barber S, Recker RR: A prospective study of quantitative ultrasound in children and adolescents. J Clin Densitom 2000;3:167–175.
73 Rupich RC, Specker BC, Lieuw AFAM, Ho M: Gender and race differences in bone mass during infancy. Calcif Tissue Int 1996;58:395–397.
74 Alfram PA, Bauer GCH: Epidemiology fractures of the forearm. J Bone Joint Surg Am 1962;44:105–114.
75 Landin L, Nilsson BE: Bone mineral content in children with fractures. Clin Orthop 1983;178: 292–296.
76 Bailey DA, Wedge JH, McCulloch RG, Martin AD, Bernhardson SC: Epidemiology of fractures of the distal end of the radius in children as associated with growth. J Bone Joint Surg Am 1989;71:1225–1231.
77 Hu JF, Zhao XH, Jia JB, Parpia B, Campbell TC: Dietary calcium and bone density among middle-aged and elderly women in China. Am J Clin Nutr 1993;58:219–227.
78 Halioua L, Anderson JJ: Lifetime calcium intake and physical activity habits: Independent and combined effects on the radial bone of healthy premenopausal Caucasian women. Am J Clin Nutr 1989;49:534–541.
79 Murphy S, Khaw KT, May H, Compston JE: Milk consumption and bone mineral density in middle-aged and elderly women. BMJ 1994;308:939–941.
80 Soroko S, Holbrook TL, Edelstein S, Barrett-Connor E: Lifetime milk consumption and bone mineral density in older women. Am J Public Health 1994;84:1319–1322.
81 Forbes RM, Weingartner KE, Parker HM, Bell RR, Erdman JW Jr: Bioavailability to rats of zinc, magnesium and calcium in casein-, egg- and soy protein-containing diets. J Nutr 1979;109: 1652–1660.
82 Forbes RM, Erdman JW Jr: Bioavailability of trace mineral elements. Annu Rev Nutr 1983;3: 213–221.
83 Fischer PR, Thacher TD, Pettifor JM, Jorde LB, Eccleshall TR, Feldman D: Vitamin D receptor polymorphisms and nutritional rickets in Nigerian children. J Bone Miner Res 2000;15: 2206–2210.
84 Heaney RP, Abrams S, Dawson-Hughes B, Looker A, Marcus R, Matkovic V, Weaver C: Peak bone mass. Osteoporos Int 2000;11:985–1009.
85 Jackman LA, Millane SS, Martin BR, Wood OB, McCabe GP, Peacock M, Weaver CM: Calcium retention in relation to calcium intake and postmenarcheal age in adolescent females. Am J Clin Nutr 1997;66:327–333.
86 Wastney ME, Martin BR, Peacock M, Smith D, Jiang XY, Jackman LA, Weaver CM: Changes in calcium kinetics in adolescent girls induced by high calcium intake. J Clin Endocrinol Metab 2000;85:4470–4475.
87 Maggiolini M, Bonofiglio D, Giorno A, Catalano S, Marsico S, Aquila S, Ando S: The effect of dietary calcium intake on bone mineral density in healthy adolescent girls and young women in southern Italy. Int J Epidemiol 1999;28:479–484.
88 Blecker U, Mehta DI, du Pont AI, Davis R, Sothern MS, Suskind RM: Fat-soluble vitamin deficiencies. Pediatr Rev 1999;20:394–395.
89 Chesney RW: Metabolic bone diseases. Pediatr Rev 1984;5:227–237.
90 Thompson GN: Determinants of serum vitamin D levels in preadolescent cystic fibrosis children. Acta Paediatr Scand 1987;76:962–965.
91 Hahn TJ, Squires AE, Halstead LR, Strominger DB: Reduced serum 25-hydroxyvitamin D concentration and disordered mineral metabolism in patients with cystic fibrosis. J Pediatr 1979;94: 38–42.

92 Congden PJ, Bruce G, Rothburn MM, Clarke PC, Littlewood JM, Kelleher J, Losowsky MS: Vitamin status in treated patients with cystic fibrosis. Arch Dis Child 1981;56:708–714.
93 Henderson RC, Lester G: Vitamin D levels in children with cystic fibrosis. South Med J 1997;90: 378–383.
94 Aarskog D, Aksnes L, Markestad T, Trygstad O: Plasma concentrations of vitamin D metabolites in pubertal girls with anorexia nervosa. Acta Endocrinol Suppl (Copenh) 1986;279:458–467.
95 Grey V, Lands L, Pall H, Drury D: Monitoring of 25-OH vitamin D levels in children with cystic fibrosis. J Pediatr Gastroenterol Nutr 2000;30:314–319.
96 Fonseca VA, D'Souza V, Houlder S, Thomas M, Wakeling A, Dandona P: Vitamin D deficiency and low osteocalcin concentrations in anorexia nervosa. J Clin Pathol 1988;41:195–197.
97 Davies PSW, Bates CJ, Cole TJ, Prentice A, Clarke PC: Vitamin D: Seasonal and regional differences in preschool children in Great Britain. Eur J Clin Nutr 1999;53:195–198.
98 Docio S, Riancho JA, Perez A, Olmos JM, Amado JA, Gonzalez-Macias J: Seasonal deficiency of vitamin D in children: A potential target for osteoporosis-preventing strategies? J Bone Miner Res 1998;13:544–548.
99 Vieth R, Carter G: Difficulties with vitamin D nutrition research: Objective targets of adequacy and assays for 25-hydroxyvitamin D. Eur J Clin Nutr 2001;55:221–222.
100 Baer MT, Kozlowski BW, Blyler EM, Trahms CM, Taylor ML, Hogan MP: Vitamin D, calcium and bone status in children with developmental delay in relation to anticonvulsant use and ambulatory status. Am J Clin Nutr 1997;65:1042–1051.
101 Kooh SW, Jones G, Reilly BJ, Fraser D: Pathogenesis of rickets in chronic hepatobiliary disease in children. Pediatrics 1979;94:870–874.
102 Tokita A, Nittono H, Mori T, Maruyama T, Hayashi M, Obinata K, Watanabe T, Yabuta K, Miyano T: Vitamin D metabolism in preoperative extrahepatic biliary atresia. Acta Paediatr Scand 1991;80:634–639.
103 Driscoll RH, Meredith SC, Sitrin M, Rosenberg IH: Vitamin D deficiency and bone disease in patients with Crohn's disease. Gastroenterology 1982;83:1252–1258.
104 Arreola F, Paniagua R, Diaz-Bensussen S, Urquieta B, Lopez-Montano E, Partida-Hernandez G, Villalpando S: Bone mineral content, 25-hydroxycalciferol and zinc serum levels in insulin-dependent (type 1) diabetes patients. Arch Invest Med (Mex) 1990;21:195–199.
105 Arikoski P, Kroger H, Riikonen P, Parviainen M, Voutilainen R, Komulainen J: Disturbance in bone turnover in children with a malignancy at completion of chemotherapy. Med Pediatr Oncol 1999;33:455–461.
106 Reed A, Haugen M, Pachman LM, Langman CB: 25-Hydroxyvitamin D therapy in children with active juvenile rheumatoid arthritis: Short-term effects on serum osteocalcin levels and bone mineral density. Pediatrics 1991;119:657–660.
107 Tonstad S, Aksnes L: Fat-soluble vitamin levels in familial hypercholesterolemia. J Pediatr 1997; 130:274–280.
108 Issa S, Rotthauwe HW, Burmeister W: 25-Hydroxyvitamin D and vitamin E absorption in healthy children and children with chronic intrahepatic cholestasis. Eur J Pediatr 1989;148:605–609.
109 Bhudhikanok GS, Lim J, Marcus R, Harkins A, Moss RB, Bachrach LK: Correlates of osteopenia in patients with cystic fibrosis. Pediatrics 1996;97:103–111.
110 Heubi JE, Hollis BW, Tsang RC: Bone disease in chronic childhood cholestasis. II. Better absorption of 25-OH vitamin D than vitamin D in extrahepatic biliary atresia. Pediatr Res 1990;27: 26–31.
111 Rajantie J, Lamberg-Allardt C, Wilska M: Does carbamazepine treatment lead to a need of extra vitamin D in some mentally retarded children? Acta Paediatr Scand 1984;73:325–328.
112 Bressot C, Meunier PJ, Chapuy MC, Lejeune E, Edouard C, Darby AJ: Histomorphometric profile, pathophysiology and reversibility of corticosteroid-induced osteoporosis. Metab Bone Relat Res 1979:1:303–311.
113 Sambrook PN, Eisman JA, Champion GD, Pocock NA: Sex hormone status and osteoporosis in postmenopausal women with rheumatoid arthritis. Arthritis Rheum 1988;31:973–978.
114 Hahn TJ, Halstead LR, Baran DT: Effects of short term glucocorticoid administration on intestinal calcium absorption and circulating vitamin D metabolite concentrations in man. J Clin Endocrinol Metab 1981;52:111–115.

115 Reid IR, Ibbertson HK: Evidence of decreased tubular reabsorption of calcium in glucocorticoid-treated asthmatics. Horm Res 1987;27:200–204.
116 Sambrook P, Birmingham J, Kelly P, et al: Prevention of corticosteroid osteoporosis. A comparison of calcium, calcitriol and calcitonin. N Engl J Med 1993;328:1747–1752.
117 Eastell R, Reid DM, Compston J, et al: A UK consensus group on management of glucocorticoid-induced osteoporosis: An update. J Intern Med 1998;244:271–292.
118 Recommendations for the prevention and treatment of glucocorticoid-induced osteoporosis: 2001 update. American College of Rheumatology Ad Hoc Committee on Glucocorticoid-Induced Osteoporosis. Arthritis Rheum 2001;44:1496–1503.
119 Jekovec-Vrhovsek M, Kocijancic A, Prezelj J: Effect of vitamin D and calcium on bone mineral density in children with CP and epilepsy in full-time care. Dev Med Child Neurol 2000;42:403–405.
120 Henderson RC, Madsen CD, Davis C, Gold SH: Longitudinal evaluation of bone mineral density in children receiving chemotherapy. J Pediatr Hematol Oncol 1998;20:322–326.
121 Halton JM, Atkinson SA, Fraher L, et al: Altered mineral metabolism and bone mass in children during treatment for acute lymphoblastic leukemia. J Bone Miner Res 1996;11:1774–1783.
122 Arikoski P, Komulainen JJ, Riikonen P, Voutilainen R, Knip M, Kroger H: Alterations in bone turnover and impaired development of bone mineral density in newly diagnosed children with cancer: A 1-year prospective study. J Clin Endocrinol Metab 1999;84:3174–3181.
123 Boot AM, van den Heuvel-Eibrink MM, Hahlen K, Krenning EP, de Muinck Keizer-Schrama SMPF: Bone mineral density in children with acute lymphoblastic leukaemia. Eur J Cancer 1999;35:1693–1697.
124 Atkinson SA, Fraher L, Gundberg CM, Andrew M, Pai M, Barr RD: Mineral homeostasis and bone mass in children treated for acute lymphoblastic leukemia. J Pediatr 1989;114:793–800.
125 Specker BL, Valaris B, Hertzberg V: Sunshine exposure and serum 25-hydroxyvitamin D concentration in exclusively breast-fed infants. J Pediatr 1985;107:372–376.
126 Standing Committee on the Scientific Evaluation of Dietary Reference Intakes. Dietary Reference Intakes: Calcium, Phosphorus, Magnesium, Vitamin D and Fluoride. Washington, National Academy Press, 1997.
127 Bischoff HA, Stahelin HB, Urscheler N, Ehrsam R, Vonthein R, Perrig-Chiello P, Tyndall A, Theiler R: Muscle strength in the elderly: Its relation to vitamin D metabolites. Arch Phys Med Rehabil 1999;80:54–58.
128 Boucher BJ: Inadequate vitamin D status: Does it contribute to the disorders comprising syndrome 'X'? Br J Nutr 1998;79:315–327.
129 Kinuta K, Tanaka H, Moriwake T, Aya K, Kato S, Seino Y: Vitamin D is an important factor in estrogen biosynthesis of both female and male gonads. Endocrinology 2000;141:1317–1324.

Ze'ev Hochberg, MD, DSc
Pediatric Endocrinology
Meyer Children's Hospital, Rambam Medical Center
POB 9602, Haifa 31096 (Israel)
Tel./Fax +972 4 8542157, E-Mail z_hochberg@rambam.health.gov.il

Abbreviations

AAP	American Academy of Pediatrics
ADHR	Autosomal-dominant hypophosphatemic rickets
AF-2	Activation factor 2
AI	Adequate intake
CaSRs	Calcium-sensing receptors
CaT1	Calcium transporter-1
CTE	C-terminal extension
DBD	DNA-binding domain
7-DHC	7-Dehydrocholesterol
DHT	Dihydrotachysterol
FGF	Fibroblast growth factor
FISH	Fluorescence in situ hybridization
FRP	Frizzled-related protein
GH	Growth hormone
HREs	Hormone response elements
HVDRR	Hereditary vitamin D-resistant rickets
IH	Idiopathic hypercalciuria
LBD	Ligand-binding domain
LBP	Ligand-binding pocket
LBW	Low birthweight
MED	Minimal erythema dose
mRNA	Messenger RNA
NEP	Neutral endopeptidase
NLS	Nuclear localization signals

NPT2a	Type 2a sodium-phosphate cotransporter
NR	Nuclear receptor
ODIF	Osteoclast differentiation/inhibitory factor
$1,25(OH)_2D$	1,25-Dihydroxyvitamin D
25(OH)D	25-Hydroxyvitamin D
OI	Osteogenesis imperfecta
OPG	Osteoprotegerin
PC-1	Plasma cell membrane glycoprotein-1
PCR	Polymerase chain reaction
PDDR	Pseudo-vitamin D-deficiency rickets
P_i	Inorganic phosphate
PMCA1	Plasma membrane calcium adenosine triphosphatase-1
PP_i	Inorganic pyrophosphate
PTH	Parathyroid hormone
PTHrP	Parathyroid hormone-related peptide
RAR	Receptors for all-trans-retinoic acid
RDA	Recommended dietary allowance
RR	Relative risk
RXR	Retinoic acid X receptor
SPF	Sun protection factor
TIO	Tumor-induced osteomalacia
TmP/GFR	Maximal tubular reabsorption of phosphate
TNAP	Tissue-nonspecific isoenzyme of alkaline phosphatase
TNF	Tumor necrosis factor
TR	Thyroid hormone
VDDR-I	Vitamin D-dependent rickets, type I
VDDR-II	Vitamin D-dependent rickets, type II
VDR	Vitamin D receptor
VDRE	Vitamin D response element
VEGF	Vascular endothelial growth factor
VLBW	Very low birthweight
XLH	X-linked hypophosphatemic rickets/osteomalacia

Subject Index